Every Woman's Guide to Eating During Pregnancy

EVERY WOMAN'S GUIDE TO

Eating

During

Pregnancy

Martha Rose Shulman
and **Jane L. Davis**, M.D.

Houghton Mifflin Company
Boston   New York
2002

This book is not intended to replace medical advice or substitute for ongoing care given by a physician. As part of good obstetrical care, women should have regular checkups. They should direct any questions or concerns regarding their pregnancy to the physician who is caring for them.

Copyright © 2002 Martha Rose Shulman and Jane L. Davis, M.D.

Table for Estimating Body Mass Index reprinted from *Nutrition During Pregnancy*. Copyright © 1990 by the National Academy of Sciences. Reprinted by permission of the National Academy Press.

Quick Spinach and Tomato Lasagna from *Light Basics Cookbook* by Martha Rose Shulman. Copyright © 1999 by Martha Rose Shulman. Reprinted by permission of HarperCollins Publishers, Inc.

For information about permission to reproduce selections from this book, write to Permissions, Houghton Mifflin Company, 215 Park Avenue South, New York, New York 10003.

Library of Congress Cataloging-in-Publication Data
Shulman, Martha Rose.
    Every woman's guide to eating during pregnancy / Martha Rose Shulman and Jane L. Davis.
      p. cm.
    Includes bibliographical references and index.
    ISBN 0-395-98660-5
    1. Pregnancy—Nutritional aspects.   2. Mothers—Nutrition.
3. Prenatal care.   I. Davis, Jane L., M.D.   II. Title.

RG559 .S55 2002
618.2'4—dc21   2001051889

Book design by Anne Chalmers
Typefaces: Minion, Barbera, Mercury

Printed in the United States of America

VB 10 9 8 7 6 5 4

To Our Families

BILL AND LIAM

EDDIE, MICHAEL, AND MADDIE

Contents

Foreword:
TWO PERSONAL PERSPECTIVES viii

Introduction ❖ 1

Before You Conceive ❖ 5

Determining Your Needs
HOW MUCH WEIGHT SHOULD YOU GAIN? 7

Eating by Trimester ❖ 12

The Recipes ❖ 30

BREAKFAST FOODS   30

SNACKS, DIPS, CONDIMENTS, AND BEVERAGES   47

SANDWICHES   70

SOUPS   88

SALADS   108

MAIN DISHES   166

GRAIN AND VEGETABLE DISHES   236

DESSERTS   268

Eating Plans for Individual Needs ⊸ **283**

    Lower-Carb, High-Protein Plan   288

    Higher-Carb, High-Protein Plan   298

    Vegetarian Plans   305

       Ovo-Lacto Vegetarian Plan   305

       Vegan Plan   305

    Plan for the Noncook or the Reluctant Cook   317

**Eating Plans for Special Needs
and High-Risk Pregnancies** ⊸ **326**

    Calcium-Rich Plan for the Lactose-Intolerant   326

    Plan for Multiples   333

    Plan for Gestational Diabetes   341

    Eating While on Bed Rest   356

Eating Plans for the Trimesters ⊸ **359**

    The First Trimester: Menus for the
       Nauseous and Tired   359

    The Second Trimester: Menus for the Hungry   364

    The Third Trimester: Little Meals   370

Eating Plan for Nursing Mothers ⊸ **373**

A Nutrition Primer ⊸ **381**

Selected Bibliography ⊸ **400**

Index ⊸ **403**

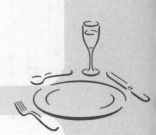

Two Personal Perspectives

FROM THE DOCTOR

I'm a doctor who loves to cook. As an OB/GYN at a busy Los Angeles hospital, I know how important diet is, not only for maintaining your health and ensuring the health of your baby during pregnancy but also for your continued well-being beyond pregnancy. A healthy diet can help lower your risk for serious medical problems such as heart disease, diabetes, osteoporosis, and several types of cancer. Pregnancy presents an opportunity for you to learn sound nutritional habits that can last a lifetime and to share that knowledge with your family.

Ideally, I like to see my patients for counseling *before* they conceive. It's best to correct poor nutritional practices that can result in conditions such as obesity, or at least be on the road to correcting them, before you become pregnant. Although many factors contribute to the ultimate health of your baby and their interplay is complex, certain aspects of diet and nutrition are very important.

Poor nutrition—whether from a surfeit of calories or a deficit—can put you and your baby at risk. Time and again, I have seen complications that could have been avoided if my patient had had a better diet. Two actual cases from my practice graphically illustrate how nutrition can affect you and your baby. Too little weight gain can result in infants with a low birth weight, while too much can lead to a multitude of health risks, such as diabetes and infection after a cesarean section.

K.L., a seventeen-year-old from an adolescent prenatal clinic that I oversee, gained just 15 pounds during her pregnancy. Her baby weighed only 4¾ pounds. Her pregnancy was complicated by poor growth of the baby in utero. The pregnancy required intensive monitoring, and K.L. eventually had to have her labor induced three weeks before her due date because an ultrasound detected some abnormalities. The baby had to stay in the hospital longer than most babies. Although she is currently developmentally normal, there are concerns about her future development, as there are for all babies known as small for gestational age (SGA).

Because K.L. lacked money to buy food, her social worker provided her with information regarding the federally subsidized Special Supplemental Nutrition Program for Women, Infants, and Children (WIC). Unfortunately, K.L. did not take advantage of this program, ate minimally, and smoked throughout her pregnancy. Without doubt, K.L.'s poor nutrition and smoking had profound effects on the outcome of her pregnancy.

❧

L.J. recently delivered her second child. She began her first pregnancy weighing 248 pounds and gained more than 60 pounds over the next nine months. She developed gestational diabetes, and because her baby was too large to fit through the birth canal, she needed to have a cesarean section. The child weighed 9¾ pounds, and L.J. developed an infection in her incision after the operation.

Before her second pregnancy, and after receiving much nutritional counseling, L.J. was able to lose 80 pounds. With her second pregnancy, she gained 33 pounds and delivered a healthy baby weighing 7½ pounds. With the second pregnancy, L.J. did not develop gestational diabetes, probably because she had lost so much weight following her first pregnancy. The weight loss also contributed to the smaller birth weight of her second child and her ability to have a successful vaginal delivery.

❧

Even in the earliest days after conception, before your first missed period and before you even suspect pregnancy, how much and what you eat are important. A balanced diet includes a variety of foods from the different food groups — breads and cereals (preferably whole grain), fresh fruits and vegetables, dairy products, and protein-rich foods of plant or animal origin.

Your nutritional needs will change throughout the nine months. Along with a nutrition primer to help you understand the basic elements of the foods that go into your body, we've provided a range of menu plans and suggestions that cover a variety of needs and appetites, from the early weeks of morning sickness to the final days before childbirth to the postpartum period when you are breastfeeding. There are higher-carb and lower-carb diet plans here, strategies for women expecting multiples, plans for vegetarians and diabetics, and menus for nursing mothers. We've also included practical information about prepared foods for people who don't cook or for those times when you're unable or not inclined to do so.

Food, we believe, is meant to be enjoyed — including during pregnancy — and a healthy diet needn't be a boring or bland one, as the recipes in this book prove. My experiences with my own pregnancies — I have a wonderful son and daughter — and my work helping other women with theirs are among the true joys of my life. Food is also a joy for my family. In this book, we help you celebrate both. Congratulations on your pregnancy!

— JANE L. DAVIS, M.D.

FROM THE COOK

When I became pregnant — at forty-seven — I needed dietary guidance, even though I had devoted my twenty-five-year career to writing cookbooks with a healthy focus. I was considered high-risk, because I was over forty. "High-risk for what?" I asked my doctor.

"Oh, we routinely put that on charts for women over forty," he said. "But don't be concerned; you're in great shape. Just yesterday I delivered healthy twins from a fifty-year-old woman, and the day before I delivered a forty-eight-year-old. Everybody was fine."

But I did worry. For the first time in my life, I worried about what I ate. How was my diet going to affect my long-awaited baby-to-be? Was I eating enough? Or too much? Was I getting enough protein and other nutrients?

It didn't help that during my first trimester, I had little appetite, except a desperate need to eat when my stomach was empty. Food was uninteresting to me for the first time in my life — an occupational hazard! I needed crackers within reach at all times, and restaurants were hard to stomach. And everybody was on my back, telling me to *eat, eat, eat*. During the early weeks of my pregnancy, I dropped to below my prepregnancy weight — not unheard-of, but I was still concerned. My doctor told me I needed to gain 30 to 35 pounds because I'd started out underweight. I was supposed to get 1,800 calories a day, but I wasn't hungry. When I tried to fulfill those caloric requirements, I felt bloated. Later on in my pregnancy, when I'd caught up on my weight gain, with a few pounds to spare, my doctor alarmed me again when he said, "Watch the carbs."

The books I read were bossy: *Don't* eat sugar, *don't* eat ice cream, *don't* eat white bread, *don't* eat bagels, they told me, at a time when I was panicked about the fact that I didn't feel like eating *anything*. *Don't* have caffeine, drink *only* nonfat milk, they warned me, when only 1% and 2% milk were appetizing. *Don't* get less than 75 grams of protein a day; watch out for dangerous additives in meat, for heavy metals in certain kinds of fish, for dangerous pesticides on vegetables. Rather than help me figure out what to eat, they made me afraid that everything I was or was not doing might be compromising the health of my baby.

I began to keep a food diary and devise menus that were based not only on my own cooking but on prepared foods and take-out as well — meals that my husband and I could throw together when neither of us had the energy to cook, that both of us would like when one of us had odd cravings. I filled my freezer with pot stickers and tortellini and bran muffins, and I used my microwave more than ever. During those early months, we ate lots of tuna sandwiches on toasted rye with lettuce and tomato, poached and scrambled eggs, and, yes, pickles. Tofu with soy sauce became my favorite first-trimester lunch (it still is, and my son, Liam, loves it, too). As Liam began to take shape, so did this book.

In the end, I needn't have worried so much. I finally stopped counting calories and protein grams and waited for my appetite to come back. It did, as the medical literature had predicted, during my fourth month of pregnancy. Then I began to enjoy all kinds of food again. I even went to Europe on a gastronomic tour of Provence and felt great the whole time. When I was six months pregnant, I participated in one of the finest Christmas dinners I've ever experienced — a group effort prepared with a number of my cookbook author colleagues.

By the time I was nine months pregnant, I had gained 25 pounds — not as much as the doctor had ordered, but enough to produce a robust, bright-eyed, 7½-pound boy. I felt terrific right through to the end, and Liam, now four, is as healthy as they come.

Whereas my pregnancy concerns had to do with bulking up after years of swimming and careful eating, most women have the opposite problem. But no matter what your personal nutritional needs and challenges are, the goal is the same for all of us: to eat well and enjoy it while we are pregnant and to maximize what our foods can do for our babies and ourselves.

The menu plans we've devised will help those of you who need to keep your carbohydrates and fat calories down, as well as those of you who, because you may be carrying more than one baby, will need significantly more calories. Select from the meal plans and recipes here and know that you will find something good to eat and that it will nourish you and your growing baby well. It is my hope that whatever you choose to eat, it will never have tasted better.

—MARTHA ROSE SHULMAN

Introduction

If you've just picked up this book and begun to read, chances are you're in your first trimester of pregnancy. You may be nauseous or starving or intermittently one or the other, and possibly for the first time in your life, you have begun to think about — and maybe worry about — what you eat. Perhaps you've been eating well up until this point, or maybe you haven't. Whatever your dietary habits, you don't want to be bossed around or punished for the way you eat. You just want some practical information. Well, you've come to the right place.

Even if you haven't ever thought much about food or your weight, now that you're pregnant, you'll find that you obsess about these matters. This is because every month at your prenatal checkup, you'll be put on the scale and told that you're doing fine or that you're gaining too much weight or not enough. If you experience morning sickness, queasiness, or fatigue, if your tastes and aversions change every week, your diet can become a challenge.

Each phase of your pregnancy will present new hurdles. During the first trimester, you may experience morning sickness or feel tired. But even if you have no energy to cook, you *can* make choices about the foods you buy. Luckily, although the *quality* of the food you eat is crucial during the early months, it is not essential that you gain a lot of weight. During the second trimester, you may feel ravenous all the time. As you near the end of your pregnancy, you will find it miraculous that there is any room for food in there at all, and little meals will suit you best during this time.

Pregnancy can be a time when you take tremendous pleasure in eating, not only because you may enjoy food more but also because you know that it is nourishing both you and your baby. It

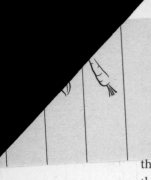

a time when you eat foods that you once considered an in-
e. Or if you have always been plagued by weight problems,
difficult time, because you may feel a conflict between the
f your baby and your own weight and appearance.

may have been given conflicting information about what
ld and shouldn't eat and about how much you should eat.
ne hand, you may hear that protein is all-important and
that you need 45 grams a day. On the other hand, you may be told
that you shouldn't eat much red meat — a very good source of
protein — because of all the saturated fat. So you turn to beans
and grains, only to hear that you should watch your carbohydrate
intake. You also may be barraged with lists of food groups, portions, calories, and grams. Suddenly, eating is not about pleasure
and satisfying hunger; it becomes a math class, with the calculator
replacing the fork and knife.

$\mathcal{L}\mathfrak{a}$

With this book, you can throw out the calculator and reach again
for your plate. We've devised a number of eating plans for you,
based on good, uncomplicated food. There's something for everyone here: if you like to cook, you'll find plenty of great recipes; if
you're too tired to cook, you'll find a number of very quick dishes;
and if you don't cook at all, there are meal plans based on healthy,
tasty packaged and frozen foods, with some fresh vegetables and
fruits thrown in for good measure. We've already done the work
for you, so you don't have to figure out how to put together your
meal strategy. Just choose the one that suits you.

Because we think it might be easier for you to understand
how the foods you eat affect your weight and health, as well as the
health of your baby, if you understand the basics of nutrition,
we've included a nutrition primer in this book. That way, when we
talk about a balanced diet — about protein, carbohydrates, and
fats; vitamins, minerals, and other nutrients — you'll know what
we mean. We also tell you what the best sources of the different
nutrients are. We've listed the key nutrients that you will be getting
in every recipe, and the nutrition section will allow you to bone up
on what these nutrients are actually doing for you and your baby.

If you already have sound eating habits, you're well on your
way to a healthy pregnancy. You will need to increase your caloric

intake, but not by much (100 to 300 calories is recommended, and you can find those in a couple of glasses of milk, a milk shake or smoothie, or a few pieces of fruit). If you need to improve the quality of your diet, this is the time to do it. The beneficial effects on the health of your baby will be the most immediate outcome, but changing your diet for the better will also have lasting effects on your own health and therefore on your quality of life.

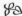

What, you may ask, are sound eating habits? The most important aspect of a good diet is balance. Whether you are a vegetarian or a meat-eater (or a little of both), a fast-food addict or committed to organic foods, lactose intolerant or diabetic, you need to have a range of nutrients in your diet: complex carbohydrates, which can come from whole grains (including breads and pasta), beans, and fresh produce; protein, from animal or plant sources; fats in moderation, with an emphasis on monounsaturates (such as olive oil) and omega-3s (see page 385). A balanced, healthy diet, one that includes lots of fresh fruits and vegetables, will also provide you with a range of micronutrients — vitamins, minerals, tiny nutrients called phytochemicals — all of which help in very specific ways to make the body function properly. And if your body is working well, in all likelihood so will your baby's. Your baby is, after all, totally dependent on what you are eating for his or her own nutrition from the time you conceive until the moment the umbilical cord is cut — and well beyond that if you nurse. Moreover, recent studies have shown that the way the baby is nourished in utero can have a lasting effect on his or her own health. Overweight babies, for example, are more likely to have weight problems in adulthood. And because a baby's taste buds and olfactory senses develop by the third trimester, your child may be more likely to want to eat good, healthy foods such as broccoli, carrots, and greens if you eat plenty of them while you're pregnant.

Remember that it's normal and healthy to accumulate fat during pregnancy. You even produce special hormones that tell the body to store fat. Your body needs those fat stores, both for your developing baby and your own energy needs, as well as to prepare for lactation. But for some people, controlling the amount of that fat may be a challenge.

This is when knowing something about nutrition can come in handy. For instance, simple carbohydrates—sugars—are often the source of many useless calories during pregnancy. Low energy and fatigue, depression, and mood swings often result in a craving for sweets. If you're gaining weight too quickly or are already overweight, these cravings can be problematic. If you're sensitive to carbohydrates, certain types, such as refined baked goods, can encourage your body to store too much fat. Fats, however, are the most insidious source of calories. Gram for gram, fats have more than twice as many calories as protein or carbohydrates (9 as opposed to 4), so if your diet is high in fat, it will be too high in calories. Fats also contribute to two other pregnancy afflictions: morning sickness and heartburn.

ॐ

You may love cooking or hate it, but everybody has to eat, especially during pregnancy. Whether you are twenty-five or forty-five, whether your pregnancy is going swimmingly or you are feeling challenged, you'll find something in these pages that you can use. It may be a lower-carb menu plan, a vegan menu plan, or one for a multiple pregnancy. It may be a list of recommended packaged foods from the supermarket. Perhaps it'll be a few of the recipes, such as grilled chicken breasts, buttermilk pancakes, do-ahead lasagna, banana bread, or bran muffins. (These happen to be ones that are most regularly requested by our own children.) These are healthful and delicious dishes, drawn from a repertoire that we and our families have been savoring for years. The recipes, each one with a key-nutrients profile, are followed by eating plans with a week's worth of menus. You can follow them to a tee if you want to, or simply use them as guidelines. Whatever you decide to cook and eat, rest assured that you and your family will enjoy it. Our menus may be designed with pregnancy in mind, but this is not "pregnancy food." It's just good, simple cooking, developed with a cook's and a mother's touch.

Before You Conceive

Doctors today place a great deal of emphasis on preconception counseling and health care. If you're thinking of becoming pregnant, it's a good idea to make an appointment with your physician or OB/GYN. Because your baby will begin to develop vital organs within three weeks of conception — before you even know you're pregnant — now is the time to begin thinking about your eating habits. If you make sure now that your diet includes plenty of fresh fruits, vegetables, and whole grains, you won't worry later about whether your vitamin intake was sufficient during the early weeks of pregnancy. Since this is the time when malformations can occur, it's wise to start making certain changes, if they are necessary, before conception.

↣ **GIVE UP SMOKING, RECREATIONAL DRUGS, AND ALCOHOL.**

↣ **BEGIN TAKING FOLIC ACID SUPPLEMENTS.** Folic acid (folate or folacin, see page 15) is crucial during the first three months of pregnancy for the prevention of neural tube defects. The U.S. Public Health Service recommends that all women capable of bearing children take 0.4 mg of folacin a day. If you are already taking a multivitamin, you're getting that amount. During pregnancy, your doctor probably will prescribe a prenatal supplement. Most of these supplements contain 1 mg of folic acid. If you have had a child who is affected with a neural tube defect, be sure to tell your physician, preferably before you conceive. The recommended folic acid dosage for women with a previously affected child is 4 mg per day for four weeks prior to pregnancy and for the first three months of pregnancy.

↣ **TREAT EATING DISORDERS.** If you suffer from an eating disorder, you should make it a priority to seek psychological, medical, and nutritional intervention before you become pregnant.

✒ **CONSIDER YOUR EATING HABITS.** Now is the time to improve your diet if you need to — to move away from fried fast foods and sugary soft drinks and instead develop a taste for fresh produce, grains, and legumes.

✒ **START EXERCISING.** Exercise is important for maintaining health and preventing too much weight gain during pregnancy. If you don't exercise regularly, it's best to begin some kind of low-impact exercise program — it can be as simple as walking or swimming for 20 to 30 minutes three times a week — before you become pregnant. Beginning an exercise regimen during pregnancy can be difficult and is not recommended by many doctors.

Here are some other topics that you should discuss with your doctor during a prepregnancy visit.

✒ **YOUR WEIGHT.** If your doctor observes that you are severely overweight, he or she will recommend that you lose weight before you become pregnant. Weight reduction before conception is particularly important to reduce the risk of complications during pregnancy, such as gestational diabetes and high blood pressure. Ask your health care provider for a referral to a dietitian specializing in weight-reduction programs. If you are underweight, you may find it difficult to conceive. Make sure that you are obtaining adequate calories for a developing baby.

✒ **PREEXISTING MEDICAL CONDITIONS.** If you have preexisting insulin-dependent diabetes, for example, it's essential to lower your blood-sugar level before you become pregnant. If your glucose level is under control, your risk of miscarriage and major birth defects is no higher than average. However, if your blood sugar is too high, the risks can be great. Pregnancy also can increase vision problems related to diabetes.

✒ **PRESCRIPTION DRUGS.** Discuss all prescriptions that you may be taking in order to avoid drugs that may cause birth defects. Your doctor may be able to prescribe alternative therapies that are safer for the fetus.

✒ **OVER THE COUNTER PHARMACEUTICALS AND VITAMINS.** Be sure to discuss any other medications and vitamins you are taking. High doses of certain vitamins can be harmful, particularly vitamin A, which in high doses can cause birth defects.

Determining Your Needs
How Much Weight
Should You Gain?

Are you afraid of gaining too much weight or not enough? Are you putting on weight too quickly or too slowly? Or are you just looking for an all-around, well-balanced diet for a healthy pregnancy and baby?

Your prepregnancy body weight can tell you a great deal about what sort of diet will be best for you during your pregnancy and how much weight you should ideally gain. If your weight is in the normal range, health professionals recommend that you put on 25 to 35 pounds during your pregnancy; you should gain about 3 1/2 pounds during your first trimester and about a pound a week during the second and third. If you're underweight, doctors like to see you gain a little more — between 28 and 40 pounds, with an increase of about 5 pounds during the first trimester. If your weight is high, doctors will encourage you to gain less — 15 to 25 pounds, depending on how high your weight is, with only a 2-pound gain during the first trimester. Putting on this extra weight does not require many additional calories; nutritionists generally recommend that you increase your intake by 100 to 300 calories a day.

If you are underweight and eat a low-calorie diet when you become pregnant; if you're a young adolescent (you may still be growing yourself), a smoker, an African American, or a single mother; or if you have a low income, you may need to work harder to gain adequate weight. You can meet your nutritional needs more easily if you eat a diet that is higher in carbohydrates, taking suggestions from the diet plan beginning on page 298. A low weight gain during pregnancy may result in a low-birth-weight baby (one that weighs less than 5 1/2 pounds at birth), and small babies have a much higher incidence of health and developmental problems.

If you're heavy, you'll want to concentrate on a diet that is higher in protein and lower in carbohydrates. Rather than snacking on muffins, try a smoothie or vanilla yogurt. Eat fish, poultry, meat, or tofu for dinner rather than pasta, and have as many vegetables as you want. You'll find lots to choose from in the lower-carb menus beginning on page 288, and the results will be good for your own health as well as your baby's.

How do you determine whether your weight is low, normal, or high? The Institute of Medicine has come up with an index that assigns values to weight-to-height ratios, called the body mass index, or BMI. Each BMI falls into one of four categories: Obese, High, Normal, and Low. By using the chart below, you can quickly assess your status. Find the intersection of your weight and height coordinates, and you will see which category applies to you.

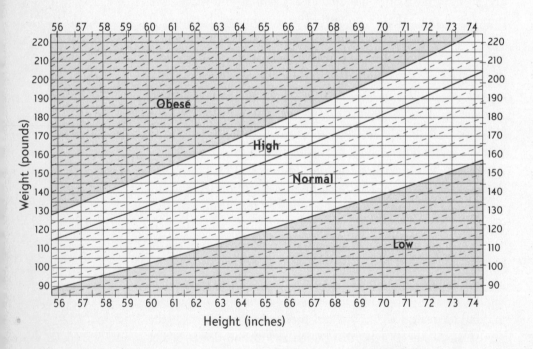

Beverage Chart*

If you're gaining too much weight but avoiding sweets, junk food, and fried foods, the extra calories may be coming from fruit juices. Though healthful, fruit juices can be high in naturally occurring simple sugars and calories. By contrast, vegetable juices, such as tomato juice and V8, are low in calories and carbohydrates. Although soda is much lower in both calories and carbs than many juices, remember that it has no nutritive value. Here's a look at the caloric content of some of the most popular beverages. Values for all the juices are for 8 fluid ounces (1 cup).

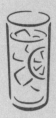

BEVERAGE	CALORIES	CARBOHYDRATES
Apple juice (bottled)	117	29 g
Apple cranberry juice (bottled)	120	30 g
Apricot nectar	141	36 g
Grape juice	154	37.8 g
Grapefruit juice from concentrate	101	24 g
Fresh grapefruit juice	96	22.7 g
Orange juice from concentrate	112	26.8 g
Fresh orange juice	112	25.8 g
Pineapple juice (canned)	140	34.4 g
Prune juice (canned)	182	44.7 g
Tomato juice (Campbell's)	50	9 g
V8	50	10 g
Budweiser, 12 fluid ounces (1 can or bottle)	147	11.4 g
for 8 ounces	110	8.5 g
Bud Light, 12 fluid ounces (1 can or bottle)	110	6.6 g
for 8 ounces	82	4.95 g
Coca-Cola, 12 fluid ounces (1 can)	146	41 g
for 8 ounces	97	27 g

*Bowes & Church's *Food Values of Portions Commonly Used,* 17th ed., revised by Jean A. T. Pennington (Philadelphia: Lippincott Williams & Wilkins, 1998), pp. 3–4, 6, 139–40.

Determining

Your

Needs

Twin and Multiple Pregnancies

Whether you are underweight, overweight, or normal weight, if you are pregnant with twins or more, you'll need to (and inevitably will) gain more weight than if you're having a single baby. According to recent studies, if you're having twins, you should gain between 35 and 45 pounds. During the second and third trimesters, you should put on about 1½ pounds a week. If you're carrying triplets, you'll need to gain even more weight — 50 to 60 pounds. The requirements go up with the number you are carrying. Since gestation periods for multiples tend to be shorter than for singleton pregnancies, averaging 37 to 38 weeks rather than 40, you'll need to gain a good portion of that weight sooner.

In fact, early weight gain — before 24 weeks — has been shown to influence the babies' growth after 24 weeks. The weight you put on during the early part of your pregnancy will result in fat stores that the babies will draw on later in your pregnancy, when their nutritional demands are tremendous. Also, it will become much more difficult to keep up with caloric demands as your pregnancy progresses, because you simply won't have much room for a lot of food — another reason to put on weight early.

As in singleton pregnancies, prepregnancy weight has a lot to do with the weight gain you should aim for. If you are underweight to begin with, you need to gain at the upper end of the scale, or maybe even more (doctors at the University of Michigan Multiples Clinic recommend a weight gain of 50 to 60 pounds for a woman who was 10 pounds underweight before conceiving twins), so you'll want to include lots of healthy carbs in your diet.

Pregnancy in Women over Forty

Most of the research done on pregnancies in older women has been directed at women over thirty-five. These days many women in their forties are becoming pregnant, often with the help of fertility treatments.

The caloric needs for pregnant women in their forties are no different than those of younger women; they do not need to eat more or less. But if you are older, you may be more set in your ways, and making dietary changes may be more difficult for you. Women tend to store more fat the older they get, so if too much weight is an issue for you, you will have to be vigilant during pregnancy. A lower-carbohydrate, lower-fat diet will probably be most suitable. If years of good habits have made you lean, however, you may have to bulk up. After all those years of buying nonfat dairy products, it may take a leap of the imagination to change to the 2% or even full-fat versions. But it will pay off. Eat more avocados and almonds, have a steak, have a bowl of ice cream, and enjoy!

Once you have some idea of what your nutritional needs will be during your pregnancy, you can use our meal plans to help you decide what you're actually going to eat. We think you'll be encouraged by how many choices you'll have.

Where Those Pounds Go

Because you're so focused on the developing person inside you, and because your belly grows so large, it's easy to imagine that everything you eat goes to the fetus. In reality, the fetus accounts for only about 25% of a pregnant woman's weight gain on average. About 6% of the weight gain is amniotic fluid, and about 5% is placenta. The other roughly two thirds is due to the expansion of your own tissues—increases in uterine and mammary tissues, volume of blood (10% of the total weight gain), fluid (the amount of fluid retained varies greatly among women), and fat stores. It is normal to accumulate fat stores during pregnancy. Their purpose may be an evolutionary need for an energy reserve during pregnancy and lactation should food supplies run short.

Eating by Trimester

The enormous and amazing changes that occur in your body throughout pregnancy can be thrilling — and sometimes annoying. They affect your appetite in different ways at different times. Knowing what is actually happening with your developing baby and what your body is doing to accommodate that development will help you understand why you feel the way you do at various times and why diet is so important.

The First Trimester

From the moment you conceive, your body begins to change at an often dizzying pace. During the early weeks of pregnancy, the fertilized egg (called a zygote) travels down the fallopian tube to your uterus, where it implants in the uterine wall. The cells of this embryo divide rapidly, and by the end of the first week, they're beginning to differentiate into organs, skin, hair, bone, and muscle. By the end of four weeks, the embryo, about the size of a grain of rice, has a heartbeat and the beginnings of a digestive system, backbone, spinal cord, and limb buds. After eight weeks, the embryo, now about an inch long (nearly half of it the head) and weighing a quarter of an ounce, has formed major organs and systems, the beginnings of legs and arms, a brain, and a face. From the ninth week on, the embryo is called a fetus. By the third month, nails have formed and the baby can open and close its hands and suck its fingers. By the end of the trimester, all of your baby's organs and tissues are formed, its kidneys are beginning to produce urine, and tooth buds for the baby teeth are appearing. All this in a fetus that is only about 3 inches long and weighs about 1½ ounces!

To accommodate these miraculous events, your body produces increased levels of hormones — more than thirty of them — in varying amounts throughout the course of your pregnancy.

Your progesterone level is ten times its prepregnancy level. This hormone helps maintain pregnancy in its earliest phases, keeping your uterus from contracting and encouraging the growth of blood vessels and glands in the uterine lining. By the seventh week, a complex relationship has been established between the embryo and the placenta, causing the placenta to produce as much estrogen in a single day as your body makes in three years when you aren't pregnant. The estrogen is necessary for changes and growth to occur in your uterus, cervix, vagina, and breasts and for metabolic changes that affect your salt and water balance, insulin secretion, and metabolism of sugars and carbohydrates. The emotional swings you may experience during your pregnancy are often the result of these high estrogen levels.

Your placenta also produces two other hormones, human chorionic gonadotropin (HCG) and human placental lactogen (HPL). HCG is the hormone that is measured to determine pregnancy. It is thought to prevent the mother from rejecting the embryo as foreign tissue, and it is probably also one of the factors that cause morning sickness. Lactogen acts as a growth hormone for your baby, changing your metabolism so that sugars and proteins are more available to it. It is also responsible for preparing your breasts for lactation.

With all of these changes going on, it's no wonder that you can feel odd at best, wiped-out and nauseous at worst.

If you aren't feeling much like eating, it will comfort you to know that caloric needs during the first trimester are the same as they were before you became pregnant, because your energy requirements during this time don't increase substantially. The changes in your body that require more calories, such as increased blood volume and fat stores, are just beginning to take place, and the fetus is tiny. Actual weight gain is less important than in the subsequent two trimesters. It's recommended that you gain between 2 and 5 pounds — about $3^{1}/_{2}$ pounds if you're of average weight, 5 pounds if you're underweight, and just 2 pounds if you're overweight. But some women gain no weight at all during the first trimester, and some actually lose weight, with no harm done to the developing baby. The important thing is to eat nutritious, unadulterated foods. If you're really sick, eating any food at all can alleviate your nausea enough to allow you to enjoy more nutritious foods. You can catch up and gain weight during subsequent trimesters.

If nausea isn't a problem and the adage "now you are eating for two" has gone to your head, you may gain too much weight during the first trimester. Cravings can be a problem if sweets are what you want. Often these carb cravings are a result of low blood sugar, which is a function of insufficient, or the wrong sort of, food intake. This is not to say that your cravings are not real, but if you are concerned about weight gain, your best strategy is to eat an adequate, balanced diet — regular meals and snacks at regular intervals — so that your blood sugar stays at an even level. Breakfast is particularly important, and many nutritionists recommend eating whole grains at every meal, as well as plenty of fruits and vegetables. If you are overweight to begin with or are concerned about gaining too much weight, be extra careful during the early months of pregnancy, when weight gain is not as important.

COMMON FIRST-TRIMESTER PROBLEMS

Fatigue

Some people experience fatigue — a tiredness unlike any they've ever felt— during the early months of pregnancy. This usually disappears after the first trimester, but it can be difficult to cope with and can certainly affect your desire or ability to eat well. If your life allows it (and it may not), give in to the fatigue; take as many naps as you feel you need. Live on the prepared foods suggested on pages 317–25, or let your partner wait on you. Do make sure, though, that your intake of food and essential nutrients is adequate, because poor nutrition will definitely contribute to fatigue. Try to avoid quick fixes like caffeine and sweets, because after a short burst of energy, you will experience a sharp drop in blood-sugar level. Finally, force yourself to exercise; it will be energizing.

One cause of fatigue can be iron deficiency anemia. Early on in your pregnancy, you will have a complete blood count (CBC), and if iron deficiency anemia is suspected, further tests, such as a serum iron, will be ordered. A more sensitive indicator of iron deficiency anemia is a test called a serum ferritin, which reflects tissue iron stores and can detect the early stages of iron deficiency anemia. You might want to ask your doctor about the ferritin test, as this is not the one that is routinely ordered.

Key Nutrients for the First Trimester

See A Nutrition Primer (page 381) for the best food sources of these nutrients.

FOLATE

Very important for cell reproduction and division and for neural development. Deficiency has been shown to be a factor in a neural tube defect called spina bifida.

ZINC

Zinc deficiencies early in pregnancy have been associated with preterm deliveries.

MANGANESE

For all of the developing organs, particularly the hearing apparatus.

POTASSIUM

Your own stores can be seriously depleted if you are vomiting frequently.

VITAMIN A

For cell growth and development, tissue growth, and eye development.

VITAMIN B$_6$

Several recent studies have shown vitamin B$_6$ to be an effective therapy for nausea and vomiting in pregnancy.[*]

[*]V. Sahakian, M.D., et al. "Vitamin B$_6$ Is Effective Therapy for Nausea and Vomiting of Pregnancy: A Randomized, Double-Blind Placebo-Controlled Study," *Obstetrics & Gynecology* 78, no. 1 (July 1991); T. Vutyavanich, M.D.; S. Wontra-ngan, M.D.; and R. Ruangsri, "Pyridoxine for Nausea and Vomiting of Pregnancy: A Randomized, Double-Blind, Placebo-Controlled Trial," *American Journal of Obstetrics and Gynecology* 173, (September 1995): 881–84.

Nausea

There are different degrees of "morning sickness," which is a misnomer, since the nausea is constant for most women who suffer from it. Some women feel slightly nauseous; others can't keep anything down. The average duration of morning sickness is 14 to 17 weeks, but some women experience nausea throughout their pregnancies.

There is no cure for pregnancy-related nausea, but there are coping mechanisms. Certain things help, such as keeping dry crackers or other foods you can stomach by the bed, in your desk, and in your purse and eating lots of snacks so that your stomach is never empty. It's extremely important to keep yourself hydrated if you are throwing up often, and sweet or sweet-tart drinks such as ginger ale, or lemonade or apple juice with lime, can be very set-

Coping with Nausea

The first trimester is a good time to experiment with different taste and texture sensations. Giving in to cravings immediately may prevent or alleviate nausea. Some of these suggestions for preventing queasiness may work for you.

- ✦ Keep appealing foods by your bed (crackers, matzo, almonds, hard candy such as lemon drops, pretzels, or apple juice or carbonated fruit drinks in an ice bucket), and eat or drink some of it before rising.
- ✦ Don't drink citrus juice first thing in the morning.
- ✦ Have a snack before going to sleep. This will help keep nausea at bay during the night.
- ✦ Eat lots of small meals.
- ✦ Alternate liquid snacks and solid snacks.
- ✦ Eat foods with a high liquid content, such as watermelon.
- ✦ Avoid greasy, rich foods; they're more difficult to digest.
- ✦ Never leave the house without food.
- ✦ Avoid sources of odors, such as refrigerators, trash cans, dirty diapers, pet products and boxes, gas stations, public restrooms, and coffeepots. Have somebody else open the refrigerator door and dispose of the trash whenever possible, and enlist someone else to change diapers.
- ✦ Ask your partner, a friend, or a relative to prepare food or bring home take-out meals.
- ✦ Use air-conditioning; heat and humidity exacerbate nausea.
- ✦ Rely on warm clothes and keep the use of artificial heaters to a minimum; these accelerate fluid loss.
- ✦ Avoid poor-quality computer screens and videos, which can cause nausea-producing dizziness.
- ✦ Keep lemons on hand to smell; their scent has proved useful as an antidote to nausea-provoking odors. Rinsing your mouth with fresh lemon juice and water also may alleviate symptoms.
- ✦ Experiment with Sea Bands (wristbands for seasickness, sold in pharmacies), acupressure, and hypnosis.
- ✦ Get up slowly.

Play It Safe

Doctors recommend taking the following measures to help ensure a healthy pregnancy.

✧ Abstain from alcohol.

✧ Reduce caffeine consumption to a minimum.

✧ Abstain from eating shark, swordfish, king mackerel, or tilefish. The Environmental Protection Agency warns that these fish may contain hazardous amounts of chemical pollutants and should not be consumed by pregnant and nursing women or by young children.

✧ Follow local health department advisories concerning fish caught in local waters. In any event, do not eat more than 6 ounces a week of cooked fish from local waters, because those waters may contain hazardous levels of chemical pollutants. You can safely eat up to 12 ounces a week of other types of cooked fish.

✧ Outside the United States, avoid eating lamb, which can carry *Toxoplasma gondii* bacteria.

✧ Avoid eating the following foods:

   ✦ Raw fish and raw shellfish.

   ✦ Fish from the Great Lakes: they may harbor dangerous levels of chemical pollutants.

   ✦ Raw meat.

   ✦ Fish soups and stews that contain mussels and clams (including pureed fish soups). One bad mussel can make you ill, and shellfish with cracked shells often go overlooked by kitchen help.

   ✦ Unpasteurized milk and milk products.

   ✦ Soft cheeses: these can carry *Listeriosa monocytogenes* bacteria.

   ✦ Pâtés and cold deli meats (unless you know that they have been safely refrigerated), which can cause food poisoning if bacteria have been able to grow.

   ✦ Where drinking water may be unsafe, fruits and vegetables that cannot be peeled.

   ✦ Raw eggs.

   ✦ Unpasteurized fruit juices and cider.

tling. In her book *No More Morning Sickness*, Miriam Erick emphasizes the importance of breaking the nausea cycle by eating whatever foods might appeal to you, be it potato chips or Popsicles, and then gradually working in more nutritious foods.

Cravings and Aversions

Most of us, whether we suffer from morning sickness or not, experience cravings and particularly aversions during pregnancy. They

Eating by

Trimester

can be surprising, too. You may have been a confirmed meat-eater before you were pregnant, but you can't imagine eating it now. No need to worry, as you can fill your protein needs with dairy products, eggs, fish, and beans. Often foods that you should avoid during pregnancy, such as coffee and alcohol, are unappealing, which makes it easy to swear off them. Other foods that may be dangerous to eat, such as raw seafood or oysters, are often unsavory. Cravings are often quite healthy — women report eating lots of grapefruit and oranges, melon, fresh greens, ice-cold milk, and simply cooked, light meats such as grilled chicken breasts. A craving for red meat could signify low iron.

Throughout your pregnancy (and from one pregnancy to the next), particularly during the early months, types of cravings and aversions may change regularly. One week you can't imagine eating tuna fish or drinking milk; the next week that's all you want. Another week you can't get enough citrus fruits. If you can manage to find foods with nutritional value to satisfy these desires, there is no reason not to give in to them. And remember, if you are suffering from nausea, any craving that will allow you to eat enough to break through your nausea should be honored.

The Second Trimester

By the end of the fourth month, your energy returns, and so does your appetite, often in a big way. As your caloric needs rise, you'll gain more weight — about a pound a week — than in the first or third trimester. This isn't surprising, since it's during the second trimester that your blood stores, fat stores, breast tissue, and water volume increase considerably. During the fourth month, you begin to produce amniotic fluid at a constant rate, and your baby's intestinal tract develops — although it doesn't completely mature until later — as the baby swallows and excretes fluid.

At the beginning of the second trimester, your baby is 3 to 3½ inches long and weighs about ¾ to 1 ounce. Then he or she has a rapid growth spurt, mostly the body and limbs. Fatty tissues that keep your baby warm develop during the fifth month, eyelashes and hair grow, and oil glands begin to secrete a fatty substance that mixes with dead cells to form a coating on the skin that will protect it from its long exposure to amniotic fluid. Your baby's hands can open and close, and he or she can suck. By the end of the sixth

The Foods We Crave

- Salty (potato chips, corn chips, pretzels, tuna, V8 juice, pickles, food sprinkled with salt, soy sauce). One of the causes of morning sickness may be low sodium in the blood, a result of increased blood plasma volume (the water portion of blood), which affects the sodium balance in your body. This also may be why you crave pickles.

- Tart, sour, and sweet-and-sour (lemonade, lemon wedges, grapefruit, lime wedges, pickles, marmalade, grapefruit juice, tonic water, apple juice with lime, vinegar, tart apples, mustard). The dill in dill pickles may be soothing to the intestinal tract.

- Sweet and juicy (citrus fruits, melon, grapes, frozen grapes, canned peaches, canned pears, canned mixed fruit).

- Crunchy (apples, carrots, celery, cucumbers, toast, chips, nuts, pickles, crackers, granola or other cereal, popcorn, biscotti).

- Bland (tofu, mashed potatoes, pasta, rice, custard, hot cereal, matzo, cottage cheese, milk, bagels with cream cheese, rice cakes).

- Soft and comforting (ice cream, frozen yogurt, flavored yogurt, mashed potatoes, Jell-O, custard, noodles, tortellini, roasted sweet potatoes, cereal with milk and fruit, milk).

- Warm (soup, tea, ginger tea, cocoa, latte).

- Sweet (hard candy such as Atomic FireBalls, cookies, ice cream, sherbet, frozen yogurt, sugared cereal, honey, canned fruit, juice, flavored yogurt, dried fruit, Power Bars, granola bars, muffins, gingerbread, graham crackers).

- Fruity/Wet (Popsicles, fresh fruit, frozen fruit, sparkling water, juice mixed with sparkling water, carbonated fruit drinks, ginger ale, fruit slush, smoothies, ice chips, Gatorade).

- Ginger (ginger ale, pickled ginger, ginger preserves). Ginger may relieve nausea symptoms, but avoid concentrated ginger capsules or supplements, since too much ginger may be harmful to the fetus.

month, the baby weighs in at 1½ to 2½ pounds and measures 11 to 14 inches long. Whereas the head accounted for half your baby's size when the second trimester began, by now the body has a newborn's proportions. The baby's skeleton turns from cartilage to bone during this period, and fingers and toes develop pads with their own unique prints. The lungs develop: tiny air sacs called alveoli begin to form in the lungs, and by the end of the month,

Eating by

Trimester

How to Make Cravings Work for You

Cravings for sweets are often driven by a drop in blood sugar. To prevent that, make sure you eat regular meals and snacks and include plenty of whole grains. Many sweets have food value, such as the following:

- Frozen yogurt or low-fat ice cream instead of regular ice cream
- Tofutti or sherbet instead of regular ice cream
- Low-fat or nonfat vanilla or fruit-flavored yogurt
- Angel food cake instead of regular cake
- Bran Muffins (page 48), Banana Bread (page 52), or Molasses Bread (page 53) instead of cake or doughnuts
- Cocoa or chocolate milk instead of chocolate candy or bars
- Fruit Popsicles
- Carbonated fruit drinks or juice diluted with sparkling water instead of soda
- Cold grapes or frozen grapes
- Cold watermelon, cantaloupe, or honeydew melon
- A cold orange or apple
- A Power Bar or granola bar
- Dried fruit, such as figs, prunes, raisins, or apricots
- Whole grain toast with jam
- Almond biscotti
- Cereal or granola with milk and fruit
- Roasted sweet potato
- Banana
- Rice Pudding (page 280)
- Bread Pudding with Apples and Peaches (page 269)

Try substituting a high-carbohydrate food that isn't sweet, such as fat-free tortilla chips, a bean quesadilla, a bean and rice burrito, or popcorn. If your craving for sweets is really a craving for carbohydrates of any kind, this may satisfy it.

If you crave potato chips but want something lower in fat, try:

- Pretzels
- Bagel chips
- Salted microwave popcorn
- Tamari-roasted almonds or trail mix
- Fat-free tortilla chips with salsa
- Dry-roasted peanuts
- Pickles
- Tuna fish; tuna sandwich on toasted rye bread with lettuce
- Seasoned rice cakes
- Edamame (fresh green soybeans) with salt or soy sauce
- Whole grains, noodles, or vegetables with soy sauce

If you crave bland foods, try:

- Basmati rice or brown rice
- Steamed new potatoes
- Poached or grilled chicken breast
- Baked or steamed sole
- Macaroni and cheese
- Tofu with soy sauce
- Avocados
- Steamed or microwaved frozen vegetables, such as green beans or carrots (these tend to be bland in comparison to fresh vegetables)
- Rice cakes

the blood vessels that will permit the exchange of oxygen and carbon dioxide are formed on the outside. Your baby's nostrils open, and he or she begins to make breathing movements. At the same time, the brain starts to display wave patterns similar to those of a full-term baby, reflecting visual and hearing activity.

Meanwhile, your own blood volume is increasing tremendously — more now than in the first or third trimester. At term, your blood supply will have increased by more than one half, from about $3\frac{1}{2}$ quarts to $5\frac{1}{2}$ quarts. And that doesn't even include the baby's blood. About a quart of the blood volume is red blood cells — a third more than you have when you're not pregnant. All of these red blood cells require iron, which is why your iron requirements increase so much during pregnancy. If iron stores are depleted, your red blood cell count will fall below normal.

Not surprisingly, your heart must work much harder to pump all this extra blood. It beats faster, resulting in a total output that is about a third higher than before pregnancy. No wonder you need extra calories!

Eating by

Trimester

Key Nutrients for the Second Trimester

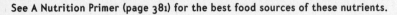

See A Nutrition Primer (page 381) for the best food sources of these nutrients.

PROTEIN

Needed for your own expanding blood volume and breast and uterine tissues, and for the growing tissues of the fetus and placenta.

IRON

Crucial four increased blood volume, and for the baby, who begins to store iron during the second trimester.

POTASSIUM

Needed for the transmission of nerve impulses. If you suffered from morning sickness during the first trimester, you may have depleted your stores of potassium.

CHROMIUM

Important in the regulation of blood sugar. A deficiency may contribute to gestational diabetes, which can occur during the second trimester.

VITAMIN C

Vital for the production of collagen, a component of connective tissue that binds together skin, blood vessels, nerves, and muscles.

This is the time when most women report feeling the best. You may have energy to cook again, and it becomes easier for you to exercise. Your belly is definitely growing but has not yet become cumbersome. If you're free of nausea, you can recoup calories and nutrients that you were too sick to consume during the early months. If you feel incredibly hungry and find yourself eating so much that you are gaining too much weight, make sure that you aren't eating too many carbohydrates and you're getting enough protein. Your protein needs are high at this time, because of all of the growth occurring in both you and your baby. Your calcium and iron needs are also peaking, as your baby's skeleton takes shape and your blood stores increase. If you're still suffering from fatigue, have your iron monitored. You may need supplementation.

COMMON SECOND-TRIMESTER PROBLEMS

The most common discomforts that occur during the second trimester have to do with digestion. The high degree of hormonal activity in your body can cause changes in your intestinal tract.

You are probably hungrier now, and if you are also struggling with digestive problems, you may want to eat many small meals rather than a few big ones.

Heartburn

Several factors contribute to heartburn, which can occur during the first trimester but more often begins during the second and may worsen during the third. Progesterone and estrogen, particularly progesterone, have a softening effect on the muscle tone of your smooth muscles — virtually all of the muscles and valves of your digestive tract. Motility — the movement of food through your digestive system — decreases, as does pressure on the sphincter that connects your stomach and esophagus. Your sphincter also works less efficiently as your uterus expands and begins to push the intestines and the stomach up and to the side, changing the angle at which the esophagus enters the stomach. This can result in reverse peristalsis — food moving backward instead of downward — which causes gastric acids combined with food to move into your esophagus. The burning sensation can be exacerbated by increased gastric acidity during pregnancy.

You may not be able to avoid heartburn altogether, but you may be able to alleviate its severity by eating small meals and avoiding gassy foods such as beans and cabbage, as well as fatty or highly spiced foods, particularly those that are fried or deep-fried. Discuss the use of antacids with your doctor. If your doctor approves, take them several hours before or after you take iron supplements and an hour before or after iron-rich meals, as they will impede iron absorption.

Constipation, Hemorrhoids, and Diarrhea

Constipation can result from progesterone's softening effect on muscle tone. The motion of the smooth muscles of your digestive tract is slowed down, and with it the transit time of food. At the same time, levels of a digestive hormone called motilin, which stimulates the movement of food through your intestines, drop. As stools sit in the lower intestine, water is absorbed, causing stools to harden. Constipation can be further exacerbated by your growing uterus, which crowds your lower intestine and rectum. Iron supplements can be another cause of constipation. Eating a fiber-rich diet — whole grains, fruits, vegetables, and legumes — and drink-

Coping with Heartburn

⮑ Eat small meals.

⮑ Do not eat dinner close to bedtime.

⮑ Avoid rich foods.

⮑ Avoid spicy foods.

⮑ Avoid gassy foods such as beans.

⮑ Do not lie down after meals. Some women sleep propped up on pillows.

⮑ Drink fluids between meals rather than with meals, but avoid carbonated beverages.

⮑ Suck on hard candy or chew sugarless gum to stimulate saliva, which helps neutralize stomach acids in the esophagus.

⮑ Avoid tight clothing.

⮑ Try to keep your weight gain in the moderate range (25 to 35 pounds). The more weight you're carrying, the more pressure there will be on your esophagus.

ing lots of fluids can help alleviate this situation. Also try to avoid caffeine, as it has a diuretic effect.

If your diet was not high in fiber before you became pregnant, introduce dietary changes slowly. If you change your diet too quickly, your enzymes won't be able to cope with all of the fiber, and you will suffer from gas. Flatulence can plague you during the second and third trimesters. If it does, eat small meals, and eat them slowly. Any foods that give you gas should be eliminated. Beans are great for you, but they're not worth eating now if they are making you uncomfortable. Find other sources of protein and fiber.

Hemorrhoids, enlarged veins in your rectum, are the result of both constipation and your increased blood supply. The same hormones that decrease motility in your lower intestine are to blame. By avoiding constipation, you can avoid hemorrhoids.

Some women experience the opposite problem, diarrhea. This also can be related to a hormone released by the placenta, called relaxin. It relaxes smooth muscle contractions, which in turn can relax your digestive tract, so that food moves through too quickly. If your diet was low in fiber before you became pregnant and you switch too quickly to high-fiber foods, flatulence and diarrhea can result, so make changes gradually.

The Third Trimester

The baby continues to grow rapidly during the last three months of pregnancy — and so do you! Weight gain is very important. Whereas during the second trimester, much of your weight gain represented the expansion of your own tissues, during the final trimester, the weight is almost all baby: he or she doubles in size during this period.

By the end of the seventh month, your baby could live outside the womb but would need some help with breathing. The baby's weight increases during this month by about a pound, and his or her length can increase by up to 3 inches. Bones begin to harden as the baby stores calcium, and muscle tone increases. You will be well aware of this, as the frequent movements often feel like hard kicks. Subcutaneous fat, called white fat, forms during the seventh month, smoothing out the baby's wrinkled skin, and the fine hair that covered the entire fetus disappears from most areas except the back and shoulders. Bone marrow takes on the production of red blood cells, and in male babies the testes descend into the scrotal sac from the abdomen. The baby also stores other minerals, such as iron, putting further demands on your own iron needs.

This is a crucial time for the baby's brain and nervous system development. The brain grows tremendously during the third trimester, acquiring many new cells and taking on the folded shape of a fully mature brain. The brain accounts for 20% of your baby's energy consumption at this time. By the end of the seventh month, it will have the capacity of a newborn's: a baby born prematurely at this time will be able to see, hear, smell, and learn. During this trimester, the baby also begins to produce a fatty sheath called myelin, which surrounds nerve fibers and functions in the transmission of nerve impulses.

A recent study indicated that the baby's taste buds and olfactory senses are working by the third trimester. Your baby may actually develop tastes for the things you eat, because flavors from your diet are transmitted to your amniotic fluid and swallowed by the fetus.[1]

During the eighth and ninth months, your baby continues to

[1] Julie A. Menella, Coren P. Jagnow, and Gary K. Beauchamp, "Prenatal and Postnatal Flavor Learning by Human Infants," *Pediatrics* 107, no. 6 (June 2001).

Eating by

Trimester

acquire fat. The lungs are still developing, forming a substance which allows them to inflate and deflate. Your baby is storing calcium, phosphorus, and iron and becoming stronger. Movements are frequent and can be quite powerful. As you near the end of term, your baby continues to gain about half a pound a week, most of it fat. The baby's movements slow as he or she drops down into your pelvis, but you will still feel the baby moving, particularly after meals. Although you may not be sleeping much at this point, your baby has adopted a sleep pattern.

Your diet during the third trimester is important not only for the developing person inside you but also for preparing you for labor and delivery and for nursing. Being in shape can make a world of difference; you will need stamina. You also will lose quite a bit of blood, and your tissues will be taxed, especially if you have a cesarean delivery, so getting extra nourishment now is crucial.

COMMON THIRD-TRIMESTER PROBLEMS

The discomforts that occur during the third trimester have to do less with hormonal changes than with the size of your baby.

Fatigue

The final months of pregnancy can be tiring. It's not the kind of fatigue you may have experienced during the first trimester, but one that grows out of physical exertion. The weight you are carrying can make movement difficult and can make you feel sluggish. You'll probably wake up several times a night to urinate, since your bladder has so little room now. And if you are suffering from heartburn, you may be sleeping — or trying to sleep — propped up on pillows. Comfort yourself with the idea that the disturbed sleep is good training for the first year of motherhood. It's important to continue to get exercise at this time so that you keep in shape for labor and delivery. If you have not been exercising, however, do not start now. Swimming or water exercises, Pilates, and yoga are easier than weight-bearing exercises.

Heartburn

This condition can begin or worsen during the last trimester. Eating small meals and avoiding rich, gassy, greasy, and spicy foods can help, as can delaying lying down until at least two hours after a

Key Nutrients for the Third Trimester

See A Nutrition Primer (page 381) for the best food sources of these nutrients.

CALCIUM
The baby's bones calcify during the last trimester. You need extra stores of calcium for yourself so that the baby doesn't draw from your own bones. This is particularly important if you are older.

IRON
The baby builds up iron stores, which protect him or her from anemia during the first few months of life. You need extra reserves to compensate for blood loss during delivery. Lack of iron can cause fatigue, and you will need stamina for labor and delivery.

PROTEIN
Protein needs are great at this time because of the baby's rapid growth rate.

OMEGA-3 FATTY ACIDS
Important for the baby's brain development.

ZINC
Another key nutrient in brain development. Also important for recovery after childbirth, since it helps in healing wounds.

VITAMIN B$_6$
Necessary for the metabolism of protein and the formation of hemoglobin and of neurotransmitters in the brain. The higher your protein needs, the higher your vitamin B$_6$ needs are.

VITAMIN C
A key nutrient in tissue repair and recovery after delivery. Also important for the immune system.

VITAMIN A
Necessary for recovery after delivery. Also helps repair the tissue that lines the vagina and uterus.

VITAMIN E
Aids in tissue repair and recovery after delivery.

PANTOTHENIC ACID
Aids in tissue repair and recovery after delivery.

meal. One way of making small meals convenient is to divide a regular meal into two portions and eat them a couple of hours apart.

Constipation and Hemorrhoids

See page 23 for a more detailed discussion of these conditions. Your digestive tract continues to be crowded by the baby, so constipation and hemorrhoids can be a problem. Eat a fiber-rich diet — don't forget about prunes and dried figs — and remember to drink lots of liquids.

Frequent Urination

This is a condition of pregnancy, especially during the final months, when your uterus is crowding your bladder. Try to drink most of your liquids early in the day. Practice Kegel exercises, which you learn in childbirth classes, to increase control.

Insomnia

Usually as a result of all of the problems listed above, most women sleep badly during the last trimester. It has been suggested that a high-carbohydrate snack before bed helps, because carbohydrates trigger the release of a brain chemical called serotonin, which aids sleep.

Leg and Pelvic Area Cramps

These can be painful and also contribute to sleep deprivation, since leg cramps usually occur at night or in the early morning when you're in bed. Experts used to say that leg cramps were a result of calcium deficiency, but this is no longer believed to be a factor. Poor circulation is probably a more accurate explanation of why these occur. Cramps and painful twinges — often excruciating — in the upper thighs and pubic area have to do with the baby pressing on nerves and the softening of pelvic joints in preparation for delivery.

Pregnancy and Food Safety

When you're pregnant, you're not at any greater risk than others for food-borne illnesses, but these illnesses can have dire consequences. Infection with the bacteria that cause listeriosis and toxoplasmosis, in particular, can result in stillbirth, miscarriage, or birth defects. The same measures that should be taken to prevent these diseases will also prevent other types of food poisoning.

- Reheat ready-to-eat meat and poultry products until steaming. Do not eat meat, poultry, or fish products that cannot be reheated.
- Wash your hands thoroughly before handling foods; after touchng meat, poultry, and ready-to-eat deli foods; and after using the bathroom. Get into the habit of washing your hands often to prevent infections you might pick up simply by holding on to subway rails, handling children, and the like. Use hot soapy water and wash your fingertips well.
- Wash all cutting boards, dishes, and utensils thoroughly with hot soapy water after handling meats, poultry, fish, and ready-to-eat foods.
- Wash your refrigerator shelves thoroughly with hot soapy water if juices drip from meat, poultry, or prepared foods. Bacteria can grow in the refrigerator.
- To prevent cross-contamination, keep raw meat, poultry, seafood, and ready-to-eat foods away from other foods (fruits, vegetables, breads, leftovers, cheese) in the refrigerator.
- Double-wrap meat and poultry in the refrigerator and freezer to prevent contamination of other foods with their juices.
- Chill or freeze perishable foods and leftovers within 2 hours.
- Cook foods to safe temperatures.
- Avoid soft cheeses, such as Brie, Camembert, and vacherin, and other cheeses and products made with raw, unpasteurized milk.
- Pay close attention to expiration dates for ready-to-eat and perishable packaged foods.
- Make sure your refrigerator is below 40°F and your freezer is at or below 0°F.
- Wash all fruits and vegetables thoroughly, including prewashed salad greens and precut vegetables.
- Never use eggs that have cracked shells. Cook eggs for at least 3 minutes, or if you are not cooking them, make sure an acid such as lemon juice or vinegar is included in the recipe; the acid will destroy any bacteria. Wash utensils in hot soapy water after working with raw eggs.

BREAKFAST FOODS

Microwave Oatmeal with Milk and Raisins 31

Couscous with Oranges and Dates 32

Muesli 33

Quick Individual Omelets, Flat or Folded 34

Scrambled Tofu 37

French Toast 38

Buttermilk Pancakes 39

Fried Eggs with Spicy Cooked Tomato Sauce
(Huevos Rancheros) 40

Dried Fruit Compote 42

Scandinavian Fruit Soup 43

Smoothies 44

Apple-Cinnamon Tofu Spread 46

Microwave Oatmeal with Milk and Raisins

ADVANCE PREPARATION
This will keep, covered, for a couple of days in the refrigerator.

In the morning, speed is everything. You're hungry and often nauseous, and the quicker you can get nutritious food into your stomach, the better. Cereals of all kinds are a great vehicle for milk, and oatmeal is especially comforting, particularly in the winter. You can make this the night before and reheat it in the morning, or make it in the morning. The longer it sits after cooking, the more the oatmeal swells and softens. Make sure to use a large Pyrex cup or bowl for this, as the water will bubble up considerably.

$\frac{1}{2}$ cup old-fashioned rolled oats or oatmeal
1 tablespoon dark or golden raisins
  Salt to taste
$\frac{3}{4}$ cup water
1 teaspoon honey or brown sugar (optional)
$\frac{1}{2}$ cup milk or soy milk
  Fresh fruit for serving (optional)

1. Combine all the ingredients except the milk and fruit in a 4-cup Pyrex measure or 1-quart Pyrex bowl. Cover with plastic wrap and pierce the plastic to vent the bowl. Place in the microwave and cook at 100% power, or high, for 3 minutes. Let sit for 1 minute, remove the plastic (take care not to burn yourself), and stir. Replace the plastic and cook for 1 minute more. Let sit for 1 minute, then carefully remove the plastic and stir in the milk. The oatmeal will swell as it absorbs the milk.

2. Transfer to a serving bowl. (If you are making this the night before, refrigerate. In the morning heat for 30 seconds in the microwave at 100% power, or high.) Serve as is or with fresh fruit, if desired. I like grated apple or sliced peaches in season.

KEY NUTRIENTS
Vitamin B_{12}
Riboflavin (if using
    regular or 1% milk)
Calcium
Iron
Manganese
Phosphorus

Breakfast Foods

ADVANCE PREPARATION

This can be made several hours ahead of serving and held at room temperature or chilled. You can make the couscous, up to adding the oranges, a day or two before serving and keep it in the refrigerator. Let it come to room temperature, then add the cut-up oranges up to a few hours before serving.

Couscous with Oranges and Dates

This is a typical Tunisian way of preparing couscous. It's delicious for breakfast, and it can also be dessert. You can find orange flower water in Middle Eastern groceries.

2¼ cups water
¼ cup sugar
2 tablespoons orange flower water (optional)
2 tablespoons unsalted butter
1½ cups couscous
½ cup dried apricots, cut in half or chopped
¼ cup dried currants or golden raisins
1 teaspoon ground cinnamon
Generous pinch of salt
3 navel oranges
10 dates, quartered lengthwise and seeds removed

1. Combine the water and sugar in a medium saucepan and bring to a boil. Reduce the heat and boil slowly for 10 minutes, until the mixture thickens slightly. Stir in the orange flower water, if using, and remove from the heat. Stir in the butter until it is melted.

2. Place the couscous in a large bowl. Stir in the dried apricots, currants or raisins, cinnamon, and salt. Pour on the syrup. Let sit for 20 minutes, stirring from time to time with a wooden spoon to break up any clumps.

3. Line a steamer basket with a clean kitchen towel and dump the couscous on top of the towel. Place the basket in a saucepan with 1 inch of simmering water. Cover and steam for 15 minutes, making sure that the water is well below the couscous. Turn out into a large bowl.

KEY NUTRIENTS
Beta Carotene
Vitamin A
Vitamin B$_6$
Folacin
Niacin
Thiamin
Vitamin C
Copper
Iron
Magnesium
Manganese
Potassium

4. Remove the skin and pith from the oranges, holding them above the couscous so that any juice escapes into the couscous. Cut 2 of the oranges in half crosswise, then into small pieces. Neatly divide the third orange into sections. Toss the steamed couscous with the 2 cut-up oranges.

5. Transfer to a wide serving bowl or platter and mold into a cone-shaped mound. Decorate the top with the orange sections and dates. Serve warm or at room temperature.

Muesli

One of my favorite ways to enjoy oatmeal, this delicate combination gets texture and sweetness from nuts and grated apple.

  2 cups quick-cooking (not instant) oatmeal
¹/₄ cup chopped almonds, sunflower seeds, or ground flax
     seeds
  1 tart apple, such as Granny Smith, peeled, cored, and
     grated
¹/₄ cup dried currants
     Milk for moistening
     Brown sugar or honey for sweetening (optional)

1. Preheat the oven to 375°F. Put the oatmeal and almonds or seeds on a baking sheet and bake for 8 to 10 minutes, just until lightly toasted.

2. Remove from the oven and toss with the apple and currants in a medium bowl. Moisten with milk. Sweeten, if you wish, with brown sugar or honey and serve.

Makes about 2 cups, or 4 servings

ADVANCE PREPARATION
You can toast the oatmeal and nuts or seeds and keep them for weeks in the refrigerator.

KEY NUTRIENTS
Fiber
Iron
Manganese
Phosphorus

Breakfast Foods

ADVANCE
PREPARATION
Make the omelet with-
out folding it, then let
cool. Cut it into
wedges and take them
to work or on a picnic.
All the fillings except
the cheese are good
cold or at room tem-
perature.

Quick Individual Omelets, Flat or Folded

Omelets, whether flat or folded, make an incredibly easy, nutritious, and fast meal. You can fill them with vegetables or
cheese, working different food groups into your breakfast,
lunch, or dinner.

2 large eggs, or 1 large egg and 2 large egg whites
Salt (a good pinch) and freshly ground pepper to taste
1 teaspoon milk
Filling of your choice (recipes follow)
1 1/2 teaspoons olive oil or butter

1. Using a whisk or fork, beat the eggs, or egg and egg
whites, in a small bowl. The whites and yolks should be nicely
amalgamated. Add the salt and pepper and milk. You can stir the
filling into the eggs now or place it down the middle of the omelet
as it cooks in the pan.

2. Heat the olive oil or butter in an 8-inch nonstick skillet
over medium-high heat. Hold your hand over the pan; it should
feel hot. Drizzle in a bit of egg; if it sizzles and cooks at once, the
pan is ready.

3. Pour in the egg mixture and tilt and swirl the pan to coat
the bottom evenly. Using a spatula, gently lift the cooked edges of
the omelet and tilt the pan to let more uncooked egg run underneath. Shake the pan constantly but gently and continue to lift and
tilt to allow the uncooked egg to run underneath the cooked egg.
When the top of the omelet is just about set, place the filling down
the middle (if you haven't stirred it into the eggs), and fold the
omelet over. Heat for 30 to 60 seconds, then slide the omelet onto
a plate, folding it over. You can also slide the omelet out without
folding it.

KEY NUTRIENTS
Protein
Vitamin A
Vitamin B$_{12}$
Folacin
Riboflavin
Iron
Phosphorus
Omega-3s (if using high-
omega eggs)

EVERY WOMAN'S

GUIDE TO EATING

DURING PREGNANCY

4. Serve at once or keep warm in a 250°F oven while you make more omelets.

FILLINGS

KEY NUTRIENTS
SWISS CHARD OR
SPINACH
Beta Carotene
Vitamin A
Vitamin B$_6$
Folacin
Riboflavin (spinach)
Vitamin C
Vitamin E
Calcium
Copper (except spinach)
Iron
Magnesium
Manganese
Potassium

Swiss Chard or Spinach

$^1/_2$ cup chopped cooked Swiss chard or spinach
   Salt to taste
1 garlic clove, minced or pressed (optional)

KEY NUTRIENTS
BROCCOLI
Beta Carotene
Vitamin A
Vitamin B$_6$
Folacin
Vitamin C
Manganese
Potassium

Steamed Broccoli or Asparagus

$^1/_3$–$^1/_2$ cup cooked chopped asparagus or broccoli, to taste
  1–2 teaspoons chopped fresh chives or parsley, to taste
    (optional)

KEY NUTRIENTS
ASPARAGUS
Beta Carotene
Vitamin A
Vitamin B$_6$
Folacin
Vitamin C
Vitamin E
Copper
Manganese
Potassium

Tomato

3–4 tablespoons tomato sauce for pasta (homemade or
    commercial) or chopped fresh tomato, to taste
  1 teaspoon slivered fresh basil leaves
  2 tablespoons freshly grated Parmesan cheese (optional)

KEY NUTRIENTS
TOMATO
Vitamin A
Vitamin C
Vitamin E

(VARIATIONS CONTINUED ON NEXT PAGE)

KEY NUTRIENTS
MUSHROOMS
Niacin
Folacin
Riboflavin
Copper
Iron
Phosphorus
Potassium

Mushrooms

1 teaspoon olive oil or butter
1 garlic clove, minced or pressed
½ cup sliced fresh mushrooms
  Salt and freshly ground pepper to taste
1–2 teaspoons chopped fresh herbs, such as parsley, chives, or thyme, to taste

Heat the oil or butter in a small nonstick skillet over medium heat and add the garlic. As soon as it begins to sizzle, add the mushrooms and a bit of salt. Cook, stirring, until the mushrooms release their liquid. Continue to cook until the liquid has evaporated and the mushrooms are tender, 5 to 10 minutes. Add the salt and pepper and herbs, and remove from the heat. Let cool for a few minutes before adding to the omelet.

KEY NUTRIENTS
CHEESE
Vitamin A
Vitamin B$_{12}$
Folacin
Riboflavin
Calcium
Magnesium
Phosphorus
Zinc

Cheese

1 ounce Gruyère, cheddar, or Monterey jack cheese, grated (about ¼ cup)

Sprinkle the cheese down the middle of the omelet as it begins to set in the pan.

Scrambled Tofu

Silken tofu can be cooked like scrambled eggs and has a similar high protein content. It will absorb the flavors of whatever you add to the dish. The tastier those ingredients are, the better.

1 tablespoon olive or canola oil
1 pound medium or firm silken tofu
Salt or soy sauce and freshly ground pepper to taste

Heat the oil in a medium or large nonstick skillet over high heat. Crumble in the tofu and season with the salt or soy sauce and pepper. Cook, stirring, until the tofu firms up and is heated through. Serve immediately, or store and reheat.

VARIATION

Scrambled Tofu with Herbs

Begin cooking the tofu, and when it begins to firm up, stir in ¼ cup chopped fresh herbs, such as parsley, tarragon, dill, basil, chives, or marjoram. Stir together for 30 to 60 seconds, then serve.

VARIATION

Scrambled Tofu with Onion

Before adding the tofu to the pan, chop 1 medium onion and cook until tender, about 5 minutes. Add the tofu and proceed as directed.

VARIATION

Mexican Scrambled Tofu

Prepare the filling for Soft Tacos with Tofu and Tomatoes (page 211) and serve.

ADVANCE PREPARATION

Unlike scrambled eggs, scrambled tofu can be cooked ahead and reheated. Keep it in the pan on the stove if you're not holding it for too long, or refrigerate for up to 2 days.

KEY NUTRIENTS (ALL VERSIONS)
Protein
Calcium
Iron

KEY NUTRIENTS MEXICAN
Protein
Vitamin A
Vitamin C
Calcium
Iron

ADVANCE
PREPARATION
If you are not serving
the French toast right
away, keep them warm
in a 200°F oven for up
to 30 minutes.

French Toast

This is eggs, toast, and milk all in one dish. Traditional French toast is made with an eggy bread like challah or brioche, which is quite rich. I like it just as well made with a whole wheat or mixed-grain sandwich bread. Make sure not to saturate the bread so much that it breaks up before you put it in the pan. Unsweetened preserves, a fruit puree, and maple syrup make nice accompaniments.

4 large eggs
1 cup milk
1 tablespoon sugar (optional)
Pinch of salt
Pinch of freshly grated nutmeg
2 tablespoons butter
8 thick slices slightly stale bread
1 teaspoon powdered sugar for dusting (optional)

1. Beat together the eggs, milk, sugar (if using), salt, and nutmeg in a large, wide bowl.

2. Heat 1 tablespoon of the butter in a large, heavy nonstick skillet over medium heat until bubbling. Take 4 slices of bread and dip each one into the batter; flip it over. The batter should moisten both sides of the bread, but the bread should hold its shape. Place the bread in the skillet, reduce the heat to medium-low, and cook slowly until golden brown, 5 to 7 minutes. Turn and cook on the other side. Heat the remaining 1 tablespoon butter in the skillet and proceed with the remaining 4 slices bread.

3. To serve, dust with powdered sugar, if you wish.

KEY NUTRIENTS
Protein
Vitamin A
Vitamin B$_{12}$
Folacin
Riboflavin
Calcium
Iron
Phosphorus

WHITE BREAD
Niacin
Riboflavin
Thiamin
Iron
Manganese
Phosphorus

WHOLE WHEAT BREAD
Vitamin B$_6$
Niacin
Folacin
Riboflavin
Thiamin
Copper
Iron
Magnesium
Manganese
Phosphorus

Buttermilk Pancakes

Even when they're made with regular whole wheat flour, these pancakes are light. The buttermilk contributes a tangy flavor, and the vanilla adds sweetness. The trick to making light pancakes is to stir the batter as little as possible.

1 cup whole wheat flour or whole wheat pastry flour
1/2 cup all-purpose flour
1 tablespoon sugar
2 teaspoons baking powder
1 teaspoon baking soda
1/2 teaspoon salt
2 large eggs
1 1/2 cups buttermilk, or 1 cup yogurt mixed with 1/2 cup milk
3 tablespoons canola oil
1 teaspoon pure vanilla extract

1. Mix together the flours, sugar, baking powder, baking soda, and salt in a medium bowl.

2. Beat together the eggs, buttermilk or yogurt-milk mixture, oil, and vanilla in a medium bowl. Add the dry ingredients and mix together quickly, stirring as little as possible.

3. Heat a large, heavy nonstick or cast-iron skillet or griddle over medium-high heat. When a drop of batter sizzles upon contact, reduce the heat to medium. Ladle 1/4-cup portions of the batter onto the hot skillet and cook until tiny bubbles break through the surface, 2 to 3 minutes. Flip over and cook for about 1 minute more, until browned. Serve at once or transfer to a platter and keep warm in a 200°F oven until all the pancakes are done.

ADVANCE
PREPARATION
Although the pancakes are best served immediately, I have kept them, well wrapped in plastic, in the freezer for a month or in the refrigerator for a few days. I just thaw or heat them in the microwave as needed. Heat refrigerated pancakes for 20 to 30 seconds on high. Use the reheat or thaw button for frozen.

KEY NUTRIENTS
Vitamin B_6
Vitamin B_{12}
Folacin
Niacin
Riboflavin
Thiamin
Calcium
Copper
Iron
Magnesium
Manganese
Phosphorus

Breakfast Foods

ADVANCE
PREPARATION
The sauce can be made
a day or two ahead and
stored, covered, in the
refrigerator.

Fried Eggs with Spicy Cooked Tomato Sauce
(Huevos Rancheros)

Although these zesty eggs with tortillas are listed with the breakfasts, there's no reason you can't eat this dish for dinner or lunch as well. Use store-bought salsa if you don't want to make your own.

FOR THE SALSA

2 pounds tomatoes, peeled and coarsely chopped
2–3 serrano peppers or 1–2 jalapeño peppers (or more to taste), seeded for a milder sauce and chopped
½ small onion, chopped
2 garlic cloves, minced or pressed
1 tablespoon canola oil
Salt to taste (about ½ teaspoon)

FOR THE TORTILLAS AND EGGS

8 corn tortillas, plus more to pass at the table
1–2 teaspoons canola oil
4–8 large eggs
Salt and freshly ground pepper to taste
1 tablespoon chopped fresh cilantro

KEY NUTRIENTS
Protein
Vitamin A
Vitamin B₁₂
Folacin
Riboflavin
Vitamin C
Vitamin E
Calcium
Iron
Phosphorus

1. FOR THE SALSA: Place the tomatoes, peppers, onion, and garlic in a blender and puree just long enough to retain a bit of texture. Heat the oil in a large, heavy nonstick skillet over medium heat. Drop a bit of puree into the skillet, and if it sizzles, add the rest. Cook, stirring, for 5 to 10 minutes, until the sauce thickens and begins to stick to the pan. Add salt to taste. Keep warm while you heat the tortillas and fry the eggs. (If you are using store-bought salsa, bring to a simmer in a saucepan.)

2. FOR THE TORTILLAS AND EGGS: Warm the tortillas in any of the following ways: wrap in aluminum foil and heat through in a 350°F oven for 15 minutes; heat 1 or 2 at a time in a dry nonstick skillet over medium-high heat until flexible; place in a steamer basket set in a saucepan with 1 inch of simmering water, cover, steam for 1 minute, and remove from the heat; wrap in wax paper or a clean dishtowel and heat in the microwave on high power for 1 minute.

3. Have 4 plates ready. Heat 1 teaspoon of the oil in a large nonstick skillet over medium heat and carefully break in 4 of the eggs. Cook sunny-side up, until the whites are cooked through and the yolks are still runny. Sprinkle with salt and pepper and turn off the heat.

4. Place 2 warm tortillas, overlapping, on each plate. Top each with 1 or 2 fried eggs. Keep warm. Repeat with the remaining 1 teaspoon oil and 4 eggs, if using.

5. Spoon the hot sauce over the whites of the eggs and the tortillas, leaving the yolks exposed. Sprinkle with the cilantro and serve at once, passing additional tortillas at the table.

ADVANCE
PREPARATION
The compote will keep
for 2 to 3 weeks in the
refrigerator. The fruit
will eventually lose
much of its flavor, but
the syrup will become
sweeter.

Dried Fruit Compote

This compote serves two purposes: it makes morning yogurt wonderfully appetizing, without all the sugar in flavored yogurts, and it's a great source of fiber. Pregnancy-related constipation was never a problem for me as long as I had this on hand. The compote keeps for weeks in the refrigerator, and a little goes a long way. All you need to do is stir a little syrup and fruit into some yogurt. Have it for breakfast or an afternoon snack.

^{1}/$_2$ pound mixed dried fruit, such as cherries, apricots, figs, prunes, or raisins
Water as needed
2 tablespoons fresh lemon juice
3 wide strips lemon zest
1 2-inch cinnamon stick
^{1}/$_4$ cup sugar
Plain yogurt for serving

1. Place the dried fruit in a bowl and cover with hot water. Let sit for 4 hours or overnight. Drain through a strainer set over a bowl.

2. Measure the soaking liquid from the dried fruit and add enough water to make 3 cups. Combine with the fruit, lemon juice, lemon zest, cinnamon stick, and sugar in a medium saucepan and bring to a simmer. Cook for 15 minutes, then strain over a bowl. Return the syrup to the saucepan and transfer the fruit to the bowl.

KEY NUTRIENTS
Fiber
Beta Carotene
Vitamin A
Vitamin B$_6$
Niacin
Riboflavin
Thiamin (raisins)
Vitamin E
Copper
Iron
Magnesium
Manganese
Phosphorus
Potassium

3. Bring the syrup to a boil and cook until thick and reduced by about a third, 5 to 8 minutes. Pour over the fruit. Let cool, then cover and chill.

4. Stir a little fruit and syrup into the yogurt and serve.

Scandinavian Fruit Soup

ADVANCE
PREPARATION
This will keep for at
least a week in the re-
frigerator but will re-
quire thinning with
water or juice.

This thick, sweet soup is really a tapioca-thickened compote, made primarily from dried fruit. It's good hot or cold and is great for breakfast or dessert. Stirred into a bowl of plain or vanilla yogurt, this makes a nutritious snack.

3 tablespoons regular or quick-cooking tapioca
1 cup dried apricots, cut in half
1 cup pitted prunes, cut in half
1/2 cup golden raisins
1/2 cup dried cherries
2 3-inch cinnamon sticks
4 cups apple, cranberry, or pear juice, plus more if needed
2 cups water, plus more if needed
2 tart apples, such as Granny Smith, peeled, cored, and chopped
1–2 tablespoons sugar, to taste
Sour cream or Yogurt Cheese (page 65) for topping (optional)

1. If using regular tapioca, soak it overnight in water to cover.

2. Drain the tapioca and combine with the dried fruit, cinnamon sticks, fruit juice, and water in a large soup pot or saucepan. Bring to a boil, reduce the heat to low, cover partially, and simmer for 45 minutes to 2 hours (depending on the type of tapioca used), until the tapioca is clear, the soup is smooth, and the fruit is soft. Stir from time to time to be sure nothing is sticking to the bottom of the pot, and add more juice or water if the mixture becomes too thick. Add the apples and continue to cook until just tender, about 10 minutes. Taste and add the sugar.

3. Serve hot, topped with a dollop of sour cream or thickened yogurt, if desired. Or let cool, refrigerate, and serve cold.

KEY NUTRIENTS
Fiber
Beta Carotene
Vitamin A
Vitamin B_6
Niacin
Riboflavin
Thiamin
Vitamin C
Vitamin E
Copper
Iron
Magnesium
Manganese
Phosphorus
Potassium

Breakfast Foods

ADVANCE PREPARATION

These are best served right away.

Smoothies

These filling fruit milk shakes make great, quick breakfasts and nutritious snacks. You can use milk, yogurt, or buttermilk. Or use soy milk for a nondairy version.

KEY NUTRIENTS
DAIRY-BASED
SMOOTHIES
Protein
Vitamin B$_{12}$
Riboflavin
Calcium
Phosphorus

SOY-BASED
SMOOTHIES
Protein
Iron
Isoflavins

BANANAS
Vitamin B$_6$
Folacin
Vitamin C
Potassium
Magnesium

MANGOES
Beta Carotene
Vitamin A
Vitamin C
Vitamin E

PEACHES
Vitamin A
Vitamin C

Banana Smoothie

1 large ripe banana
1 cup cold milk, yogurt, buttermilk, or soy milk
1 teaspoon sugar or honey, or more to taste (optional)
2–3 ice cubes

Banana Strawberry Smoothie

1 small or 1/2 large ripe banana
1 heaped cup fresh strawberries, hulled
1 cup cold milk, yogurt, buttermilk, or soy milk
1 teaspoon honey or sugar (optional)
2–3 ice cubes

Mango Smoothie

1 cup chopped, peeled ripe mango (1 medium mango)
1 cup cold milk, yogurt, buttermilk, or soy milk
1 tablespoon fresh lime juice
1 teaspoon sugar (optional)
2–3 ice cubes

Peach Smoothie

2 medium sweet, juicy, ripe peaches, peeled and pitted
1 cup cold milk, yogurt, buttermilk, or soy milk
1 teaspoon honey
2–3 ice cubes

Strawberry Smoothie

STRAWBERRIES
Folacin
Vitamin C
Manganese

2 cups fresh strawberries, hulled
1 cup cold milk, yogurt, buttermilk, or soy milk
2 teaspoons honey
2-3 ice cubes

Optional Additions

2 teaspoons ground flax seeds
1-2 tablespoons protein powder, to taste
1 tablespoon brewer's yeast
1-3 teaspoons toasted wheat germ, to taste

Place all the ingredients and additions of your choice (if using) in a blender jar with 2 or 3 ice cubes. Blend at high speed until smooth. Pour into a tall glass and serve.

ADVANCE
PREPARATION
This will keep for a
week in the refrigera-
tor.

Apple-Cinnamon Tofu Spread

This sweet spread is great any time of day, but it's particularly good on toast. The blended tofu and applesauce, sweetened with a bit of honey and spice, firms up as it bakes. It's sort of like a tofu cheesecake — and indeed, you could eat it for dessert.

$^1/_2$ pound soft, medium, or firm silken tofu
 1 cup unsweetened applesauce
 2 tablespoons mild-flavored honey (such as clover) or
     maple syrup
 1 tablespoon fresh lemon juice
 1 tablespoon sesame tahini
 1 teaspoon pure vanilla extract
 1 tablespoon unbleached or all-purpose flour
$^1/_2$ teaspoon ground cinnamon
$^1/_4$–$^1/_2$ teaspoon freshly grated nutmeg, to taste
 $^1/_4$ teaspoon salt

1. Preheat the oven to 350°F. Butter or oil a 1-quart baking dish or bread pan.

2. Puree all the ingredients in a food processor until very smooth. Scrape into the prepared baking dish. Bake for 30 to 40 minutes, until firm and just beginning to brown.

3. Cool and use as a spread for toast. Store, refrigerated, in a covered container.

KEY NUTRIENTS
Protein
Calcium
Iron

SNACKS, DIPS, CONDIMENTS, AND BEVERAGES

Bran Muffins 48

High-Protein Muffins 50

Banana Bread 52

Molasses Bread 53

Deviled Eggs 54

Crudités with Thai Peanut Sauce 55

Jicama with Lime Juice and Salt 56

Cheese-Stuffed Figs or Prunes 56

Hummus 57

White Bean or Black-Eyed Pea Pâté 58

Tofu with Dipping Sauces 60

Curried Yogurt Dip 61

White Bean Puree 62

Fresh Tomato Salsa 63

Low-Fat Mayonnaise 64

Yogurt Cheese 65

Tofu Mayonnaise 66

Tofu Green Goddess 67

Blueberry Peach Frappe 68

Limeade or Lemonade, Sparkling or Flat 69

Ginger Tea 69

ADVANCE
PREPARATION

These will keep in a
cool place for 3 or 4
days and freeze well.

Bran Muffins

Most commercially made muffins are oversized and over-caloric. These are easy to make and will provide you with lots of fiber. Though not supersweet, they will satisfy your sweet cravings. Let the batter sit overnight or for several hours during the day to allow the bran to swell, which gives these muffins a very nice, moist texture. They freeze well, and I find that they're just the thing for an afternoon or midmorning snack.

1 cup dark or golden raisins or chopped dried figs or apricots
1³/₄ cups boiling water
2 cups unprocessed bran
2 large eggs
¹/₃ cup canola oil
¹/₃ cup mild-flavored honey (such as clover) or dark brown sugar
2 tablespoons regular or blackstrap molasses
1 cup buttermilk or plain yogurt
¹/₂ cup milk
1¹/₂ cups whole wheat flour or whole wheat pastry flour
1 cup unbleached or all-purpose flour
2¹/₂ teaspoons baking soda
¹/₂ teaspoon salt

KEY NUTRIENTS
Fiber
Vitamin B_6
Vitamin B_{12}
Folacin
Niacin
Riboflavin
Thiamin
Copper
Iron
Magnesium
Manganese
Phosphorus
Potassium

1. Place the dried fruit in a small bowl and pour the boiling water over it. Let sit for 5 minutes, then stir in the bran. Let sit for 10 minutes.

2. In a large bowl, beat together the eggs, oil, honey or brown sugar, and molasses. Stir in the buttermilk or yogurt and milk. Stir in the dried fruit and bran mixture and combine well.

3. In a medium bowl, sift together the flours, baking soda, and salt. Fold into the wet ingredients and combine quickly. Cover with plastic wrap and refrigerate for several hours or overnight.

4. Preheat the oven to 400°F. Oil or spray 18 to 24 muffin cups.

5. Stir the batter and fill each cup two-thirds full. Bake for 20 to 30 minutes, until the muffins are puffed and browned. Let cool in the tins for 15 minutes, then remove from the tins and cool on a rack.

6. Serve cooled. Store in a cool place in plastic bags. If freezing, transfer the muffins to zipper-lock freezer bags. Thaw in the microwave or toaster oven before serving.

ADVANCE
PREPARATION
These will keep in a
cool place for 5 days
and freeze well.

High-Protein Muffins

These are power-packed muffins, with a high-protein grain
(rye or barley flakes), whole wheat flour, and yogurt and eggs.
You can make them sweeter if you wish; just add another tablespoon or two of sugar or honey.

2 large eggs
1 cup plain yogurt
1/2 cup milk
1/4 cup canola oil
1–2 tablespoons mild-flavored honey (such as clover), to
        taste
2 tablespoons nonfat dry milk
1 cup stone-ground whole wheat flour
1/3 cup unbleached or all-purpose flour
1/3 cup soy flour or rye flour
1/3 cup stone-ground cornmeal
3 tablespoons sugar
1 tablespoon baking powder
1/2 teaspoon salt
2/3 cup dried cherries or cranberries
1/3 cup barley flakes or rye flakes

1. Preheat the oven to 375°F. Oil or spray a 12-cup muffin
tin.

KEY NUTRIENTS
Protein
Vitamin B$_6$
Folacin
Niacin
Riboflavin
Thiamin
Copper
Iron
Magnesium
Manganese
Phosphorus

2. In a large bowl, beat together the eggs, yogurt, milk, oil,
honey, and nonfat dry milk.

3. In a medium bowl, sift together the flours, cornmeal,
sugar, baking powder, and salt. Stir into the wet ingredients with
just a few strokes. Fold in the dried cherries or cranberries and
barley or rye flakes.

4. Spoon the batter into the muffin cups, filling each about two-thirds full. Bake for 25 minutes, or until the tops brown and a toothpick inserted in the center of a muffin comes out clean. Let cool in the tin for 15 minutes, then remove from the tin and cool on a rack.

5. Serve cooled. Store in a cool place in plastic bags. If freezing, transfer the muffins to zipper-lock freezer bags. Thaw in the microwave or toaster oven before serving.

ADVANCE
PREPARATION
This will be better the
day after you bake it.
Wrap it tightly in foil
once it has cooled
completely. It will keep
for 5 to 7 days.

Banana Bread

The bread makes a marvelous snack or dessert. You can use the same recipe to make 12 muffins. Fill the muffin cups three-quarters full and bake for 20 to 25 minutes. Let cool in the tin for 10 minutes, then remove from the tin and let cool on a rack.

1 cup whole wheat flour
1 cup unbleached or all-purpose flour
1/2 cup packed light brown sugar
1 teaspoon baking soda
1 teaspoon ground cinnamon
1/2 teaspoon freshly grated nutmeg
1/2 teaspoon salt
2 large eggs
1/2 cup plain yogurt or buttermilk
1/4 cup canola oil
2 medium or 3 small ripe bananas, mashed (about 1 cup)
1 teaspoon pure vanilla extract
1 cup chopped walnuts

1. Preheat the oven to 375°F. Oil or butter an 8- or 9-inch loaf pan.

2. Sift together the flours, brown sugar, baking soda, cinnamon, nutmeg, and salt in a medium bowl.

3. In another medium bowl, beat together the eggs, yogurt or buttermilk, oil, bananas, and vanilla. Quickly stir the wet ingredients into the dry ingredients and mix well without overbeating. Fold in the walnuts.

4. Scrape the batter into the pan. Bake for 50 to 60 minutes, until the bread is firm when lightly pressed and a toothpick inserted in the middle comes out clean. Let cool in the pan for 10 to 15 minutes, then turn out onto a rack to cool completely.

KEY NUTRIENTS
Vitamin B_6
Folacin
Niacin
Riboflavin
Thiamin
Vitamin C
Copper
Iron
Magnesium
Manganese
Phosphorus
Potassium
Omega-3s

Molasses Bread

ADVANCE
PREPARATION
This is a good keeper.
Wrap it tightly in foil,
and it will keep for a
week at room tempera-
ture.

This dark, rich, sweet bread is iron-rich and one of my favorite snacks. It's great with a glass of milk or topped with a little plain yogurt or applesauce. You can also make 12 muffins from this recipe, filling the cups three-quarters full and baking them for 20 to 25 minutes.

1 cup whole wheat flour
1 cup unbleached or all-purpose flour
1 teaspoon baking powder
1 teaspoon ground ginger
³/₄ teaspoon salt
¹/₂ teaspoon baking soda
2 large eggs
¹/₄ cup packed dark brown sugar
1 cup plain yogurt or buttermilk
¹/₂ cup regular or blackstrap molasses
¹/₄ cup canola oil
³/₄ cup dark or golden raisins

1. Preheat the oven to 350°F. Oil or butter an 8- or 9-inch loaf pan.

2. Sift together the flours, baking powder, ginger, salt, and baking soda in a medium bowl.

3. In another medium bowl, beat together the eggs, brown sugar, yogurt or buttermilk, molasses, and oil. Quickly whisk or fold the wet ingredients into the dry (this can be done with an electric mixer on low speed). Fold in the raisins.

4. Scrape the batter into the pan. Bake for 50 minutes, or until a tester inserted in the middle comes out clean. Let cool in the pan on a rack for 10 to 15 minutes, then turn out onto the rack and let cool completely before slicing.

KEY NUTRIENTS
Vitamin B₆
Folacin
Niacin
Riboflavin
Thiamin
Calcium
Copper
Iron
Magnesium
Manganese
Phosphorus
Potassium

Snacks, Dips,

Condiments,

and Beverages

ADVANCE
PREPARATION
Deviled eggs will keep
for 3 to 4 days in the
refrigerator.

Deviled Eggs

This delicious snack relies on less mayonnaise than traditional recipes call for. It doesn't compromise the flavor at all.

6 hard-cooked eggs (see page 155)
2 tablespoons plain yogurt
4 rounded teaspoons Hellmann's or Best Foods mayonnaise
1 teaspoon Dijon mustard
1 teaspoon fresh lemon juice
Salt and freshly ground pepper to taste
Paprika and chopped fresh parsley for garnish

Peel the eggs, cut them in half lengthwise, and carefully remove the yolks from the whites. Mash the yolks with a mortar and pestle or with a fork in a small bowl. Add the yogurt, mayonnaise, mustard, and lemon juice and mash together until smooth. Season with salt and pepper. Spoon into the egg whites. Cover and refrigerate until ready to serve. Just before serving, sprinkle on the paprika and parsley.

KEY NUTRIENTS
Protein
Vitamin A
Vitamin B_{12}
Folacin
Riboflavin
Iron
Phosphorus
Omega-3s (if using high-
omega eggs)

EVERY WOMAN'S

GUIDE TO EATING

DURING PREGNANCY

Crudités
with Thai Peanut Sauce

ADVANCE
PREPARATION
The sauce will keep for
a few days in the
refrigerator.

Use whatever vegetables appeal to you. Carrots sticks (for convenience, you can buy baby carrots that are ready to eat), celery, red bell peppers, jicama, and cucumbers are easy to keep on hand. You can find a number of delicious commercial Thai peanut sauces on supermarket shelves, where the Asian foods are stocked. If you want to make your own sauce, this one is not quite as rich as commercial brands. It also makes a nice sauce for tofu and a good topping for grains.

¹/₄ cup plain yogurt
3 tablespoons all-natural smooth peanut butter
2 tablespoons hot water, plus more for thinning
1 tablespoon rice wine vinegar
1 tablespoon fresh lime juice
2–3 teaspoons soy sauce, to taste
2 teaspoons light brown sugar
1–2 teaspoons grated or minced fresh ginger, to taste
      (optional)
Pinch of cayenne pepper, or more to taste
Raw or cooked vegetables, as desired

Combine all the ingredients, except the vegetables, in a small bowl. Thin with additional water as desired. Serve with the raw or cooked vegetables of your choice.

KEY NUTRIENTS
Vitamin B₆
Folacin
Niacin
Thiamin
Vitamin E
Copper
Iron
Magnesium
Manganese
Phosphorus
Potassium
Zinc

Snacks, Dips,

Condiments,

and Beverages

ADVANCE
PREPARATION
The peeled, sliced
jicama will keep for a
couple of days in a
covered bowl in the re-
frigerator.

Jicama with Lime Juice and Salt

Jicama is a sweet, juicy root vegetable that is widely eaten in Mexico and found in most large supermarkets. It makes a refreshing snack or salad, sprinkled with salt and lime juice.

KEY NUTRIENT
Vitamin C

1 medium or ¹/₂ large jicama, peeled and sliced
Salt to taste
Chili powder to taste (optional)
Juice of 1–2 limes, to taste

Cut the jicama slices into 1-inch-wide pieces. Sprinkle with salt and chili powder (if using), and then toss with lime juice just before serving.

Cheese-Stuffed Figs or Prunes

KEY NUTRIENTS
FIGS
Vitamin B₆
Calcium
Copper
Iron
Magnesium
Manganese
Potassium

PRUNES
Fiber
Beta Carotene
Vitamin A
Vitamin B₆
Niacin
Riboflavin
Vitamin E
Copper
Iron
Magnesium
Manganese
Phosphorus
Potassium

This makes a filling and energizing snack.

2–5 dried figs or pitted prunes, cut in half
1–3 tablespoons ricotta or mashed cottage cheese
Honey or freshly grated nutmeg for topping (optional)

Arrange the figs or prunes on a small plate. Spoon a scant 1 teaspoon of cheese onto the cut surface of each fruit. If you wish, drizzle on a tiny amount of honey or sprinkle with nutmeg.

Makes about 2 cups,
or 10 servings
as a starter

Hummus

ADVANCE
PREPARATION
Hummus will keep for a
few days in the refrig-
erator, but it will be-
come more pungent.

Hummus is easy to find, not only in delis and Middle Eastern stores but also in natural food stores and markets. It's quite easy to make at home, so if you find that you want to eat it all the time, make a batch using this recipe. This is a low-fat version of the traditional dip, with much less tahini and oil.

2 garlic cloves
2 cups cooked chickpeas, drained and rinsed
$1/2$ teaspoon ground cumin
    Salt to taste
$1/4$ cup fresh lemon juice
3–4 tablespoons plain yogurt or cooking liquid from the
        chickpeas (if you cooked them; do not use liquid from
        the can), plus more for thinning if desired
2 tablespoons olive oil
3 tablespoons sesame tahini

Turn on the food processor and drop in the garlic. When it is chopped and adhering to the sides of the machine, stop the food processor and scrape down the sides of the bowl. Add the chickpeas, cumin, and salt and turn on the machine for about 30 seconds. Stop the machine, scrape down the sides, and start the machine again. With the machine running, add the lemon juice, yogurt or cooking liquid, and oil and blend until smooth. Add the tahini and blend again. Thin with additional yogurt or liquid, if desired. Taste and adjust the salt before serving. (Hummus requires a fair amount of salt.)

KEY NUTRIENTS
Protein
Folacin
Thiamin
Copper
Iron
Magnesium
Manganese
Phosphorus
Potassium
Zinc

Snacks, Dips,

Condiments,

and Beverages

ADVANCE
PREPARATION
This is best if it has a
day to mature in the
refrigerator, where it
will keep for 4 days. It
also can be frozen.

White Bean or
Black-Eyed Pea Pâté

This savory spread is ideal for vegetarian sandwiches and also
makes a nice snack or hors d'oeuvre, spread on crackers or
bread.

1 heaped cup dried white beans or black-eyed peas,
   washed, picked over, and soaked in 1 quart water for
   6 hours or overnight (black-eyed peas require no
   soaking)
4 cups water
1 medium onion, chopped
5 large garlic cloves, 2 crushed, 3 minced or pressed
1 bay leaf
   Salt to taste (about 2 teaspoons)
1 tablespoon olive oil
2 large eggs
2 tablespoons fresh lemon juice
$1/2$ cup fresh bread crumbs
$1/4$ teaspoon dried thyme
   Freshly ground pepper to taste (about 10 twists of the
   mill)

1. Drain the beans and combine with the water in a large
saucepan or bean pot. Bring to a boil and skim off any foam that
rises to the surface during the first few minutes. Add half of the
onion, the crushed garlic, and the bay leaf. Cover, reduce the heat,
and simmer for 1 hour. Season with salt (about 1 teaspoon) and
continue to cook for 30 to 60 minutes more, until the beans are
very tender.

2. While the beans are cooking, heat the oil in a heavy nonstick skillet over medium heat. Add the remaining onion and cook,
stirring, until tender, 3 to 5 minutes. Add the minced or pressed

KEY NUTRIENTS
Protein
Vitamin B$_6$
Folacin
Thiamin
Copper
Iron
Magnesium
Manganese
Phosphorus
Potassium

garlic and cook, stirring, until fragrant, about 1 minute. Remove from the heat and transfer to a medium bowl. Oil a pâté tureen or bread pan. Preheat the oven to 400°F.

3. Remove the beans from the heat and drain through a colander placed over a large bowl. Measure out ⅓ cup of the cooking liquid and set aside. Remove and discard the bay leaf. Puree the beans in a food processor until smooth. Scrape down the sides and add the eggs, lemon juice, and salt (about 1 teaspoon). Turn on the machine and add the reserved cooking liquid with the machine running. Process until completely smooth. Scrape into the bowl with the onions. Stir in the bread crumbs, thyme, and pepper. Pour or scrape the mixture into the tureen or bread pan and cover tightly with foil or a lid. Bake for 50 to 60 minutes, until the top is just beginning to color. Let cool in the pan. Serve warm, or refrigerate and serve cold.

ADVANCE
PREPARATION
The dipping sauces can
be made 2 to 3 days in
advance.

Tofu with Dipping Sauces

If you like tofu, you might find it's a godsend during those first
months of pregnancy, when bland food can really hit the spot.
Keep one or more of these dipping sauces on hand in the refrigerator for quick tofu fixes.

3–4 ounces firm tofu (1 thick slice or several thinner slices or
strips)
Dipping sauce of your choice (recipes follow)

Simple Soy Ginger Dipping Sauce

The stock or water reduces the saltiness in this easy sauce.

¹/₄ cup soy sauce
1 tablespoon grated or minced fresh ginger
¹/₂ cup chicken or vegetable stock or water (optional)

Combine the soy sauce and ginger in a small bowl. Thin
with water or stock, if desired.

Tahini Soy Dipping Sauce

This sauce also makes a particularly nice sandwich spread.

¹/₄ cup soy sauce
¹/₄ cup sesame tahini
1 teaspoon grated or minced fresh ginger (optional)
Water (optional)

KEY NUTRIENTS
(TOFU ONLY)
Protein
Calcium
Iron

Combine the soy sauce, tahini, and ginger (if using) in a
small bowl. Thin with water, if desired. Spread on tofu, or spread
on bread and top the bread with tofu and lettuce.

Teriyaki Dipping Sauce

Don't worry about the alcohol here. When the mixture boils, the alcohol boils off, leaving only the flavors of the sake and mirin.

3 tablespoons sake
3 tablespoons mirin (sweet Japanese rice wine)
3 tablespoons soy sauce
1¹/₂ teaspoons sugar

Mix together all the ingredients in a small saucepan and bring to a boil. Boil, stirring, until the sugar is dissolved. Remove from the heat and let cool before serving.

Curried Yogurt Dip

Makes 1 cup

ADVANCE
PREPARATION
The dip can be made
1 day ahead.

This is great to keep on hand as a dip for vegetables, a sandwich spread, or a salad dressing.

³/₄ cup plain yogurt or Yogurt Cheese (page 65)
2 tablespoons Hellmann's or Best Foods mayonnaise
2 tablespoons fresh lime juice
1 tablespoon sherry vinegar
1 teaspoon Dijon mustard
1 teaspoon curry powder
Pinch of cayenne pepper
Salt to taste

Mix together all the ingredients in a small bowl. Refrigerate in a covered container until ready to serve.

KEY NUTRIENTS
Vitamin B_{12}
Riboflavin
Calcium
Phosphorus

Snacks, Dips,

Condiments,

and Beverages

White Bean Puree

This zesty white bean puree is quickly assembled and is suitable for vegans. Spread it on croutons, use it as a dip for vegetables, or spread it on bread for sandwiches.

$1/2$ pound dried white beans, washed, picked over, and
    soaked in 1 quart water for 6 hours or overnight, or
    two 15-ounce cans white beans, drained and rinsed
 6 cups water (omit for canned beans)
 1 bay leaf (omit for canned beans)
2–4 garlic cloves (to taste), minced or pressed
    Salt to taste
 2 tablespoons olive oil
 2 tablespoons fresh lemon juice
2–4 tablespoons milk, soy milk, or cooking liquid from the
    beans as desired

1. For the dried beans, drain the beans and combine with the water in a large pot. Bring to a boil and skim off any foam. Add the bay leaf and 1 of the garlic cloves. Cover, reduce the heat, and simmer for 1 hour. Add the salt (1 teaspoon or more), cover, and simmer for another 30 to 60 minutes, until the beans are very tender. Drain through a strainer set over a bowl. If you're using canned beans, simply drain and rinse.

2. Puree the beans in a food processor. Add the remaining garlic, the olive oil, and lemon juice. Thin as desired with the milk, soy milk, or cooking liquid. Taste and adjust the seasonings. Serve warm or cold.

KEY NUTRIENTS
Vitamin B_6
Folacin
Riboflavin
Niacin
Thiamin
Copper
Iron
Magnesium
Manganese
Phosphorus

Fresh Tomato Salsa

ADVANCE
PREPARATION
The salsa is best served
the day it's made, but
you can make it a few
hours ahead, or at
least chop the ingredi-
ents.

With all of the salsas on the market today, you certainly don't have to make your own. But if you want a wonderful fresh flavor, this one is hard to beat. The vinegar or lime juice is necessary if the tomatoes are unexciting, but not if you can find sweet, juicy, locally grown ones.

    1 pound ripe fresh tomatoes, finely chopped
  1/4 small red onion, minced and rinsed with cold water
  1-3 jalapeño or serrano peppers (to taste), seeded for a
        milder salsa and minced
  1/4 cup chopped fresh cilantro, or more to taste
    2 teaspoons red wine vinegar, balsamic vinegar, or fresh
        lime juice (optional)
      Salt and freshly ground pepper to taste

Toss together all the ingredients in a medium bowl. Let stand at room temperature for 15 to 30 minutes so that the flavors blend and ripen, then serve.

NOTE: Rinsing the onions helps remove the long-lasting raw-onion flavor. Place in a bowl, cover with cold water, drain, and rinse again.

VARIATION
Salsa with Avocado

To the above salsa, add 1 ripe but firm avocado, finely diced. This is especially good if you need extra calories.

KEY NUTRIENTS
Vitamin A
Vitamin C
Vitamin E

KEY NUTRIENTS
WITH AVOCADO
Vitamin B$_6$
Folacin
Niacin
Copper
Magnesium
Potassium

Snacks, Dips,

Condiments,

and Beverages

ADVANCE
PREPARATION
This will keep in the re-
frigerator up to the
expiration date on the
cottage cheese.

Low-Fat Mayonnaise

A little bit of mayonnaise goes a long way to give a mayon-
naise-like flavor to this mixture, which is mostly cottage
cheese. Keep it on hand to use in place of mayonnaise for sandwiches and dips.

1 cup low-fat or nonfat cottage cheese
¼ cup Hellmann's or Best Foods mayonnaise
¼ cup low-fat or nonfat plain yogurt
Salt to taste

Place the cottage cheese in a food processor and blend until
smooth. Add the mayonnaise and yogurt and blend until there is
no longer a trace of graininess. Season with salt and serve.

ADVANCE
PREPARATION
This will keep for a
couple of days in the
refrigerator. The green
color will darken after
a day.

VARIATION

Low-Fat Green Mayonnaise

To the above ingredients, add the following items.

1 garlic clove (optional)
¼ cup chopped fresh parsley or spinach (cooked or
    uncooked)
1 tablespoon chopped fresh tarragon

Turn on the food processor and drop in the garlic, if using.
Scrape down the sides of the bowl. Add the parsley or spinach and
tarragon and process to finely chop. Add the cottage cheese and
proceed as directed above.

KEY NUTRIENTS
(BOTH VERSIONS)
Vitamin B₁₂
Riboflavin
Phosphorus

Yogurt Cheese

ADVANCE
PREPARATION
This will last through
the sell-by date on
your yogurt. It will
continue to give up
water in the container,
which you can simply
pour off.

Yogurt cheese is simply drained yogurt. Let it sit in a cheese-cloth-lined strainer over a bowl for a few hours so that it loses half of its water content and becomes thick and spreadable, almost like fresh cheese in consistency. You can serve it plain, or seasoned with herbs or garlic, as a spread, dip, or topping. Or sweeten it with honey and serve it with desserts. It makes a fine low-fat alternative to sour cream or cream cheese if you need to control your weight. For a nonfat version, use nonfat yogurt, but check the label and buy a brand that does not contain gums, which may prevent the yogurt from draining properly.

2 cups plain yogurt

Line a wire strainer with a double thickness of cheesecloth and set it over a bowl. Or use a large coffee filter or double thickness of paper towels. Place the yogurt in the strainer and refrigerate for at least 1 hour, preferably 4 hours or overnight. Transfer to a covered container and refrigerate. Serve cold.

VARIATION

Herbed Yogurt Cheese

ADVANCE
PREPARATION
Can be made up to a
day ahead.

This makes a good sandwich spread, dip, or topping for baked potatoes.

1 cup Yogurt Cheese
1 garlic clove, minced or pressed
1/4–1/2 cup chopped fresh herbs, such as parsley, tarragon, dill, thyme, or basil, to taste
Salt and freshly ground pepper to taste

KEY NUTRIENTS
(BOTH VERSIONS)
Protein
Vitamin B$_{12}$
Riboflavin
Calcium
Phosphorus

Mix together all the ingredients in a small bowl. Taste and adjust the seasonings. Transfer to a covered container and refrigerate. Serve cold.

Snacks, Dips,

Condiments,

and Beverages

ADVANCE
PREPARATION
This will keep for a few
days in the refrigera-
tor.

Tofu Mayonnaise

Silken tofu is the best tofu to use here, as it gives a silky texture to this blended mayonnaise. It's a super choice for a tasty, low-fat dip or spread, and it's great for vegans.

1/2 pound (1 package) silken tofu
2 tablespoons fresh lemon juice
2 tablespoons plain yogurt, soy milk, mayonnaise, or buttermilk, plus more for thinning if desired
2 tablespoons extra-virgin olive oil or canola oil
2 tablespoons Hellmann's or Best Foods mayonnaise (optional)
1 tablespoon vinegar (red or white wine, sherry, cider, or, for a slightly sweet flavor, rice wine vinegar)
1–2 teaspoons soy sauce, to taste
1 teaspoon Dijon mustard
1 garlic clove, minced or pressed (optional)
1/4 teaspoon salt

Combine all the ingredients in a blender or food processor and blend until completely smooth. Thin with additional yogurt, soy milk, mayonnaise, or buttermilk, if desired.

KEY NUTRIENTS
Protein
Calcium
Iron

Tofu Green Goddess

Makes 1¼ cups

This creamy, vibrant sauce is perfect with salmon and makes a fabulous dip or sauce for asparagus, artichokes, and other crudités. It's also great for sandwiches, and you can thin it for use as a dressing.

¹/₂ pound silken tofu
2 tablespoons fresh lemon juice
2 tablespoons plain yogurt, soy milk, or buttermilk, plus more for thinning if desired
2 tablespoons extra-virgin olive oil or canola oil
2 tablespoons Hellmann's or Best Foods mayonnaise (optional)
1 tablespoon vinegar (red or white wine, sherry, cider, or, for a slightly sweet flavor, rice wine vinegar)
1–2 teaspoons soy sauce, to taste
1 teaspoon Dijon mustard
¹/₄ cup chopped fresh parsley or spinach (cooked or uncooked)
1–2 tablespoons chopped fresh tarragon, to taste
¹/₄ teaspoon salt

Combine all the ingredients in a blender or food processor and blend until completely smooth. Thin with additional yogurt, soy milk, or buttermilk, if desired.

ADVANCE PREPARATION
This will keep for a couple of days in the refrigerator.

KEY NUTRIENTS
Protein
Calcium
Iron

Snacks, Dips,

Condiments,

and Beverages

Blueberry Peach Frappe

This indulgence has plenty of things going for it. The blueberries are packed with phytochemicals — tiny compounds found in plants that help the body fight disease-causing agents such as carcinogens. The vanilla frozen yogurt gives the frappe the illusion of being made with ice cream, yet there is very little fat, especially if you use 1% milk. The milk offers plenty of calcium and protein. And it tastes wonderful.

> 1 cup frozen blueberries
> 1/2 ripe peach, pitted
> 1 cup milk
> 2 scoops (1/2–2/3 cup) vanilla frozen yogurt

Put all the ingredients in a blender and blend at high speed until thick and smooth. Serve immediately.

VARIATION
Blueberry Frappe
Omit the peach.

KEY NUTRIENTS
Vitamin B$_{12}$
Riboflavin
Vitamin C
Calcium
Phosphorus

Limeade or Lemonade, Sparkling or Flat

Makes 5 or 6 servings

Some women have reported getting relief from morning sickness from lemon juice. If it helps you, make a pitcher of this and keep it on hand in the refrigerator. Take a water bottle of it with you to work.

1¹/₃ cups fresh lime or lemon juice
¹/₂ cup sugar, or more to taste
4 cups sparkling water or flat water
   Ice cubes

Combine the lime or lemon juice and sugar in a medium bowl. Stir until the sugar is dissolved. Transfer to a pitcher or carafe, add the water, and stir. Pour over ice in individual glasses and serve.

OTHER SPRITZERS: Combine 1 part juice, such as apple juice, with 1 part sparkling water.

ADVANCE PREPARATION

The sweetened citrus juice can be kept in the refrigerator for several days. If you prefer the sparkling version, it's best to add the water just before serving. If you use flat water, you can make up the lemonade or limeade and keep it in the refrigerator.

KEY NUTRIENT
Vitamin C

Ginger Tea

Makes 4 servings

Drink this soothing tea hot in winter, iced in summer. Ginger improves circulation and can cool you down on a hot day. It's also good for colds. If you're serving this iced, you can also add a little sparkling water.

1 2-inch piece fresh ginger, peeled and grated or minced
4 cups water
   Honey or sugar to taste
   Ice cubes (optional)
   Fresh lemon juice to taste (optional)

Place the ginger in a teapot or large Pyrex measuring cup. Bring the water to a boil and pour over the ginger. Let steep for 5 minutes, then strain. Sweeten each cup with honey or sugar. If you're making iced tea, sweeten the entire pot, then pour over ice and add fresh lemon juice, if desired.

KEY NUTRIENT
Potassium

Snacks, Dips,

Condiments,

and Beverages

69

SANDWICHES

Club Sandwich 72

Chicken Breast and Red Pepper Sandwich 73

Tuna for the Week 74

Avocado Sandwich 75

Sardine Spread and Cucumber Sandwich 76

My Egg Salad Sandwich 77

Roast Beef Sandwich 78

Peanut Butter and Banana Sandwich 78

Simple, Quick Tofu Sandwich 79

Tofu and Spinach Pita Pocket 80

Barbecued Tempeh Sandwich 81

White Bean or Black-Eyed Pea
    Pâté Sandwich 82

Hummus Pita Pocket 82

Grilled Portobello and Cheese (or Miso)
    Sandwich 83

Grilled Cheese Sandwich 84

Tomato, Mozzarella, and Basil Sandwich 85

Bruschetta 86

Wraps

If you're watching your carbohydrates but you love sandwiches, you might try wrapping something around the filling, rather than putting the filling between two slices of bread. To hold the filling, try a lettuce leaf, grape leaf, rice-flour wrapper, or corn tortilla.

LETTUCE LEAVES

Lettuce leaf wraps can be crisp — and used more like a scoop or taco shell than a wrapper — or if they are slightly wilted, they can be wrapped like little packages. You can use one big leaf or several smaller leaves. Boston lettuce is flexible and delicate; romaine is sturdy. If you are not wilting the leaves, it's best to use inner ones, which are easier to fill and won't have such a stiff center rib.

For more flexible packets, use large romaine leaves, medium Swiss chard leaves, or savoy cabbage leaves. Blanch them for 30 seconds in boiling water. Remove the leaves with tongs and immediately transfer them to a bowl of ice water. Drain and blot with paper towels. Put the leaves rib side down on your work surface and place a couple of spoonfuls of filling on the bottom half of each leaf. Fold the two sides of the leaf over, then roll it up and place seam side down on a plate.

GRAPE LEAVES

Grape leaves are available in jars in most supermarkets. Look in the imported foods section. Take a few leaves from the jar and rinse with cold water. Place the leaves on your work surface, cut away the stem, and fill as you would lettuce leaves.

RICE-FLOUR WRAPPERS

These are the wrappers used for Vietnamese spring rolls. They need just a short soak in warm water, then you can fill them like an egg roll. They come in large and small sizes. Place 1 wrapper at a time in a bowl of hot water for about 30 seconds, until just softened. Remove from the water, blot dry with paper towels, and place on your work surface. Place the filling in the center of the bottom half of the wrapper, then fold the sides over and roll up.

CORN TORTILLAS

These are slightly lower in carbohydrates than wheat bread. Warm each tortilla in a dry skillet or for 20 seconds in the microwave — just enough so it's flexible. Place the filling on top and fold over or roll up.

ADVANCE
PREPARATION
The chicken or turkey
and bacon can be
cooked hours ahead
(the chicken or turkey
will keep for 3 days in
the refrigerator). Once
assembled, the sand-
wich should be served
immediately.

Club Sandwich

Here's a good way to get grains, protein, and vegetables in one dish. A club sandwich is easy to come by in practically any restaurant. If you make it at home, use whole grain or rye bread. Classic club sandwiches are made with three slices of bread, which make the sandwiches so thick that they're awkward to eat. In this version, I've replaced the middle slice of bread with a little more chicken or turkey.

2 slices whole wheat, whole grain, or rye bread
1 tablespoon mayonnaise, Low-Fat Mayonnaise (page 64), or a mixture of mayonnaise and plain yogurt
2–4 Bibb, Boston, or romaine lettuce leaves (depending on the size), or a handful of arugula, watercress, or baby salad greens, rinsed
2½ ounces thinly sliced cooked chicken or turkey breast
2–3 slices ripe but firm tomato
3–4 slices bacon, cooked until crisp and drained on paper towels

Toast the bread lightly and spread one side of each slice with mayonnaise or a mixture of mayonnaise and yogurt. Top one slice with half the lettuce or greens and all the chicken or turkey. Top with the remaining lettuce, the tomato slices, and bacon. Cut the remaining slice of toast in half on the diagonal and place the pieces, mayonnaise side down, on top of the bacon. Cut the sandwich in half, running the knife down between the two cut halves of toast. Hold the sandwich together with toothpicks.

VARIATION

Club Sandwich with Avocado

After spreading the top slice of bread with mayonnaise, spread it with ¼ ripe avocado.

KEY NUTRIENTS
(BOTH VERSIONS)
Vitamin B$_6$
Vitamin B$_{12}$
Folacin
Niacin
Riboflavin
Thiamin
Calcium (if using white
    bread)
Copper
Iron
Magnesium
Manganese
Phosphorus

Chicken Breast
and Red Pepper Sandwich

ADVANCE
PREPARATION
Cooked chicken breasts
will keep for 3 days in
the refrigerator.
Homemade roasted red
peppers will keep for a
week or more if cov-
ered with olive oil. Bot-
tled will keep a little
longer.

If you buy a package of chicken breasts and poach them all,
you'll have a few days' worth of chicken for sandwiches and
salads. I like to serve this sandwich on lightly toasted
mixed-grain bread.

$^1/_2$ boneless, skinless chicken breast (3–4 ounces), poached
    (see page 156) or pan-cooked (see page 169)
2 slices whole grain bread
2 teaspoons mayonnaise, plain yogurt, or mustard, or a
    combination
2–3 wide slices bottled, canned, or homemade roasted red
    pepper (see page 119)
    Salt and freshly ground pepper to taste
    A few fresh basil leaves (optional)
    Lettuce leaves or arugula (optional)

Cut the chicken breast crosswise (across the grain) into thin
slices. Spread the bread with mayonnaise, yogurt, or mustard (or a
combination). Top one slice with chicken. Sprinkle lightly with salt
and pepper. Lay the roasted pepper slices over the chicken and top
with the basil and lettuce or arugula, if desired. Top with the other
slice of bread. Cut the sandwich in half and serve.

VARIATIONS
Chicken, Red Pepper,
and Avocado Sandwich

Add $^1/_4$ ripe avocado. Either slice the avocado and lay it over
the red pepper, or spread it on the bread.

Chicken Sandwich
with Lettuce and Tomato

Omit the roasted pepper. Add about 4 tomato slices and a
few lettuce leaves.

KEY NUTRIENTS
Protein
Beta Carotene
Vitamin A
Vitamin B$_6$
Vitamin B$_{12}$
Folacin
Niacin
Riboflavin
Thiamin
Vitamin C
Copper
Iron
Magnesium
Manganese
Phosphorus
Potassium (avocado)

Sandwiches

ADVANCE
PREPARATION
This will keep for 5
days in the refrig-
erator.

Tuna for the Week

During my first three months of nausea, there were times
when the only thing I found appetizing was a tuna sandwich. I
got the sandwiches from delis (with extra pickles), or I made
them at home. The tuna was great for protein, and the bread
added needed calories. As my nausea subsided, I still craved a
tuna sandwich for lunch at least once a week, and tuna salads
of various types were a frequent, quick dinner. If you make up
the tuna portion and keep it in the refrigerator, you can easily
assemble a sandwich or salad when hunger strikes.

    2 6-ounce cans water-packed tuna
 1/4 cup plain yogurt, mayonnaise, or Low-Fat Mayonnaise
        (page 64)
    2 tablespoons fresh lemon juice
  1-2 teaspoons Dijon mustard, to taste
      Freshly ground pepper to taste

    OPTIONAL ADDITIONS
  1-2 celery stalks, chopped
  1/2 cucumber, peeled, seeded, and chopped
    1 red or green bell pepper, seeded and chopped
  1-2 dill pickles, chopped

Drain the tuna and mash together with the yogurt or mayonnaise, lemon juice, mustard, and pepper. Add any of the additions of your choice and mix well. Cover tightly and refrigerate for
up to 5 days. Use for sandwiches or salads.

VARIATION

Tuna Sandwiches

Toast 2 slices of whole wheat or rye bread and spread each slice
with nonfat yogurt or a little mayonnaise. Then top with tuna, a
few leaves of crunchy lettuce (romaine or iceberg), and, if they're
in season, a couple of tomato slices.

KEY NUTRIENTS
(TUNA SALAD FOR
THE WEEK)
Protein
Vitamin B$_6$
Vitamin B$_{12}$
Niacin
Iron
Magnesium
Phosphorus
Potassium

Tuna Salad Combinations

TUNA AND ANY GREEN SALAD

TUNA AND BEANS (WHITE BEANS, CHICKPEAS, OR LENTILS)

TUNA AND BROCCOLI

TUNA, BROCCOLI, AND BEANS

TUNA, BROCCOLI, AND POTATOES

TUNA, GREEN BEANS, POTATOES, AND HARD-COOKED EGGS

TUNA, TOMATO, AND FRESH BASIL

Avocado Sandwich

Makes 1 sandwich

ADVANCE
PREPARATION
It's best to eat this
soon after it's made.

When you spread ripe avocado on warm toast, it melts into the bread like butter. If you use crusty country bread for this sandwich, I think it's easier to eat the sandwich if it's open-faced. Use the tomato only if you can find locally grown ones in season.

2 slices whole grain bread or crusty country bread
1/2 large ripe avocado, preferably Hass
  Salt to taste
1/4 cup cottage cheese (optional)
4 slices ripe fresh tomato (optional)
  A few fresh basil leaves (optional)
2 medium romaine lettuce leaves

KEY NUTRIENTS
Vitamin A
Vitamin B$_6$
Folacin
Niacin
Riboflavin
Thiamin
Vitamin C
Vitamin E
Copper
Iron
Magnesium
Manganese
Phosphorus
Potassium

Lightly toast the bread. While still warm, mash half of the avocado over one side of each slice. Sprinkle with salt and top with the cottage cheese, tomato slices, and basil, if using. Finish off with the lettuce leaves. Serve open-faced or as a traditional sandwich.

Sandwiches

Sardine Spread
and Cucumber Sandwich

Sardines are very high in calcium, especially if you eat the bones. They're also a great source of omega-3 fatty acids, which can protect people against heart disease and diabetes, and are important for brain development and function in the fetus (see page 27). This pleasing puree can give you a real taste for the fish. Water-packed sardines should be easy to find.

2 slices rye or whole wheat bread
Mayonnaise or plain yogurt for the bread
3–4 tablespoons Sardine Spread (recipe follows)
Several cucumber slices or pickles

Spread the bread with the mayonnaise or yogurt. Top one slice with the Sardine Spread and layer with cucumber slices or pickles. Top with the other slice of bread. Cut the sandwich in half without pressing down too hard, so that the spread doesn't run out. Serve immediately.

Sardine Spread

Makes ¾ cup

1 3.75-ounce can water-packed sardines
1 tablespoon fresh lemon juice, or more to taste
1 tablespoon Hellmann's or Best Foods mayonnaise
1 tablespoon plain yogurt
1 teaspoon Dijon mustard
1 small garlic clove, minced or pressed (optional)
1 tablespoon chopped fresh herbs, such as chives, dill, or
    parsley (optional)
Salt and freshly ground pepper to taste

KEY NUTRIENTS
Protein
Vitamin B_6
Vitamin B_{12}
Folacin (if using whole
    wheat bread)
Niacin
Riboflavin
Thiamin
Calcium
Copper (if using whole
    wheat bread)
Iron
Magnesium
Manganese
Phosphorus
Potassium
Omega-3s

Drain the sardines and put them in the bowl of a food processor. Process until finely chopped. Add the lemon juice, mayonnaise, yogurt, and mustard and process until smooth. Stir in the garlic and herbs, if using, and season with salt and pepper. Use as a sandwich spread or a topping for bruschetta. Serve at room temperature or cold.

My Egg Salad Sandwich

Makes 1 sandwich

This is a vibrant, healthier version of the classic, made with my low-fat, high-flavor egg salad (page 146).

2 slices whole grain bread
  Plain yogurt or mayonnaise for the bread
⅓ cup Egg Salad (page 146)
  Lettuce leaves or arugula
  Tomato slices (optional)

Spread the bread with yogurt or mayonnaise. Top one slice with the Egg Salad, lettuce or arugula, and tomato slices (if using). Top with the other slice of bread and serve immediately.

ADVANCE PREPARATION
The Egg Salad will keep for a few days in the refrigerator, but the herbs will lose their color.

KEY NUTRIENTS
Protein
Vitamin A
Vitamin B_6
Vitamin B_{12}
Folacin
Niacin
Riboflavin
Thiamin
Copper
Iron
Magnesium
Manganese
Phosphorus

ADVANCE
PREPARATION
This sandwich will keep
for a few hours in the
refrigerator.

KEY NUTRIENTS
Protein
Vitamin B$_6$
Vitamin B$_{12}$
Folacin
Niacin
Riboflavin
Thiamin
Copper
Iron
Manganese
Magnesium
Phosphorus
Potassium
Zinc

Roast Beef Sandwich

My favorite roast beef sandwich is an open-faced one that is
served on thin slices of sourdough bread at a café I used to frequent in Paris. You can make yours this way or put the meat
between the bread.

2 slices whole grain or sourdough bread
  Mustard to taste
2 ounces thinly sliced roast beef
  Tomato slices, pickles, and lettuce leaves (optional)

Spread the bread with mustard. Make 2 open-faced sandwiches with several slices of roast beef on each slice of bread, or
put all the roast beef on one slice of bread for a traditional 2-slice
sandwich. Top the beef with tomato slices, pickles, and lettuce
leaves, if desired. Serve immediately.

ADVANCE
PREPARATION
This keeps for a few
hours and is a good
one to take to work.

KEY NUTRIENTS
Vitamin B6
Folacin
Niacin
Riboflavin
Thiamin
Vitamin C
Vitamin E
Copper
Iron
Magnesium
Manganese
Phosphorus
Potassium
Zinc

Peanut Butter
and Banana Sandwich

This high-calorie sandwich may sound like kid food, or a meal
from the sixties — and it is! But it also makes quite a nutritious, satisfying lunch, and it's a real energy booster. This
makes a particularly good snack if you are carrying multiples.

  2 slices whole grain bread
  1 teaspoon honey (optional)
1^1/$_2$ tablespoons all-natural peanut butter, smooth or
      crunchy
 ^{1}/$_2$ ripe banana, thinly sliced

Spread one slice of bread with the honey, if you wish.
Spread the other slice of bread with the peanut butter. Top with
banana slices and the first slice of bread. Cut in half and serve.

Simple, Quick Tofu Sandwich

ADVANCE PREPARATION
The dipping sauces can be made in advance, but the sandwich should be made just before serving, so the bread does not get soggy.

If you are a tofu eater, this highly nutritious sandwich may become your most frequent pregnancy lunch, especially if meat, cheese, and spicy foods have little appeal.

2 slices whole wheat or rye bread, toasted if desired
1–3 teaspoons plain yogurt, mayonnaise, mustard, or sesame tahini, or a combination
3 ounces firm tofu, plain, pan-cooked (see page 223), or broiled or grilled (see page 224), sliced
Dipping sauce of your choice (see pages 60–61) or soy sauce
Lettuce leaves and tomato slices (optional)

Spread the bread with yogurt, mustard, mayonnaise, or tahini (or a combination), depending on your taste and caloric requirements. (If you need to watch the calories, use the yogurt or mustard rather than the mayonnaise or tahini.) Top with the tofu. Douse or spread the tofu with the dipping sauce, or simply sprinkle with soy sauce. Top with lettuce leaves and tomato slices, if desired, and the other slice of bread. Cut in half and serve immediately.

KEY NUTRIENTS
TOFU
Protein
Calcium
Iron

WHOLE WHEAT BREAD
Vitamin B6
Folacin
Niacin
Riboflavin
Thiamin
Copper
Iron
Magnesium
Manganese
Phosphorus

VARIATION

Tofu Sandwich with Avocado and Tomato

Add ½ ripe avocado, sliced or mashed, to the sandwich. Top the tofu with tomato slices.

KEY NUTRIENTS
AVOCADOS
Vitamin B6
Folacin
Niacin
Vitamin C
Copper
Magnesium
Potassium

TOMATOES
Vitamin A
Vitamin C
Vitamin E

Sandwiches

ADVANCE
PREPARATION
You can keep the filling
in the refrigerator for
a couple of days, but it
will discolor slightly.

Tofu and Spinach Pita Pocket

This is an easy and delicious way to obtain a rich assortment of nutrients and protein from several different food groups. The tofu-spinach mixture will keep for a couple of days in the refrigerator, so you can double or triple this recipe and have great lunches in minutes. Use packaged baby spinach for convenience.

A generous handful (about 1 ounce) baby spinach or
    fresh spinach leaves, stemmed, washed thoroughly,
    and dried
1/4 pound medium or firm tofu
3–4 tablespoons mayonnaise, Low-Fat Mayonnaise (page 64),
    Tofu Mayonnaise (page 66), or any creamy salad
    dressing
1 teaspoon soy sauce, or more to taste
1 whole wheat pita bread
Dijon mustard (optional)
Tomato and/or cucumber slices (optional)

1. Chop the spinach finely in a food processor. Add the tofu and pulse to mash. Add 2 tablespoons plus 1 teaspoon of the mayonnaise or dressing and the soy sauce. Mix well.

2. Cut the pita bread in half and open up each half. Spread with mustard, if desired (I think the mustard is a fabulous addition), then spread with the remaining mayonnaise or dressing. Fill the halves with the spinach and tofu mixture. Add the tomato and/or cucumber slices, if you wish. Serve immediately.

KEY NUTRIENTS
Protein
Beta Carotene
Vitamin A
Vitamin B$_6$
Folacin
Niacin
Riboflavin
Thiamin
Vitamin C
Vitamin E
Calcium
Copper
Iron
Magnesium
Manganese
Phosphorus
Potassium

Barbecued Tempeh Sandwich

ADVANCE
PREPARATION
You can prepare the
tempeh and marinade
several days ahead.

Tempeh, a high-protein fermented soybean product, is a staple food in Indonesia and has become popular among many vegetarians in this country.

¹/₂ cup soy sauce
¹/₂ cup water
1 tablespoon canola oil
2 garlic cloves, minced or pressed
1 1-inch slice fresh ginger, peeled and minced
¹/₂ pound tempeh, cut into 4 pieces
1 cup barbecue sauce (homemade or commercial), plus
    more for the bread if desired
4 slices whole grain bread
    Mayonnaise, plain yogurt, or mustard for the bread
    Lettuce leaves or shredded cabbage, tomato slices,
    and/or pickles (optional)

1. Combine the soy sauce, water, oil, garlic, and ginger in a small frying pan just large enough to accommodate the tempeh in one layer. Place the tempeh in the pan. Bring the liquid to a boil, reduce the heat, cover, and simmer for 8 minutes. Turn the tempeh over, cover the pan, and simmer for 8 minutes more, until all the liquid is absorbed. Cook for about 5 minutes more, turning once, until the tempeh begins to brown. Toss with the barbecue sauce in a medium bowl. Cover and refrigerate for at least 1 hour or up to several days.

2. Remove the tempeh from the marinade and grill or broil it for 5 minutes on each side. Cut the pieces crosswise into strips. Spread the bread with mayonnaise, yogurt, mustard, or more barbecue sauce. Top with the tempeh. Add lettuce leaves or shredded cabbage, tomato slices, and/or pickles, if you wish. Cut in half and serve.

KEY NUTRIENTS
Protein
Vitamin B₆
Riboflavin
Folacin
Niacin
Thiamin
Calcium
Copper
Iron
Magnesium
Manganese
Phosphorus

Sandwiches

White Bean or Black-Eyed Pea Pâté Sandwich

KEY NUTRIENTS
WITH BREAD
Vitamin B$_6$
Riboflavin
Folacin
Niacin
Thiamin
Copper
Iron
Magnesium
Manganese
Phosphorus

PÂTÉS
Protein
Vitamin B$_6$
Folacin
Thiamin
Copper
Iron
Magnesium
Manganese
Phosphorus
Potassium

If you've made one of the delicious bean pâtés on page 58, you'll be able to lunch on this satisfying sandwich.

1–2 slices whole grain bread
1 $^1/_2$-inch-thick slice White Bean or Black-Eyed Pea Pâté
(page 58)
Lettuce leaves and tomato slices

Toast the bread, if you wish. Use 1 slice for an open-faced sandwich, 2 slices for a traditional sandwich. Spread one slice with the pâté, then top with the lettuce leaves and tomato slices. For a traditional sandwich, place the other slice on top and cut in half. Serve immediately.

Hummus Pita Pocket

KEY NUTRIENTS
Protein
Vitamin B$_6$
Folacin
Niacin
Riboflavin
Thiamin
Copper
Iron
Magnesium
Manganese
Phosphorus
Potassium
Zinc

1 whole wheat pita bread
$^1/_4$ cup Hummus (page 57)
Tomato slices, cucumber slices, and/or romaine lettuce
leaves

Cut the pita bread in half and open up each half. Fill with the hummus and top with the tomato, cucumber, and/or lettuce.

Grilled Portobello and Cheese (or Miso) Sandwich

ADVANCE PREPARATION
The mushrooms can be cooked a few hours or even a day ahead, but they won't be as succulent. You can assemble the sandwich hours ahead to carry to work, and the mushrooms will stay moist.

Portobello mushrooms have a meaty texture, and these sandwiches are hefty and satisfying. If you are using the miso, remember that it is quite salty, so go easy on the salt when seasoning the mushroom slices.

    1 large portobello mushroom
    1 tablespoon olive oil
      Salt and freshly ground pepper to taste
    4 slices whole grain bread, toasted if desired
  1–2 teaspoons mayonnaise or plain yogurt or $1/4$ ripe
        avocado for the bread
    1 tablespoon miso paste or 1 ounce Gruyère cheese, thinly
        sliced
      Lettuce leaves and tomato slices (optional)

1. Cut the mushroom into thick slices, discarding the stem. Brush the slices on both sides with the olive oil, then sprinkle with salt and pepper. Heat a nonstick skillet over high heat and sear the slices for about 5 minutes per side, until they begin to release their liquid. You can also grill or broil the slices.

2. Spread the bread with mayonnaise, yogurt, or avocado. If using miso, spread it on both slices of bread. Top one slice with the mushroom. Add the cheese (if using), lettuce leaves, and tomato slices (if using). Cover with the other slice of bread, cut in half, and serve.

KEY NUTRIENTS
Vitamin B_6
Folacin
Niacin
Riboflavin
Thiamin
Copper
Iron
Magnesium
Manganese
Phosphorus
Potassium

Sandwiches

Grilled Cheese Sandwich

A classic American grilled cheese sandwich is made in a frying pan. The cheese is sandwiched between two slices of bread, and the sandwich is browned in butter until the cheese melts. There's no doubt this is delicious, but I find it easier to make my grilled cheese sandwiches in a toaster oven, especially if I'm omitting the butter.

2 slices whole wheat, whole grain, or rye bread
  Mustard, butter, plain yogurt, or mayonnaise for the bread (optional)
1–2 ounces thinly sliced or grated cheese, such as cheddar, Gruyère, fontina, Monterey jack, or dry jack, to taste
1 tablespoon butter (if frying)

TRADITIONAL METHOD: Spread the bread with mustard, butter, yogurt, or mayonnaise, if you wish. Top one slice of bread with the cheese and cover with the other slice. Heat the butter in a heavy skillet over medium heat until the foam subsides, then place the sandwich in the pan. Cook, pressing down gently with a spatula, until lightly browned. Turn the sandwich over and cook on the other side until lightly browned and the cheese begins to ooze. Remove from the heat, cut in half, and serve.

TOASTER OVEN METHOD: Toast the bread lightly. Spread with mustard, butter, yogurt, or mayonnaise, if you wish. Top one slice of bread with the cheese and cover with the other slice. Place on the oven's baking sheet and toast until the cheese begins to ooze. Remove from the toaster, cut in half, and serve.

OPEN-FACED SANDWICH: Lightly toast the bread. Top each slice with half the cheese. Place on the toaster oven's baking sheet and toast or bake until the cheese melts. Remove from the toaster and serve.

KEY NUTRIENTS
Vitamin A
Vitamin B$_6$
Vitamin B$_{12}$
Folacin
Niacin
Riboflavin
Thiamin
Vitamin C (if using tomato)
Calcium
Copper
Iron
Magnesium
Manganese
Phosphorus
Zinc

Grilled Cheese and Tomato Sandwich

Layer half the cheese on the bread and top with a few tomato slices. Cover the tomato with the remaining cheese and continue as above.

Grilled Cheese and Sage Sandwich

Layer a few fresh sage leaves, torn into pieces, on top of or between the cheese and continue as above.

Tomato, Mozzarella, and Basil Sandwich

You can use part-skim or whole-milk mozzarella for this sandwich (obviously, if you need to restrict your fat intake, go for the part-skim), or you can use string cheese. It is worth making only if you can find delicious in-season tomatoes.

2 slices whole grain bread
Mustard and/or plain yogurt for the bread
A few slices of ripe but firm tomato
Salt to taste
4–5 fresh basil leaves
1¹/₂–2 ounces mozzarella cheese, thinly sliced, or 1¹/₂–2 ounces string cheese, shredded
A few wide slices bottled, canned, or homemade roasted red pepper (see page 119; optional)

Spread the bread with mustard and/or yogurt. Top one slice with tomatoes and sprinkle lightly with salt. Add the basil, cheese, and pepper slices (if using). Cover with the other slice of bread, cut in half, and serve.

Makes 1 sandwich

ADVANCE PREPARATION
You shouldn't make this sandwich too far ahead, because the tomato juice will saturate the bread.

KEY NUTRIENTS
Protein
Vitamin A
Vitamin B₆
Vitamin B₁₂
Niacin
Riboflavin
Thiamin
Calcium
Copper
Folacin
Iron
Magnesium
Manganese
Phosphorus
Zinc

Sandwiches

ADVANCE
PREPARATION
You may keep the
bruschetta warm for 30
minutes in a 250°F
oven. Add the toppings
right before serving.

KEY NUTRIENTS
WHITE BREAD
Folacin
Niacin
Riboflavin
Thiamin
Calcium
Iron
Manganese
Phosphorus

WHOLE WHEAT BREAD
Vitamin B$_6$
Folacin
Niacin
Riboflavin
Thiamin
Copper
Iron
Magnesium
Manganese
Phosphorus

Bruschetta

Bruschetta (pronounced brus-ke-tah) are thick slices of lightly toasted country bread rubbed with garlic and brushed or drizzled with olive oil. Then they're topped with something, to make an open-faced Italian sandwich.

8–12 thick slices country bread
1–2 large garlic cloves (as needed), unpeeled and sliced in
half (optional)
1–2 tablespoons olive oil, as needed (optional)
Topping of your choice (recipes follow)

1. If you are not using a toaster or toaster oven, prepare the grill or preheat the broiler. Lightly toast the bread, or set the bread over hot coals or under the broiler, about 4 to 5 inches from the heat. The bread should be toasted on both sides but remain soft inside. This goes very quickly under a broiler (1 minute or less per side), so watch carefully.

2. Remove from the heat and immediately rub both sides with the cut garlic, if desired. Brush with the olive oil, if you wish. Cut into halves if your slices are wide. Garnish with the topping of your choice.

TOPPINGS

Tomatoes with Parmesan

Tomato-Balsamic Salsa (page 196)
2 ounces Parmesan cheese, shaved

Make the bruschetta as directed. Top with the salsa, then the Parmesan.

ADVANCE
PREPARATION
All the toppings will
hold for several hours
in the refrigerator.

KEY NUTRIENTS
Vitamin A
Vitamin C
Vitamin E

Mozzarella or Goat Cheese and Roasted Peppers

KEY NUTRIENTS
Protein
Beta Carotene
Vitamin A
Vitamin B$_6$
Vitamin B$_{12}$
Folacin
Riboflavin
Vitamin C
Calcium
Phosphorus
Zinc

4 roasted red peppers, bottled, canned, or homemade (see
    page 119), cut into wide slices
   Salt and freshly ground pepper to taste
1 tablespoon olive oil
1–2 garlic cloves (to taste), minced or pressed (optional)
2 tablespoons slivered fresh basil leaves
3 ounces mozzarella cheese, thinly sliced, or 3 ounces goat
    cheese, crumbled

Make the bruschetta as directed. If you plan to serve the
bruschetta hot, preheat the oven to 350°F. Toss the peppers with
the salt and pepper, olive oil, garlic (if using), and basil in a
medium bowl. Top the bruschetta with the seasoned peppers and
cheese. Heat through, if desired, for 10 minutes, then serve.

Beans and Sage

KEY NUTRIENTS
Protein
Vitamin B$_6$
Folacin
Thiamin
Copper
Iron
Magnesium
Manganese
Phosphorus
Potassium

1 15-ounce can white beans, drained and rinsed
6 fresh sage leaves, chopped or cut into slivers
   Salt and freshly ground pepper to taste
1–2 ounces Parmesan cheese (to taste), shaved

Make the bruschetta as directed. If you plan to serve the
bruschetta hot, preheat the oven to 350°F. Toss together the beans,
sage, salt and pepper, and Parmesan in a medium bowl. Top the
bruschetta with the bean mixture and serve, or heat through for 10
minutes and serve.

SOUPS

Chicken Noodle or Tofu Noodle Soup 89

Mexican Chicken Soup with Zucchini,
Chickpeas, and Tomatoes 90

Asian Noodle Soup with Spinach and
Salmon 92

Chicken Soup with Egg and Lemon 93

Hot and Sour Soup 94

Miso Soup with Tofu 96

Italian Spinach and Egg Soup 97

Garlic Soup with Broccoli 98

Minestrone 100

Winter Vegetable Soup 102

Lentil Soup 103

Mushroom and Barley Soup 104

Gazpacho 106

Chilled Cucumber Yogurt Soup 107

Chicken Noodle or Tofu Noodle Soup

Makes 6 servings

ADVANCE PREPARATION
The stock, cooked noodles, and poached chicken will hold for a few days in the refrigerator. The soup should be made just before serving.

When chicken soup might be all you care to eat, this comforting and nourishing version will help you a lot during the first trimester. The noodles and bits of chicken or tofu add important nutrients to the mixture.

6 cups chicken or vegetable stock
2 tablespoons soy sauce
2 teaspoons grated or minced fresh ginger
6 ounces soba, vermicelli, or angel hair pasta, cooked ahead if desired (see page 262)
$^3/_4$ pound medium or firm tofu, diced, or 1 whole skinless chicken breast, poached and shredded ($1^1/_2$–$1^3/_4$ cups; see page 156)
$1^1/_2$ cups fresh or thawed frozen peas, or $^1/_4$ pound (2 cups) snow peas, trimmed
Salt to taste
6 tablespoons chopped fresh cilantro

Combine the stock, soy sauce, and ginger in a soup pot or Dutch oven. Bring to a boil and stir in the noodles (if uncooked), tofu or chicken, and peas. Reduce the heat and simmer until the noodles are cooked, about 5 minutes. (If you cook the noodles ahead, simply divide the cooked noodles among soup bowls and ladle the soup over them.) Taste and add salt, if needed. Stir in the cilantro and serve.

KEY NUTRIENTS
Protein
Vitamin A
Vitamin B_6
Vitamin B_{12} (chicken)
Folacin
Niacin
Thiamin
Vitamin C
Calcium (tofu)
Copper
Iron
Magnesium
Manganese
Phosphorus

Soups

ADVANCE
PREPARATION
The soup can be made
ahead through step 3
and will hold for a few
days in the refrigera-
tor.

Mexican Chicken Soup with Zucchini, Chickpeas, and Tomatoes

There's plenty of protein in the form of chickpeas and chicken in this delicious, heady soup, although it's quite light.

8 cups water, plus more as needed
1 large whole chicken breast (about 1¼ pounds), skinned
2 medium onions, 1 quartered, 1 diced
4 large garlic cloves, 2 crushed, 2 minced or pressed
½ teaspoon dried oregano
1 bay leaf
 Salt to taste
1 15-ounce can chickpeas, drained and rinsed
1 large carrot, peeled and diced
1 medium or 2 small zucchini or other summer squash, diced
1 large tomato, peeled, seeded, and chopped
2 tablespoons chopped fresh cilantro
1 ripe avocado, preferably Hass, peeled, pitted, and diced
2 limes, cut into wedges, for serving

1. Combine the water, chicken, quartered onion, and crushed garlic in a soup pot or Dutch oven and bring to a simmer. Skim off any foam that rises to the top, then add the oregano and bay leaf. Partially cover, reduce the heat to low, and cook for 15 minutes, until the chicken is cooked through. Remove the chicken from the broth with a slotted spoon, and when it's cool enough to handle, bone and shred the meat and set aside in a small bowl. (If you cook the chicken the day before you plan to serve the soup, place the chicken in a small bowl, salt lightly, cover well, and refrigerate.)

KEY NUTRIENTS
Protein
Vitamin B$_6$
Vitamin B$_{12}$
Folacin
Niacin
Thiamin
Copper
Iron
Magnesium
Manganese
Phosphorus
Potassium
Zinc

2. Strain the stock through a cheesecloth-lined strainer into a large bowl. If using right away, skim off any visible fat. If using the next day or in a few hours, cover the bowl and refrigerate; the next day you can easily lift the fat off the top. Add enough water to measure 8 cups of stock.

3. Combine the stock, chickpeas, diced onion, minced or pressed garlic, carrot, squash, and tomato in the soup pot or Dutch oven, and bring to a simmer. Add salt, cover, and simmer for 20 to 30 minutes, until the vegetables are tender. Taste and adjust the seasonings.

4. Just before serving, stir in the shredded chicken and cilantro. Heat through, taste, and adjust the seasonings. Place a portion of diced avocado in each soup bowl, then ladle in the soup. Serve with a lime wedge.

VARIATION

Vegetarian Mexican Soup

Omit the chicken breast. Double the amount of carrots and squash. Substitute 8 cups vegetable stock for the chicken stock. Begin the recipe at step 3. The nutrients in the vegetarian version do not include vitamins B_6 and B_{12}.

ADVANCE
PREPARATION

The stock can be pre-
pared and the noodles
cooked (see page 262)
up to 3 days ahead.
The spinach can be
stemmed, washed, and
dried a couple of days
ahead.

KEY NUTRIENTS
Protein
Beta Carotene
Vitamin A
Vitamin B$_6$
Vitamin B$_{12}$
Folacin
Niacin
Riboflavin
Thiamin
Vitamin C
Vitamin E
Calcium
Iron
Magnesium
Manganese
Phosphorus
Potassium
Omega-3s

KEY NUTRIENTS
TOFU AND SPINACH
Protein
Beta Carotene
Vitamin A
Vitamin B$_6$
Folacin
Riboflavin
Vitamin C
Vitamin E
Calcium
Iron
Magnesium
Manganese
Potassium
Isoflavins

Asian Noodle Soup with Spinach and Salmon

This meal-in-a-bowl is a comforting mixture of broth, noo-dles, fish, and spinach.

6 cups vegetable, fish, or chicken stock
1 sliver fresh ginger, peeled
6 ounces soba, udon, or spaghettini
1 pound salmon fillets, cut into 4 equal pieces
1 pound fresh spinach, stemmed and washed thoroughly
1 bunch scallions, white parts and about $^1\!/_3$ of the green
      parts, thinly sliced separately
Salt and/or soy sauce to taste

1. Combine the stock and ginger in a soup pot or Dutch oven. Bring to a simmer, add the noodles, and cook for 5 to 7 minutes.

2. Add the salmon, spinach, and white parts of the scallions. Cover the pot and turn off the heat. Let sit without removing the lid for 5 to 8 minutes, until the salmon is just cooked through and the spinach is wilted. Taste and adjust the seasonings, adding salt or soy sauce to taste.

3. Divide the salmon, noodles, and spinach evenly among the bowls. Ladle in the broth. Sprinkle on the green parts of the scallions, and serve.

VARIATION

Asian Noodle Soup with Tofu and Spinach

Substitute $^3\!/_4$ pound firm tofu, cut into 1-inch dice, for the salmon. Simmer for 2 minutes, then turn off the heat and continue as directed.

Chicken Soup
with Egg and Lemon

ADVANCE
PREPARATION
The soup can be made
through step 1 several
hours ahead of serving
and refrigerated.

Lemon juice has been reported as an effective antidote to pregnancy-related nausea. This soup is both nourishing and comforting and may have the added virtue of helping with your morning sickness. Make sure the eggs you use are of the highest quality.

8 cups chicken stock
$^1/_2$–1 cup long-grain rice or bulgur, to taste
Salt and freshly ground pepper, to taste
4 large eggs, preferably free-range or high-omega, at
    room temperature
Juice of 2 lemons (6–8 tablespoons; to taste)
Chopped fresh parsley or dill for garnish

1. Bring the stock to a simmer in a soup pot or Dutch oven. Add the rice or bulgur and simmer, partially covered, until the grain is cooked through, 15 to 30 minutes. Taste and add salt, if needed.

2. Meanwhile, in a medium bowl, beat together the eggs and lemon juice until frothy.

3. Just before serving, gradually add about 4 ladles of hot broth to the egg and lemon mixture, beating vigorously with a whisk to avoid curdling. Turn off the heat under the soup, pour the egg-broth mixture into the soup, and stir well with a wooden spoon.

4. Serve, adding a bit of pepper to each bowl and garnishing with the parsley or dill.

KEY NUTRIENTS
Protein
Vitamin A
Vitamin B$_{12}$
Folacin
Niacin
Riboflavin
Thiamin
Vitamin C
Iron
Manganese
Phosphorus

ADVANCE
PREPARATION
This soup will keep for
several days in the re-
frigerator, but don't
add the eggs, scallions,
cilantro, and sesame oil
until you heat it
through before serving.

Hot and Sour Soup

Pork is the traditional meat used in hot and sour soup, but you
also have the option of using chicken breast. If you can't stomach meat at all or if you're a vegetarian, you can omit it and still
make a soothing, appetizing version of the soup. The Chinese
use their Shaohshing wine for this soup. You can find it in most
Asian grocery stores. Otherwise, use dry sherry.

FOR THE MARINATED PORK OR CHICKEN

4 ounces lean pork loin or boneless, skinless chicken
    breast
2 tablespoons water
1 teaspoon soy sauce
1 teaspoon Shaohshing wine or dry sherry
1 teaspoon dark sesame oil
1 teaspoon cornstarch
  Pinch of salt
  Freshly ground pepper to taste

FOR THE SOUP

10 dried shiitake or Chinese mushrooms
  Water
1 ounce bean thread noodles
6 cups chicken stock
1/2 pound firm, regular, or silken tofu, cut into matchsticks
1 teaspoon sugar
  Salt to taste (depending on the stock)
2 tablespoons soy sauce
1 tablespoon cornstarch dissolved in 1 tablespoon water
3–4 tablespoons unseasoned rice wine vinegar or cider
    vinegar, to taste
1–1 1/2 teaspoons freshly ground pepper, to taste
2 large eggs, beaten
2 tablespoons finely chopped scallions, both white and
    green parts
2 tablespoons chopped fresh cilantro
1 teaspoon dark sesame oil

KEY NUTRIENTS
Protein
Vitamin B$_6$
Vitamin B$_{12}$
Folacin
Niacin
Riboflavin
Thiamin
Calcium
Copper
Iron
Magnesium (chicken)
Phosphorus
Potassium
Zinc

1. FOR THE MARINATED PORK OR CHICKEN: Cut the pork or chicken breast into matchsticks. In a medium bowl, mix together the water, soy sauce, wine or sherry, sesame oil, cornstarch, salt, and pepper. Add the pork and toss until thoroughly coated with the marinade. Cover, refrigerate, and let marinate for 15 to 30 minutes or longer.

2. FOR THE SOUP: Soak the mushrooms in hot water to cover for 20 minutes. Drain and squeeze out any excess liquid. Cut away and discard the mushroom stems and cut the caps into slivers. Soak the bean threads in warm water to cover for 5 minutes. Drain and cut into 3-inch lengths.

3. Bring the stock to a simmer in a large soup pot or Dutch oven. Stir in the pork or chicken with its marinade, separating the strips of meat with a fork or chopsticks. Simmer for 2 minutes, until there is no trace of pink in the meat, then stir in the mushrooms, bean threads, tofu, sugar, salt, and soy sauce. Bring back to a simmer and stir in the dissolved cornstarch. Bring back to a simmer again and stir in the vinegar and pepper. Taste and adjust the seasonings. Drizzle the beaten eggs into the soup, stirring with chopsticks or a fork to create strands. Stir in the scallions, cilantro, and sesame oil. Serve immediately.

ADVANCE
PREPARATION
This is a last-minute
soup.

Miso Soup with Tofu

Miso, a fermented soybean and grain paste, makes for a highly nutritious soup or beverage. It's the ultimate in instant, healthy meals. Keep some miso at the office to have as a quick lunch or snack. The miso can be dissolved in water or the traditional Japanese broth called dashi, which you can find in Japanese groceries.

1 tablespoon miso
1 cup dashi (Japanese broth) or water, warmed
1/2 small carrot, peeled and thinly sliced
4 small or 2 large mushrooms, trimmed and thinly sliced, or 2 shiitake mushrooms, trimmed and sliced
2 ounces silken or regular tofu, drained and cut into small dice
1/2 white part of scallion, chopped or thinly sliced

OPTIONAL ADDITIONS
1 tablespoon chopped watercress
1 teaspoon snipped fresh chives
1/2 cup steamed broccoli florets

Put the miso in a small bowl and add 2 to 4 tablespoons of the dashi or water. Whisk until the miso is softened and blended with the liquid. Bring the remaining dashi or water barely to a simmer and gradually add the softened miso. Do not boil, as this changes the flavor. Add the carrots, mushrooms, tofu, scallion, and any of the additions of your choice. Bring to just below the boiling point and remove from the heat. Ladle into a bowl or cup and serve.

KEY NUTRIENTS
Protein
Folacin
Niacin
Riboflavin
Calcium
Copper
Iron
Phosphorus
Potassium

EVERY WOMAN'S

GUIDE TO EATING

DURING PREGNANCY

Italian Spinach and Egg Soup

ADVANCE PREPARATION
This is a last-minute soup.

Here's a light, luscious soup, filled with spinach and bolstered with egg, which is quickly thrown together, especially if you use prewashed baby spinach. Semolina is finely ground hard wheat, used for making pasta. You can find it in Italian and Middle Eastern groceries.

 4 large eggs
 6 cups chicken stock
 ¼ cup freshly grated Parmesan cheese
 2 tablespoons semolina flour
   Salt and freshly ground pepper to taste
1–2 garlic cloves (to taste), minced or pressed
 1 package baby spinach, rinsed

1. Beat the eggs in a medium bowl and mix in ¼ cup of the stock, the Parmesan, semolina, and salt and pepper. Set aside.

2. Bring the remaining stock to a simmer in a soup pot or Dutch oven. Add the garlic and simmer for 10 to 15 minutes. Taste and adjust the seasonings. Add the spinach and gradually drizzle in the egg mixture, stirring slowly with a long-handled wooden spoon. Simmer for 1 minute and serve.

KEY NUTRIENTS
Protein
Beta Carotene
Vitamin A
Vitamin B_6
Vitamin B_{12}
Folacin
Riboflavin
Vitamin E
Calcium
Iron
Magnesium
Manganese
Phosphorus
Potassium

Soups

ADVANCE
PREPARATION
This is a last-minute
soup.

Garlic Soup with Broccoli

Garlic soup is practically an instant soup. It can be as comforting as chicken soup, made in a fraction of the time. The garlic will not taste strong after it simmers.

       6 cups water
   4–6 large garlic cloves (to taste), minced or pressed, plus 1
           garlic clove, cut in half
$1^1/_2$–2 teaspoons salt, to taste
       1 bay leaf
$^1/_4$–$^1/_2$ teaspoon dried thyme, a few sprigs fresh thyme, or 2–3
           fresh sage leaves, to taste
     $^1/_2$ cup dried pasta, such as small shells, elbows, or fusilli
     $^1/_2$ pound broccoli crowns, broken into florets
       4 thick slices crusty country bread or French bread
       2 large eggs, beaten
       1 tablespoon olive oil (optional)
       2 tablespoons chopped fresh parsley
           Freshly ground pepper to taste
   2–3 tablespoons freshly grated Parmesan or Gruyère cheese,
           to taste, for serving

1. Bring the water to a boil in a 3- or 4-quart saucepan or soup pot. Add the minced or pressed garlic, $1^1/_2$ teaspoons of the salt, the bay leaf, and thyme or sage. Reduce the heat, cover, and simmer for 15 minutes. Taste and adjust the salt.

2. Add the pasta to the pot. Simmer for 5 minutes, then add the broccoli. Simmer for 5 minutes more, until the pasta is cooked al dente.

3. Meanwhile, toast the bread. As soon as it's done, rub both sides with the cut garlic and set aside.

KEY NUTRIENTS
Beta Carotene
Vitamin A
Vitamin B$_6$
Vitamin B$_{12}$
Folacin
Riboflavin
Vitamin C
Iron
Manganese
Potassium

4. Beat together the eggs and olive oil (if using). Spoon a ladleful of the hot soup into the eggs and stir together. Turn off the heat under the soup and stir in the egg mixture. The eggs should cloud the soup, but they shouldn't scramble. Stir in the parsley and pepper.

5. Place a garlic toast in each soup bowl. Ladle in the soup, sprinkle with cheese, and serve.

ADVANCE
PREPARATION
The soup will keep for
3 or 4 days in the
refrigerator, and it
benefits from being
cooked a day ahead of
time. However, the
pasta will absorb more
liquid, so the soup will
require thinning. A
better method is to
make the soup a day
ahead but add the
pasta the day you are
serving it.

Minestrone

I promise not to give you many other recipes with long ingredient lists like this one. You won't regret the prep time when
you taste the thick, hearty soup. Make a pot of this on the
weekend and eat it throughout the week. A cup could start a
meal or be a snack; a bowl makes a meal.

1–2 tablespoons olive oil, as needed
 2 medium onions, chopped
 2 leeks, white parts only, washed thoroughly and sliced
 2 medium carrots, peeled and chopped
 2 celery stalks, chopped
 ½ small head green cabbage, cored and shredded
 4 large garlic cloves, minced or pressed
   Salt to taste
 8 cups water
 2 medium potatoes, scrubbed and diced
 2 medium turnips, peeled and diced
 1 14-ounce can diced tomatoes
 ½ teaspoon dried oregano
 1 Parmesan rind
   A few sprigs each fresh thyme and parsley
 1 bay leaf
 1 cup fresh or thawed frozen peas
 ½ pound green beans, trimmed and cut into 1-inch lengths
     (about 2 cups)
 1 15-ounce can cannellini or borlotti beans, drained and
     rinsed
 ½ cup dried pasta, such as elbows, small shells, or broken
     spaghetti
   Freshly ground pepper to taste
 ¼–½ cup chopped fresh basil or parsley (to taste)
 ⅓ cup freshly grated Parmesan cheese for serving

KEY NUTRIENTS
Beta Carotene
Vitamin A
Vitamin B$_6$
Folacin
Niacin
Thiamin
Vitamin C
Copper
Iron
Magnesium
Manganese
Phosphorus
Potassium

1. Heat 1 tablespoon of the olive oil in a soup pot or Dutch oven over medium-low heat. Add the onions and cook, stirring, until they begin to soften. Add the leeks and continue to cook, stirring, for about 5 minutes, until the vegetables are tender and translucent but not browned. Add the carrots and celery and continue to cook, stirring often, for 5 to 10 minutes, until the vegetables are tender and fragrant. Add more olive oil, if necessary. Stir in the cabbage and half the garlic, add a little salt, and cook for about 5 minutes, until the cabbage has wilted. Add the water, potatoes, turnips, tomatoes and their juice, and oregano. Increase the heat to high and bring to a boil. Tie the Parmesan rind, thyme and parsley sprigs, and bay leaf together with kitchen string or in cheesecloth and add to the pot. Add about 2 teaspoons salt, reduce the heat to low, cover, and simmer for 45 minutes.

2. While the soup is simmering, blanch the peas and green beans. Bring a pot of water to a boil. Add 1 teaspoon salt and the peas and green beans. Boil for 5 to 8 minutes, until just tender but still bright green. Use a slotted spoon to transfer the vegetables to a colander and run it under cold water, or transfer to a bowl of ice water, then drain. Set aside. Reserve the cooking water in case you want to thin the soup later.

3. Stir the remaining garlic and the canned beans into the soup. Add the pasta and simmer for 10 minutes, until the pasta is cooked al dente. Stir the cooked peas and green beans into the soup. Grind in some pepper. Taste and adjust the seasonings. If the soup seems too thick, thin with a little cooking water from the vegetables.

4. Remove the Parmesan rind bundle from the soup, then stir in the basil or parsley. Serve in wide soup bowls, with about a tablespoon of Parmesan sprinkled on each bowl.

ADVANCE
PREPARATION
This will keep for a
couple of days in the
refrigerator and
freezes well. Whisk to
restore the texture
after freezing.

Winter Vegetable Soup

This comforting, classic European soup is made with hearty root vegetables and winter squash.

6 cups water or chicken or vegetable stock
$3/4$–1 pound russet or Yukon Gold potatoes, peeled and diced
$1/2$ pound winter squash, such as butternut, peeled, seeded, and diced
6 medium or 3 large leeks, white parts only, washed thoroughly and sliced
2 medium carrots, peeled and chopped
2 small turnips, peeled and diced
1 large onion, chopped
1 celery stalk, chopped
1–2 garlic cloves (to taste), minced or pressed
A bouquet garni made with 1 bay leaf and a couple of sprigs each fresh thyme and parsley
Salt and freshly ground pepper to taste
1 cup milk
Yogurt Cheese (page 65), chopped fresh parsley, or grated Gruyère cheese (1–2 teaspoons per serving) for garnish (optional)

1. Combine the water or stock, vegetables, and bouquet garni in a soup pot or Dutch oven and bring to a boil. Season with salt, reduce the heat, cover, and simmer for 1 hour. Remove the bouquet garni and puree the soup through the medium blade of a food mill or with a handheld, or immersion, blender. Do not use a food processor or blender, or the texture will be too smooth.

2. Return the soup to the pot and place over medium heat. Add the milk and plenty of pepper. Taste and adjust the salt. You will need quite a bit to bring up the flavors. Heat through and serve, garnishing each bowl with a dollop of Yogurt Cheese or a sprinkling of parsley or Gruyère, if desired.

KEY NUTRIENTS
Beta Carotene
Vitamin A
Vitamin B$_6$
Folacin
Niacin
Vitamin C
Copper
Iron
Magnesium
Manganese
Potassium

Lentil Soup

When you can't think of anything to eat, remember lentils. They are quickly cooked and a super-food, with a high concentration of vitamins and minerals.

For a nutritious variation, add ½ to 1 pound greens, such as beet greens, Swiss chard, or spinach, stemmed, washed thoroughly, and chopped. Reduce the amount of lentils to ½ pound (1 heaped cup), and proceed as directed, adding the greens during the final 5 minutes of cooking.

ADVANCE
PREPARATION
The soup will keep for
3 or 4 days in the
refrigerator and
freezes well. It will
thicken, so you may
wish to thin it with a
little water when you
reheat it.

  1 tablespoon olive oil
  1 medium onion, chopped
  1 carrot, peeled and chopped
  1 celery stalk, chopped
2–4 garlic cloves (to taste), minced or pressed
  1 pound (2 heaped cups) lentils, washed and picked over
  8 cups water
  1 bay leaf
  1 Parmesan rind
    Salt and freshly ground pepper to taste
  2 ounces Parmesan cheese, grated (about ½ cup), for
      serving

1. Heat the oil in a heavy soup pot over medium heat and add the onion, carrot, and celery. Cook, stirring, until the vegetables have softened, about 5 minutes. Add half the garlic and stir together. Add the lentils, water, bay leaf, and Parmesan rind and bring to a boil. Reduce the heat, cover, and simmer for 30 minutes. Add the remaining garlic and season with salt (1 to 2 teaspoons or more). Cover and simmer for 15 minutes more. Taste and adjust the seasonings, adding pepper to taste.

2. Remove the soup from the heat and remove the bay leaf and Parmesan rind. Puree all or part of the soup coarsely in batches in a blender or with a handheld, or immersion, blender. Return to the pot and heat through gently. Serve, topping each bowl with a generous spoonful of Parmesan.

KEY NUTRIENTS
Protein
Vitamin B_6
Folacin
Thiamin
Copper
Iron
Magnesium
Manganese
Phosphorus
Potassium

Soups

ADVANCE
PREPARATION
This will keep for 3 or 4
days in the refrigera-
tor. The barley will
continue to swell, so
you might need to add
a bit of water or stock
to thin it.

Mushroom and Barley Soup

This classic soup can be made with vegetable, chicken, or beef stock. It makes a filling, hearty lunch or dinner.

7 cups chicken, beef, or vegetable stock
$^1/_2$ pound mushrooms, trimmed and sliced (reserve the stems)
1 tablespoon olive oil, canola oil, or butter
1 medium onion, chopped
1 medium carrot, peeled and minced
Salt to taste
2 large garlic cloves, minced or pressed
1 teaspoon chopped fresh thyme or $^1/_2$ teaspoon dried
$^3/_4$ cup pearl barley
$^1/_4$ cup dry white wine or dry sherry
$^1/_2$ pound waxy potatoes, peeled and diced (optional)
Freshly ground pepper to taste
1 tablespoon soy sauce
1 tablespoon fresh lemon juice (optional)
1 tablespoon chopped fresh dill
1 cup Yogurt Cheese (page 65) or sour cream for serving

1. Combine the stock and mushroom stems in a large saucepan over medium heat and cook for 30 minutes. Strain.

2. Meanwhile, heat the oil or butter in a soup pot or Dutch oven over medium-low heat. Add the onion and carrot and cook, stirring, for 5 to 10 minutes, until the vegetables are tender. Add the mushrooms and a generous pinch of salt. Cook, stirring, until the mushrooms begin to release their liquid, then add the garlic and thyme. Continue to cook, stirring, until the mushrooms are tender and the mixture is fragrant, 5 to 10 minutes. Stir in the barley and wine or sherry and cook, stirring, until the liquid in the pot evap-

KEY NUTRIENTS
Protein
Vitamin B$_6$
Folacin
Niacin
Riboflavin
Thiamin
Copper
Iron
Magnesium
Manganese
Phosphorus
Potassium
Zinc

orates, about 3 minutes. Add the hot stock, potatoes (if using), and salt to taste. Increase the heat and bring to a boil. Reduce the heat again, cover, and simmer for 1 hour, until the barley is tender and the soup aromatic. Stir in the soy sauce, lemon juice (if using), and dill. Taste and adjust the seasonings with salt and pepper.

3. Remove the soup from the heat and serve, topping each bowl with a generous dollop of Yogurt Cheese or sour cream.

ADVANCE
PREPARATION
This will hold for a couple of days in the refrigerator.

Gazpacho

One of the easiest and most refreshing ways to include lots of vegetables in your daily diet is to make gazpacho, a cold tomato soup that includes cucumbers and peppers. This is a blender version, a bit different from a classic gazpacho because of the untraditional vegetables.

1½ pounds ripe tomatoes, peeled and seeded
  2 garlic cloves
½ small onion, coarsely chopped and rinsed
  1 carrot, peeled and coarsely chopped
  1 small cucumber, peeled, seeded, and coarsely chopped
  1 green bell pepper, seeded and coarsely chopped
¼ cup red wine vinegar or fresh lemon juice, or more to taste
  2 tablespoons chopped fresh basil (optional)
  2 tablespoons olive oil
  3 cups V8 juice
    Salt and freshly ground pepper to taste
    Slivered fresh basil leaves or chopped fresh parsley for garnish

OPTIONAL ADDITIONS
  1 small cucumber, peeled, seeded, and minced
  1 red or green bell pepper, seeded and minced
  2 hard-cooked eggs (see page 155), chopped
½ pound medium shrimp, shelled and cooked

1. In a large bowl, combine all the ingredients, except the slivered basil or chopped parsley and additions. Transfer to a blender in batches and blend until smooth. Return to the bowl and stir together. Taste and adjust the seasonings. Chill for several hours, if possible.

2. Place any of the additions of your choice in separate small bowls. Ladle the gazpacho into soup bowls, then garnish with slivered basil or chopped parsley. Serve, passing the additions at the table.

KEY NUTRIENTS
Vitamin A
Vitamin C
Vitamin E

SHRIMP
Vitamin B₁₂
Niacin
Copper
Iron
Magnesium
Phosphorus
Zinc

Chilled Cucumber Yogurt Soup

ADVANCE
PREPARATION
This will keep for 3
days in the refrigera-
tor.

Sometimes, if you're feeling queasy, liquid meals are easier to take than solid ones. This soup is especially refreshing in the summertime, and it takes only minutes to prepare. The garlic is traditional, but I'm making it optional here, just in case it doesn't appeal to you.

   2 regular cucumbers, peeled and seeded, or 1 European
       cucumber
1–2 garlic cloves (to taste), minced or pressed (optional)
   4 cups plain yogurt
 1/2 cup cold water
     Juice of 1 lemon, or more to taste
   2 tablespoons chopped fresh mint
     Salt and freshly ground pepper to taste
   4 thin lemon slices and several fresh mint leaves for
       garnish

1. Finely chop the cucumbers, using the pulse button of a food processor. Add the garlic (if using), yogurt, water, lemon juice, chopped mint, and salt and pepper. Blend together until the mixture is well amalgamated but still has some texture. (You can also use a blender or chop everything by hand and mix together in a bowl.) Taste and adjust the salt and lemon juice.

2. Serve immediately, over an ice cube if you wish, garnishing each serving with a lemon slice and a few mint leaves. Or refrigerate for 1 to 2 hours, until thoroughly chilled, and serve.

KEY NUTRIENTS
Fiber
Vitamin B_{12}
Folacin
Riboflavin
Vitamin C
Calcium
Phosphorus

Soups

SALADS

Baby Greens Salad 110

Baby Spinach Salad with Mushrooms 111

Arugula or Baby Greens and Beet Salad 112

Three Omega-3 Salad (Spinach Salad with
Chickpeas, Walnuts, and Feta) 114

Greek Salad 115

Tomato and Arugula Salad with Feta
Cheese 116

Beet and Orange Salad 117

Grapefruit and Avocado Salad 118

Roasted Red Pepper Salad 119

Roasted Pepper and Mozzarella Antipasto 120

Guacamole 121

Grated Carrots in Vinaigrette 122

Moroccan Cooked Carrot Salad with Cumin 123

Marinated Carrots 124

Creamy Cucumber Salad 125

Quick Cucumber Pickles 126

Coleslaw 127

Asian Coleslaw 128

Potato Salad 129

Potato and Green Bean Salad 130

Warm Potato and Goat Cheese Salad 132

Chickpea Salad 133

Bean Salad with Cumin Vinaigrette 134

French Lentil Salad, Warm or Cold 136

White Bean and Basil Salad 137

Classic Tabbouleh 138

Couscous Tabbouleh 139

Quinoa and Black Bean Salad with Lime
    Dressing 140

Broccoli and Chickpea Salad with Egg 141

Curried Mixed-Grain Salad 142

Wild Rice Salad 144

Egg Salad 146

Beef and Arugula Salad 147

Frisée, Poached Egg, and Bacon Salad 148

Niçoise Salad 150

Tuna and Bean Salad 152

Cobb Salad 154

Three Chicken Salads 156

    Curried Chicken Salad

    Asian Chicken Salad

    Mexican Chicken Salad

Asian Noodle Salad 160

Tempeh and Sesame Salad 162

Vinaigrettes 164

    Classic Vinaigrette

    Lemon Vinaigrette

    Yogurt or Buttermilk Vinaigrette

ADVANCE
PREPARATION
The dressing will keep
for several hours or
even up to a week in
the refrigerator.

Baby Greens Salad

Baby greens come packaged and practically ready to eat, requiring a quick rinse and spin in the salad spinner (even when the package says "prewashed," it's important to wash them again). They are so delicate and tasty that they go best with a very simple dressing. Use mixed salad greens, sometimes referred to as spring greens, or baby arugula here.

FOR THE DRESSING
2 teaspoons balsamic vinegar
1 tablespoon red wine vinegar or sherry vinegar, or more
    to taste
Salt and freshly ground pepper to taste
1/2 teaspoon Dijon mustard
1 small garlic clove, minced or pressed (optional)
1/4 cup extra-virgin olive oil

FOR THE SALAD
1 package (about 5 cups) baby salad greens, rinsed and
    dried

OPTIONAL ADDITIONS
A few sliced fresh mushrooms
1–2 tablespoons chopped fresh herbs, such as tarragon or
    parsley
A handful of walnuts
1 ounce Parmesan cheese, shaved

KEY NUTRIENTS
Beta Carotene
Vitamin A
Vitamin B$_6$
Folacin
Vitamin C
Vitamin E
Calcium
Copper
Iron
Magnesium
Manganese
Potassium
Monounsaturates

1. FOR THE DRESSING: Mix together the vinegars, salt and pepper, mustard, and garlic (if using) in a medium bowl. Whisk in the olive oil.

2. FOR THE SALAD: Place the salad greens in a large bowl and add any of the additions of your choice.

3. Toss the salad with the dressing and serve.

Baby Spinach Salad with Mushrooms

ADVANCE
PREPARATION
The spinach can be
rinsed and dried hours
ahead of time, then
wrapped in a clean
kitchen towel, sealed in
a plastic bag, and
refrigerated. The
mushrooms can be
sliced and tossed with
the lemon juice a few
hours ahead of time.
The dressing will hold
in the refrigerator for
a few hours.

Usually you can find packaged or bulk baby spinach. The tender, iron-rich leaves go nicely with mushrooms and a light, lemony vinaigrette.

4–6 large mushrooms, trimmed and thinly sliced
1 tablespoon fresh lemon juice
6–8 ounces baby spinach, rinsed and dried

OPTIONAL ADDITIONS
2 tablespoons chopped walnuts
1 ounce Parmesan cheese, shaved, or 1 ounce feta cheese,
    crumbled (about 1/4 cup)
1–2 hard-cooked eggs (see page 155), sliced or chopped
1–2 slices bacon, cooked until crisp and crumbled
1 small red onion, thinly sliced and rinsed
1 pear, peeled, cored, and sliced

1/2 cup Lemon Vinaigrette (page 164) or Yogurt or
    Buttermilk Vinaigrette (page 165), using a
    combination of lemon juice and vinegar

Toss the mushrooms with the lemon juice in a salad bowl. Add the spinach and any of the additions of your choice and toss to combine. Toss with the vinaigrette just before serving.

KEY NUTRIENTS
Beta Carotene
Vitamin A
Vitamin B$_6$
Folacin
Niacin
Riboflavin
Vitamin C
Vitamin E
Calcium
Copper
Iron
Magnesium
Manganese
Phosphorus
Potassium
Monounsaturates

Salads

ADVANCE
PREPARATION
The roasted beets will
keep for up to a week
in a covered bowl in
the refrigerator. The
dressing can be made
several hours ahead of
serving.

Arugula or Baby Greens and Beet Salad

If you buy baby greens or baby arugula that is prewashed, and if you roast the beets in advance, you can assemble this delicious and highly nutritious, iron-rich salad very quickly. Remember to save the beet greens for use in another dish, such as Lentil Soup with greens added (page 103).

FOR THE SALAD

4 small or medium or 2–3 large beets

1/4 cup walnut pieces (optional)

1/2 pound baby arugula or salad greens, rinsed and dried

1 ounce Parmesan cheese, shaved

1–2 tablespoons chopped fresh herbs, such as chives, tarragon, or parsley, to taste (optional)

FOR THE DRESSING

2 teaspoons balsamic vinegar

2 tablespoons sherry vinegar or red wine vinegar, or more to taste

Salt and freshly ground pepper to taste

1 small garlic clove, minced or pressed (optional)

1/2–1 teaspoon Dijon mustard, to taste

1/4 cup extra-virgin olive oil or plain yogurt

2 tablespoons walnut oil

KEY NUTRIENTS
Beta Carotene
Vitamin A
Vitamin B$_6$
Folacin
Vitamin C
Vitamin E
Calcium
Copper
Iron
Magnesium
Manganese
Potassium
Monounsaturates
Omega-3s

1. FOR THE SALAD: Preheat the oven to 425°F. Cut away the beet leaves, leaving about 1/4 inch at the stem end. (Save the leaves for another purpose.) Scrub the beets under warm water with a vegetable brush. Place in a baking dish and add about 1/4 inch of water. Cover tightly with foil or a lid and bake for 30 to 60 minutes, depending on the size of the beets. Test for doneness by sticking a knife into a beet. It should slide in easily. Remove from the oven and let cool; reduce the oven temperature to 350°F. When the beets are cool, cut off the stem ends and slip off the skins. Cut the beets in half lengthwise, then slice very thinly or cut into small wedges. Place in a salad bowl.

2. Toast the walnuts (if using) on a baking sheet in the oven for 10 to 15 minutes, until lightly browned. Transfer immediately to a plate or small bowl.

3. Add the arugula or salad greens to the beets and toss. Add the walnuts, Parmesan, and herbs (if using) and toss again.

4. FOR THE DRESSING: Mix together the vinegars, salt and pepper, garlic (if using), and mustard in a small bowl. Whisk in the olive oil or yogurt and the walnut oil. Taste; if you want the dressing to be a bit more acidic, add another teaspoon or so of sherry or wine vinegar. Thin the dressing with a little water if it's too thick.

5. Add the dressing to the salad, toss, and serve.

Three Omega-3 Salad
(Spinach Salad with Chickpeas, Walnuts, and Feta)

This salad contains three foods that are excellent vegetable sources of omega-3 fatty acids: chickpeas, walnuts, and canola oil. Greens and olive oil are also high in omega-3s.

FOR THE SALAD
1 package baby spinach, rinsed and dried
1/3 cup walnut pieces
1 15-ounce can chickpeas, drained and rinsed
1/4 cup crumbled feta cheese, or 1 ounce Parmesan cheese, shaved

FOR THE DRESSING
2 tablespoons fresh lemon juice, sherry vinegar, or red wine vinegar, or a combination
1 teaspoon Dijon mustard
1 small garlic clove, minced or pressed (optional)
Salt and freshly ground pepper to taste
3 tablespoons canola oil
3 tablespoons extra-virgin olive oil, or a mixture of plain yogurt and oil

KEY NUTRIENTS
Beta Carotene
Vitamin A
Vitamin B$_6$
Folacin
Riboflavin
Thiamin
Vitamin C
Vitamin E
Calcium
Copper
Iron
Magnesium
Manganese
Potassium
Phosphorus
Zinc
Monounsaturates
Omega-3s

1. FOR THE SALAD: Put the spinach, walnuts, chickpeas, and cheese in a salad bowl and toss to combine.

2. FOR THE DRESSING: Mix together the lemon juice and/or vinegar, mustard, garlic (if using), and salt and pepper in a small bowl. Whisk in the oils.

3. Add the dressing to the salad and toss just before serving.

EVERY WOMAN'S

GUIDE TO EATING

DURING PREGNANCY

Greek Salad

ADVANCE
PREPARATION
The onions, tomatoes,
cucumber, and pepper
can be prepared and
assembled hours before
serving. Add the re-
maining ingredients
just before serving.

This salad is incredibly easy: nothing is finely chopped, and there's no lettuce to wash. Its only stringent requirement is good, sweet, vine-ripened tomatoes.

1 red onion or sweet onion
1 teaspoon vinegar (any kind)
5 medium or large ripe tomatoes, cut into wedges (the wedges cut in half if very large)
½ European cucumber or 1 regular cucumber, peeled (if desired), cut in half lengthwise, and sliced
1 large green, red, or yellow bell pepper, seeded and cut into 1-inch squares or into rings
12–16 kalamata olives (to taste), pitted if desired
Salt and freshly ground pepper to taste
4–6 tablespoons extra-virgin olive oil, to taste
2–3 tablespoons red wine vinegar or sherry vinegar, to taste
3 ounces feta cheese, crumbled
2–3 tablespoons chopped fresh mint (to taste), or 1 teaspoon dried oregano, or a combination

1. Cut the onion in half lengthwise and slice crosswise. Place in a bowl of cold water, add the vinegar, and soak for 10 minutes or more. Drain.

2. In a salad bowl, combine the onion and all the remaining ingredients; toss well. Taste and adjust the seasonings, then serve.

KEY NUTRIENTS
Beta Carotene
Vitamin A
Vitamin B$_6$
Folacin
Vitamin C
Vitamin E
Monounsaturates

Salads

Makes 4 to 6
servings

ADVANCE
PREPARATION

Everything can be pre-
pared hours ahead of
time, but wait until the
last minute to toss the
salad together.

Tomato and Arugula Salad with Feta Cheese

Here's a summer salad that takes advantage of tomatoes when they're at their finest.

FOR THE SALAD

1½ pounds sweet, ripe but firm tomatoes, cut into wedges
   Salt, preferably coarse sea salt, to taste
 1 garlic clove, minced or pressed (optional)
 4 large fresh basil leaves, cut into slivers (optional)
 4 cups baby arugula, rinsed and dried
12 imported black olives, pitted and cut in half
 1 ounce feta cheese, crumbled (about ¼ cup), or 1 ounce
   Parmesan cheese, cut into slivers

FOR THE DRESSING

2 teaspoons balsamic vinegar
4 teaspoons sherry vinegar or red wine vinegar
¼ cup extra-virgin olive oil, or 1 tablespoon oil and 3
   tablespoons plain yogurt or buttermilk

Freshly ground pepper to taste

1. FOR THE SALAD: Toss the tomatoes with the salt, garlic (if using), and basil in a salad bowl. Add the arugula, olives, and cheese.

2. FOR THE DRESSING: Whisk together the vinegars and oil (or oil and yogurt or buttermilk) in a small bowl. Thin with water, if desired.

3. Add the dressing to the salad and toss. Sprinkle with pepper and serve.

KEY NUTRIENTS
Beta Carotene
Vitamin A
Vitamin B6
Folacin
Vitamin C
Vitamin E
Calcium
Copper
Iron
Magnesium
Manganese
Potassium
Monounsaturates

EVERY WOMAN'S

GUIDE TO EATING

DURING PREGNANCY

116

Beet and Orange Salad

ADVANCE
PREPARATION
The roasted beets will
keep for up to a week
in a covered bowl in
the refrigerator.

If you eat citrus with nonmeat foods that contain iron, you will absorb much more of the iron. This salad is a delicious way to accomplish that, and it's beautiful as well.

4 small or medium or 2–3 large beets (1 bunch)
3 navel oranges
1 tablespoon chopped fresh parsley
¼ cup extra-virgin olive oil
1 tablespoon balsamic vinegar
1 tablespoon red wine vinegar or sherry vinegar
1 teaspoon Dijon mustard
   Salt to taste
¼ pound (about 3 heaped cups) arugula, trimmed, washed, and dried (optional)

1. Preheat the oven to 425°F. Cut away the beet leaves, leaving about ¼ inch at the stem ends. (Save the leaves for another purpose.) Scrub the beets under warm water with a vegetable brush. Place in a baking dish and add about ¼ inch of water. Cover tightly with foil or a lid and bake for 30 to 60 minutes, depending on the size of the beets. Test for doneness by sticking a knife into a beet. It should slide in easily. Remove from the oven and let cool. When cool enough to handle, cut off the stem ends and slip off the skins. Slice thinly. If they are large, cut them in half lengthwise, then slice. Place in a medium bowl.

2. Peel the oranges and cut away the white pith. Cut into rounds and add to the beets. Add the parsley.

3. Mix together the olive oil, vinegars, mustard, and salt in a small bowl. Toss with the beets, oranges, and parsley.

4. If desired, line a salad bowl with the arugula and top with the beet and orange mixture. Or transfer the mixture to an unlined salad bowl. Serve immediately.

KEY NUTRIENTS
Folacin
Vitamin C
Manganese
Iron (arugula)

Salads

ADVANCE
PREPARATION
This should be served
shortly after it's as-
sembled, but you can
prepare the grape-
fruits and greens hours
ahead and keep them
in the refrigerator.

Grapefruit and Avocado Salad

I think of this light, refreshing salad as a very California or Florida dish. But you can get avocados and grapefruits anywhere. Just make sure the avocados are ripe and the grapefruits juicy.

1 bunch watercress or arugula, trimmed, washed, and dried
2 pink grapefruits, peel and pith removed, divided into sections
2 ripe but firm avocados, preferably Hass, peeled, pitted, and sliced
Salt to taste
1/4 cup extra-virgin olive oil
2 tablespoons fresh lime juice
1 teaspoon mild-flavored honey, such as clover or acacia
2–3 teaspoons snipped fresh chives (to taste) for garnish

1. Line a platter with the watercress or arugula and arrange the grapefruit and avocado slices on top. Sprinkle the avocado with salt.

2. Mix together the olive oil, lime juice, and honey in a small bowl. Season with salt, then drizzle over the salad. Garnish with the chives and serve.

KEY NUTRIENTS
Vitamin B$_6$
Folacin
Niacin
Vitamin C
Copper
Magnesium
Potassium
Monounsaturates

Roasted Red Pepper Salad

ADVANCE PREPARATION
Roasted peppers will keep for at least 5 days in the refrigerator. Cover them with a thin film of olive oil before refrigerating.

You can find good-quality roasted red peppers in jars and delis, but you can also make them yourself with little effort. I like to roast them in the oven. They'll keep for at least five days in the refrigerator. Omit the dressing if you plan on keeping these on hand for sandwiches or other dishes. Cover with a thin film of olive oil before refrigerating.

4 medium red or yellow bell peppers
Coarse sea salt and freshly ground pepper to taste

FOR THE DRESSING
1 tablespoon extra-virgin olive oil
1 tablespoon red wine vinegar or balsamic vinegar
1–2 garlic cloves (to taste), minced or pressed
2 tablespoons slivered fresh basil or thyme leaves

1. Preheat the oven to 400°F. Line a baking sheet or pan with foil. Place the bell peppers on the foil and roast for 30 to 45 minutes, turning the peppers with tongs every 10 minutes, until the peppers are soft and the skins are browned and puffed.

2. Transfer the peppers to a large bowl. Cover the bowl with a plate and let sit for 30 minutes or longer. When cool enough to handle, carefully remove the skins and seeds from the peppers, holding them over the bowl so you don't lose any of the liquid. Cut the peppers into strips. Toss with the salt and pepper in a medium bowl. Strain the pepper juice and add to the peppers.

4. FOR THE DRESSING: Combine the olive oil, vinegar, and garlic in a small bowl.

5. Add the dressing to the peppers and toss. Add the basil or thyme, toss lightly, and serve.

KEY NUTRIENTS
Beta Carotene
Vitamin A
Vitamin B$_6$
Folacin
Vitamin C

Salads

119

Roasted Pepper and Mozzarella Antipasto

This makes a quick first course or salad course if you have roasted peppers, either store-bought or homemade, on hand. The fresher the mozzarella, the better.

- 2 large red bell peppers, roasted (see page 119)
- 6–8 ounces mozzarella cheese, thinly sliced
- 2 tablespoons extra-virgin olive oil
- Salt and freshly ground pepper to taste
- A few fresh basil leaves, torn or snipped

Cut the roasted peppers into wide strips and arrange on a platter with the sliced mozzarella. Drizzle on the olive oil. Sprinkle with the salt and pepper and basil. Serve at room temperature or slightly chilled.

VARIATION

Tomato and Mozzarella Antipasto

Substitute 2 large, ripe but firm, in-season tomatoes for the peppers. Slice them into rounds. Cut the rounds in half if very large. Arrange with the mozzarella as instructed. If you wish, drizzle the tomatoes with a small amount of balsamic vinegar before drizzling on the olive oil.

Guacamole

Guacamole should be made with the knobby-skinned Hass avocados, since other types are watery. Although Mexican guacamole is often made spicy with the addition of minced fresh chile peppers, such as serranos, I like to make the heat optional — even when I'm not pregnant.

ADVANCE PREPARATION

This can be stored in the refrigerator for a couple of hours, but the color will not remain bright.

3 medium or large ripe Hass avocados
1 large or 2 small ripe but firm tomatoes, chopped
   Fresh lemon or lime juice to taste
   Salt to taste

OPTIONAL ADDITIONS
1 small garlic clove, minced or pressed
1/4 teaspoon ground cumin
1–2 serrano peppers (to taste), minced
   Chopped fresh cilantro for garnish

Cut the avocados in half, remove the pits, and scoop out the flesh. Mash with a mortar and pestle or with a fork or the back of a large spoon in a medium bowl. Do not use the food processor. Add the tomatoes, lemon or lime juice, and salt and continue to mash. Stir in the garlic, cumin, and peppers, if using. Taste and adjust the seasonings. Garnish with cilantro, if using, and serve.

NOTE: If not serving right away, the top will discolor. Cover tightly with plastic wrap and stir well before serving.

KEY NUTRIENTS
Vitamin A
Vitamin B$_6$
Folacin
Niacin
Vitamin C
Vitamin E
Copper
Magnesium
Potassium

Salads

ADVANCE
PREPARATION
This will hold for a
couple of days in the
refrigerator.

Grated Carrots
in Vinaigrette

I got hooked on grated carrot salads when I lived in France. One of the best things about them is that they are very good keepers, so you can hold them in the refrigerator for a few days.

1 pound carrots
¼ cup chopped fresh parsley
½–¾ cup Classic Vinaigrette (page 164) or Yogurt or
  Buttermilk Vinaigrette (page 165), using a
  combination of lemon juice and vinegar and omitting
  the garlic if desired
Salt and freshly ground pepper to taste

1. Peel the carrots and cut the tips off. If you're using a hand grater, leave the stem ends attached, so that you can hold on to them as you grate. If you're using a food processor, cut off the stem ends. Grate on the fine holes of a grater or in a food processor fitted with the grating blade. You should have about 4 cups grated carrots. Transfer to a salad bowl. Add the parsley.

2. Toss the vinaigrette with the carrots and parsley. Season with salt and pepper and toss again. Serve immediately, or refrigerate and serve chilled.

KEY NUTRIENTS
Beta Carotene
Vitamin A
Vitamin C
Potassium
Monounsaturates

Moroccan Cooked Carrot Salad with Cumin

ADVANCE PREPARATION
This will keep for a couple of days in the refrigerator, provided you don't add the lemon juice until shortly before serving. Bring to room temperature before serving.

In North Africa, many salads are made with cooked vegetables. This is a favorite of mine.

1 pound carrots, peeled and thinly sliced
2 tablespoons extra-virgin olive oil
1–2 garlic cloves (to taste), minced or pressed (optional)
1 teaspoon crushed cumin seeds
$\frac{1}{2}$ teaspoon salt, or to taste
$\frac{1}{2}$ teaspoon freshly ground pepper
$\frac{1}{4}$ cup chopped fresh parsley
3–4 tablespoons fresh lemon juice, to taste
Black olives for garnish (optional)

1. Place the carrots in a steamer basket set in a saucepan with 1 inch of simmering water. Cover and steam for 5 to 6 minutes, until tender. Drain.

2. Heat the oil in a large nonstick skillet over medium heat. Add the carrots, garlic (if using), cumin, salt, and pepper. Stir together for about 5 minutes, until the carrots are nicely coated with the mixture. Add the parsley and toss.

3. Transfer the carrot mixture to a salad bowl. Sprinkle with the lemon juice and toss. Taste and adjust the seasonings. Garnish with black olives, if you wish. Serve at room temperature.

KEY NUTRIENTS
Beta Carotene
Vitamin A
Vitamin C
Potassium

Salads

ADVANCE
PREPARATION
This will keep for a
week in the refrigera-
tor.

Marinated Carrots

Once you taste these lightly steamed, marinated carrots, you'll be amazed at how fast you'll go through a pound of carrots.

1 pound carrots, peeled, quartered lengthwise, and cut
    into 2- to 3-inch lengths
Salt, preferably coarse sea salt, to taste
2 tablespoons sherry vinegar
2 tablespoons extra-virgin olive oil
1 tablespoon finely chopped fresh mint or parsley
    (optional)

1. Place the carrots in a steamer basket set in a saucepan with 1 inch of simmering water. Cover and steam for 5 to 6 minutes, until just tender. Transfer to a colander and run it under cold water, or transfer to a bowl of ice water, then drain.

2. Transfer the carrots to a serving bowl and toss with the remaining ingredients. Serve at room temperature, or refrigerate and serve cold.

VARIATION
Marinated Carrots with Garlic

When you're pregnant, raw garlic might not appeal to you. But if it does, you can add a clove or two of finely minced or pressed garlic to the above recipe.

KEY NUTRIENTS
Beta Carotene
Vitamin A
Vitamin C
Potassium

Creamy Cucumber Salad

This is a perfect pregnancy salad because it's high in protein, very refreshing, and easy to make. It's also a great sandwich filling.

This will keep for a few days in the refrigerator, but the cucumbers will continue to release water, so remember to stir the mixture before you use it.

2 regular cucumbers, peeled, seeded, and minced, or 1 European cucumber, minced
Salt to taste
2 cups cottage cheese
½ cup plain yogurt
Lots of freshly ground pepper

1. Place the cucumbers in a colander in the sink and toss with a generous amount of salt. Let sit for 20 minutes. Rinse the cucumbers and drain on paper towels. Transfer to a medium bowl.

2. Blend the cottage cheese in a food processor until smooth. Add the yogurt and continue to blend until there is no trace of graininess. Mix with the cucumber in the bowl. Add a generous amount of pepper, taste, and adjust the salt. Serve immediately.

VARIATION

Creamy Cucumber Sandwich
Makes 1 sandwich

This is especially good with sourdough whole grain or dark rye bread.

2 slices whole grain, sourdough whole grain, or dark rye bread, toasted if desired
½ cup Creamy Cucumber Salad

Spread one or both slices of the bread with the cucumber salad and serve as either 1 traditional or 2 open-faced sandwiches.

KEY NUTRIENTS
Fiber
Protein
Vitamin B$_{12}$
Folacin
Riboflavin
Vitamin C
Phosphorus

KEY NUTRIENTS SANDWICH
Vitamin B$_6$
Folacin
Niacin
Thiamin
Copper
Iron
Magnesium
Manganese

Salads

ADVANCE
PREPARATION
This will keep for sev-
eral days in the refrig-
erator.

Quick Cucumber Pickles

You could call this incredibly quick, simple combination a pickle, relish, or salad. Whatever you name it, it's slightly sweet, due to the rice wine vinegar, and makes a very agreeable accompaniment to sandwiches, cottage cheese, tuna fish, and Asian dishes. Keep it on hand in the refrigerator.

1 European cucumber or 2 regular cucumbers, peeled
    (if desired) and thinly sliced
Salt
$^1/_3$ cup seasoned rice wine vinegar
Pinch of hot red pepper flakes (optional)

Place the cucumbers in a colander in the sink and toss with a generous amount of salt. Let sit for 15 to 30 minutes. Rinse the cucumbers and drain on paper towels. Transfer to a medium bowl and toss with the vinegar and pepper flakes (if using). Refrigerate for 15 minutes or longer before serving.

KEY NUTRIENTS
Fiber
Folacin
Vitamin C

Coleslaw

Calcium-rich yogurt replaces most of the mayonnaise in this tangy coleslaw.

FOR THE DRESSING
- 3/4 cup plain yogurt or Yogurt Cheese (page 65)
- 1/4 cup Hellmann's or Best Foods mayonnaise
- 2 tablespoons cider vinegar
- 2 tablespoons milk, plus more for thinning
- 1 tablespoon plus 1 teaspoon Dijon mustard or prepared horseradish
- 1/2 teaspoon sugar, or more to taste
- Salt and freshly ground pepper to taste

FOR THE SALAD
- 4 heaped cups very finely shredded green cabbage (about 1/2 medium head)
- 4 scallions, white and green parts, finely chopped (optional)
- 2 medium carrots, peeled and finely grated
- 1 green bell pepper, seeded and cut into slivers (optional)

1. FOR THE DRESSING: Mix together all the ingredients in a small bowl. If the dressing is too thick for your taste, add another tablespoon or so milk to thin it. Taste and adjust the salt and horseradish or mustard. If you like your coleslaw a little sweeter, add more sugar.

2. FOR THE SALAD: Mix together all the ingredients in a salad bowl.

3. Add the dressing to the salad and toss. Refrigerate for at least 30 minutes. Toss again and serve.

ADVANCE PREPARATION
This will keep for several days in the refrigerator.

KEY NUTRIENTS
Beta Carotene
Vitamin A
Folacin
Vitamin C
Potassium
Calcium

Salads

ADVANCE
PREPARATION

This has good staying power. It will keep for a day or two in the refrigerator.

Asian Coleslaw

This sweet-and-sour, slightly picante cabbage salad goes wonderfully with Asian meals.

FOR THE SALAD

1 medium head white, savoy, or napa cabbage, quartered, cored, and shredded (about 7 cups)
1 red bell pepper, seeded and cut into 2-inch-long slivers
1/4 cup chopped fresh cilantro
1/2–1 red Thai chile pepper or serrano pepper (to taste), minced (optional)

FOR THE DRESSING

1/3 cup rice wine vinegar
1–1 1/4 teaspoons sugar, to taste (use half this amount if using seasoned vinegar)
Salt to taste
1/4 cup peanut oil, canola oil, or plain yogurt

1. FOR THE SALAD: Toss together all the ingredients in a salad bowl.

2. FOR THE DRESSING: Mix together the vinegar, sugar, and salt in a small bowl. Make sure the sugar is dissolved. Whisk in the oil or yogurt.

3. Add the dressing to the salad and toss. Let sit for at least 15 minutes, toss again, and serve.

KEY NUTRIENTS
Beta Carotene
Vitamin A
Vitamin B$_6$
Folacin
Vitamin C

Potato Salad

ADVANCE
PREPARATION
The salad will keep for
3 or 4 days in the
refrigerator.

This potato salad is lower in fat than a classic American potato salad because it calls for some mayonnaise but more yogurt. I prefer this combination to low-fat mayonnaise, because low-fat mayo tends to be too sweet.

2 pounds waxy potatoes, such as red or new potatoes,
    scrubbed and quartered if large
1/3 cup Hellmann's or Best Foods mayonnaise
2/3 cup plain yogurt
2 tablespoons red or white wine vinegar or sherry vinegar,
    or more to taste
Salt and freshly ground pepper to taste
2 celery stalks, chopped
2–4 tablespoons minced red onion or scallions (to taste),
    rinsed with cold water and drained, or 1/4 cup snipped
    fresh chives

1. Place the potatoes in a steamer basket set in a saucepan with 1 inch of simmering water. Cover and steam until tender, 15 to 20 minutes. Meanwhile, stir together the mayonnaise and yogurt in a small bowl.

2. When the potatoes are done — you should be able to pierce them easily with a fork or knife, but they shouldn't fall apart — remove from the heat and drain. Use a dishtowel to steady the hot potatoes with one hand and cut into medium dice. Toss the potatoes with the vinegar and salt and pepper in a large bowl. Add the celery; red onion, scallions, or chives; and mayonnaise-yogurt mixture. Toss together. Taste and add more vinegar, if desired. Adjust the seasonings and serve warm or at room temperature.

KEY NUTRIENTS
Vitamin B$_6$
Niacin
Vitamin C
Copper
Iron
Magnesium
Manganese
Potassium

Salads

ADVANCE
PREPARATION

The potatoes can be
cooked and tossed with
a portion of the dress-
ing hours or even a day
before finishing the
salad.

Potato and
Green Bean Salad

This makes a great lunch, and it's wonderful to have in the refrigerator. If you're holding the salad for a couple of days, the
beans will lose their brightness because of the acid in the dressing. You can get around this by tossing the potatoes with about
a third of the salad dressing and adding the rest of the dressing
when you're ready to serve.

1½ pounds new or Yukon Gold potatoes, scrubbed and cut
    into ½- to 1-inch dice
¾ pound green beans, trimmed and broken in half if very
    long

FOR THE DRESSING
3 tablespoons wine vinegar or sherry vinegar
2 teaspoons Dijon mustard
Salt to taste
1 small garlic clove, minced or pressed (optional)
½ cup extra-virgin olive oil, or ¼ cup oil and ¼ cup plain
    yogurt or buttermilk
Freshly ground pepper to taste

Salt and freshly ground pepper to taste
¼ cup minced red onion, rinsed with cold water (optional)
2 hard-cooked eggs (see page 155), diced
1 ounce Parmesan cheese, cut into slivers, or 1 ounce goat
    cheese, crumbled (about ¼ cup)
A handful of fresh herbs, such as parsley, chives, tarragon,
    or dill, chopped

1. Place the potatoes in a steamer basket set in a saucepan
with 1 inch of simmering water. Cover and steam for about 15 minutes, until tender but firm enough to hold their shape. Remove
from the heat.

KEY NUTRIENTS
Vitamin A
Vitamin B$_6$
Folacin
Niacin
Vitamin C
Copper
Iron
Magnesium
Manganese
Potassium
Monounsaturates

EVERY WOMAN'S

GUIDE TO EATING

DURING PREGNANCY

2. Steam or blanch the beans for 5 to 6 minutes, until just tender and bright green. Transfer to a bowl of cold water, then drain.

3. FOR THE DRESSING: Meanwhile, whisk together the vinegar, mustard, and salt in a medium bowl. Add the garlic, if using, then whisk in the oil (or oil and yogurt or buttermilk). Add the pepper.

4. Drain the potatoes and transfer to a salad bowl. Add the salt and pepper and $1/4$ cup of the dressing; toss. Add the beans, onion (if using), eggs, cheese, and herbs. Add the remaining dressing and toss well. Taste and adjust the pepper. Serve warm, at room temperature, or chilled.

ADVANCE PREPARATION
This salad will hold at room temperature for a few hours and makes a great picnic dish.

Warm Potato and Goat Cheese Salad

If all you feel like is a salad for lunch or dinner, this one would be a good choice. The cheese melts when you toss it with the potatoes, and the dish is comforting and easily put together.

1½ pounds new or Yukon Gold potatoes, scrubbed

FOR THE DRESSING
3 tablespoons red wine vinegar or sherry vinegar
1 teaspoon Dijon mustard
1 small garlic clove, minced or pressed (optional)
Salt and freshly ground pepper to taste
⅓ cup plain yogurt
2 tablespoons olive oil

Salt and freshly ground pepper to taste
1 small red onion, thinly sliced and soaked in a bowl of water for 5 minutes, then rinsed
½ cup chopped fresh parsley
3 ounces goat cheese, crumbled or cut into pieces (about ¾ cup)

1. Place the potatoes in a steamer basket set in a saucepan with 1 inch of simmering water. Cover and steam until tender, 10 to 15 minutes. When the potatoes are tender but still firm, remove from the heat.

2. FOR THE DRESSING: Meanwhile, mix together the vinegar, mustard, garlic, and salt and pepper in a medium bowl. Whisk in the yogurt and olive oil.

3. Use a dishtowel to steady the hot potatoes with one hand and cut into quarters. Toss the hot potatoes at once in a large bowl with salt and pepper and half the dressing. Add the onion, parsley, goat cheese, and remaining dressing; toss. Taste and adjust the seasonings. Serve warm or at room temperature.

KEY NUTRIENTS
Vitamin B_6
Vitamin B_{12}
Niacin
Vitamin C
Copper
Iron
Magnesium
Manganese
Phosphorus
Potassium

EVERY WOMAN'S

GUIDE TO EATING

DURING PREGNANCY

Chickpea Salad

ADVANCE
PREPARATION
You can make this sev-
eral hours ahead and
keep it in the refriger-
ator.

This is a great pantry meal. The only fresh ingredients you really need are the parsley and lemon juice, and even the parsley
can be omitted. You can also omit the garlic if it doesn't agree
with you.

FOR THE SALAD

3 15-ounce cans chickpeas, drained and rinsed
1 large red bell pepper, seeded and diced, or 1 cup diced
     bottled, canned, or homemade roasted red peppers
     (see page 119)
¹/₂ cup chopped fresh parsley (optional)
1–2 garlic cloves (to taste), minced or pressed (optional)
¹/₂ teaspoon crushed cumin seeds

FOR THE DRESSING

¹/₄ cup plain yogurt
3 tablespoons fresh lemon juice
2 tablespoons extra-virgin olive oil
1 tablespoon red wine vinegar or sherry vinegar
Salt and freshly ground pepper to taste

1. FOR THE SALAD: Toss together all the ingredients in a salad
bowl.

2. FOR THE DRESSING: Whisk together all the ingredients in a
small bowl.

3. Add the dressing to the salad and toss. Serve immediately or refrigerate and serve chilled.

KEY NUTRIENTS
Protein
Beta Carotene
Vitamin A
Vitamin B$_6$
Folacin
Thiamin
Vitamin C
Copper
Iron
Magnesium
Manganese
Phosphorus
Potassium
Zinc

Salads

ADVANCE
PREPARATION
The beans will keep for
5 days in the refriger-
ator. Add the bell pep-
per and cilantro just
before serving.

Bean Salad
with Cumin Vinaigrette

Beans taste wonderful in a cumin-flavored vinaigrette. Make a
batch and keep it on hand in the refrigerator.

1 pound dried black beans, pinto beans, red beans, or
   black-eyed peas, washed and picked over
8 cups water
1 medium onion, chopped
4 garlic cloves, minced or pressed
1 bay leaf
Salt to taste

FOR THE VINAIGRETTE
1/4 cup red wine vinegar or sherry vinegar
1 garlic clove, minced or pressed
1 teaspoon Dijon mustard
1 teaspoon ground cumin
Salt and freshly ground pepper to taste
1/2 cup cooking liquid from the beans or plain yogurt if
   using canned beans
1/4 cup extra-virgin olive oil

1 medium red bell pepper, seeded and diced
1/2 cup chopped fresh cilantro
3–4 cups baby arugula or salad greens, rinsed and dried
   (optional)

1. Soak the beans in water to cover for 6 hours or
overnight. (Black-eyed peas do not require soaking.) Drain and
rinse. Combine the beans and water in a soup pot, casserole, or
Dutch oven and bring to a boil. Reduce the heat slightly and spoon
off any foam. When all the foam has been spooned off, add the
onion, garlic, and bay leaf. Reduce the heat again, cover, and simmer for 30 minutes. Add the salt (about 2 teaspoons) and continue

KEY NUTRIENTS
Protein
Vitamin B$_6$
Folacin
Thiamin
Copper
Iron
Magnesium
Manganese
Phosphorus
Potassium

to simmer for 15 minutes more, until the beans are thoroughly tender but still intact. Taste and adjust the seasonings. Drain the beans over a bowl and return them to the pot. Set aside ½ cup of the cooking liquid for the vinaigrette.

2. FOR THE VINAIGRETTE: Stir together the vinegar, garlic, mustard, cumin, and salt and pepper in a medium bowl. Whisk in the cooking liquid or yogurt and oil.

3. Add the beans to the vinaigrette and stir to combine. If serving the beans warm, add the bell pepper and cilantro. If serving cold, let the beans cool slightly and refrigerate. Shortly before serving, stir in the bell pepper and cilantro. Taste and adjust the seasonings.

4. If desired, line a big salad bowl or platter, or individual salad plates, with the arugula or salad greens. Give the beans a stir, pile them onto the greens, and serve.

NOTE: To make this with canned beans, use four 15-ounce cans of beans. Drain and rinse the beans, then transfer to a medium bowl. Proceed with recipe beginning with step 2. For a warm salad, warm the beans in a saucepan in the vinaigrette, then toss with the bell pepper and cilantro.

ADVANCE
PREPARATION
This will keep for 3
days in the refrigera-
tor, but it's best to
add the parsley or
mixed herbs just before
serving. To serve warm,
gently reheat it in a
saucepan.

French Lentil Salad,
Warm or Cold

Lentils make a high-protein soup or salad, and this French
salad is one of my favorites.

1 pound (about 2 heaped cups) dried lentils, washed and
    picked over
Water
1 medium onion, cut in half
2 cloves
2 large garlic cloves, cut in half
1 bay leaf
Salt to taste (about 2 teaspoons)

FOR THE DRESSING
1/4 cup red wine vinegar
1 tablespoon Dijon mustard
1 large garlic clove, minced or pressed
Salt and freshly ground pepper to taste
1/2 cup cooking liquid from the lentils
2 tablespoons extra-virgin olive oil

1/4–1/2 cup chopped fresh parsley (to taste), or a mixture of
    parsley and other fresh herbs, such as chives,
    tarragon, or thyme

KEY NUTRIENTS
Protein
Vitamin B$_6$
Folacin
Thiamin
Copper
Iron
Magnesium
Manganese
Phosphorus
Potassium

WITH CHEESE
Vitamin A
Riboflavin
Calcium
Zinc

1. Place the lentils in a heavy saucepan and add water to
cover by 1 inch. Stick each onion half with a clove. Add the onion
halves, garlic, and bay leaf. Bring to a boil. Reduce the heat, cover,
and simmer for 25 minutes. Add the salt and simmer for 10 to 15
minutes more, until the lentils are tender but not mushy. Remove
from the heat and drain through a strainer set over a bowl. Set
aside 1/2 cup of the cooking liquid for the dressing. Discard the
onion, garlic, and bay leaf. Transfer the lentils to a salad bowl. Taste
and adjust the salt.

2. FOR THE DRESSING: Mix together the vinegar, mustard, and garlic in a medium bowl. Add a little salt and pepper, then stir in the cooking liquid and olive oil. Taste and adjust the salt.

3. Stir the dressing into the lentils, along with the parsley or mixed herbs. Serve warm, or refrigerate and serve cold.

VARIATION

Warm Lentil Salad with Goat Cheese

Make the salad as directed and divide among 4 salad plates. Slice 3 ounces fresh goat cheese into 4 rounds. Top each portion of salad with a round and serve at once.

White Bean and Basil Salad

With canned beans on hand and fresh basil in the refrigerator, you can make this Mediterranean salad very quickly.

    2 15-ounce cans white beans, drained and rinsed
 1/4 cup slivered fresh basil leaves
 1/2 cup cherry tomatoes, cut in half if large
 1/2 pound green beans, trimmed, broken in half, and
         steamed for 5 minutes (optional)
1/2–3/4 cup Classic Vinaigrette (page 164)
 1/4 cup freshly grated Parmesan cheese
     Salt and freshly ground pepper to taste

Combine the beans, basil, tomatoes, and green beans (if using) in a medium bowl. Toss with the vinaigrette and Parmesan. Taste and adjust the seasonings with salt and pepper before serving.

Makes 4 servings

ADVANCE
PREPARATION
This will keep for a couple of days in the refrigerator, but the basil will lose its vibrant color.

KEY NUTRIENTS
Protein
Vitamin A
Vitamin B$_6$
Folacin
Thiamin
Vitamin C
Vitamin E
Copper
Iron
Magnesium
Manganese
Phosphorus
Potassium

Salads

You can keep tab-
bouleh in the refriger-
ator for a couple of
days, but the parsley
will fade and the fla-
vors won't be as vivid.

Classic Tabbouleh

This is the salad to eat if you're craving something green, tart,
and refreshing. It's almost like pure parsley, enhanced with
lemon juice and mint and fortified with a small amount of
bulgur.

$2/3$ cup boiling water
2 ounces (about $1/3$ heaped cup) fine bulgur
Juice of 3 large lemons, or more to taste
Salt to taste
4 cups flat-leaf parsley leaves (from about 4 large
  bunches), washed and spun dry
$1/4$–$1/2$ cup chopped fresh mint, to taste (optional)
4 scallions, white and green parts, chopped
3 ripe tomatoes, diced
2 tablespoons extra-virgin olive oil
Small romaine lettuce leaves and pita bread triangles for
  serving

1. Pour the boiling water over the bulgur in a small bowl
and soak for 20 minutes, until softened. Drain and squeeze out any
excess water. Return to the bowl and toss with the lemon juice and
salt. Set aside.

2. Chop the parsley in a food processor, then transfer to a
salad bowl. Add the mint (if using), scallions, tomatoes, and bulgur mixture and toss together. Add the olive oil and toss again.
Taste and adjust the lemon juice and salt. It should be quite
lemony. Chill until ready serve.

3. Serve with romaine lettuce leaves and pita bread trian
gles to scoop up the tabbouleh.

KEY NUTRIENTS
Beta Carotene
Vitamin A
Vitamin B_6
Folacin
Vitamin C
Vitamin E
Calcium
Copper
Iron
Magnesium
Manganese
Potassium

Couscous Tabbouleh

ADVANCE
PREPARATION
The salad will hold for
several hours in the re-
frigerator. It tastes
good even after the
color of the parsley
fades.

This lemony salad keeps well in the refrigerator, so you can have it on hand for quick, nutritious lunches.

1 cup couscous
$^3/_4$ cup water, plus more if needed
$^1/_2$ cup fresh lemon juice
$^3/_4$ teaspoon salt
$^1/_2$ teaspoon ground cumin
2 tablespoons extra-virgin olive oil
2 cups finely chopped flat-leaf parsley (1 large or 2
    medium bunches)
4 scallions, white and green parts, chopped
1 red or green bell pepper, seeded and finely chopped
1 pound (4 medium) tomatoes, finely chopped
1 15-ounce can chickpeas, drained and rinsed
Small romaine lettuce leaves for serving

1. Place the couscous in a salad bowl. Mix together the water, lemon juice, salt, and cumin in a small bowl. Pour over the couscous. Let sit for 30 minutes, stirring the mixture with a wooden spoon or rubbing it between your fingers and thumbs every so often so that it doesn't form clumps.

2. Stir all the remaining ingredients, except the lettuce leaves, into the couscous. Taste and adjust the seasonings. Refrigerate until ready to serve.

3. Serve with the lettuce leaves, using them as scoops for the salad.

KEY NUTRIENTS
Protein
Beta Carotene
Vitamin A
Vitamin B_6
Folacin
Niacin
Thiamin
Vitamin C
Vitamin E
Calcium
Copper
Iron
Magnesium
Manganese
Phosphorus
Potassium
Zinc

Salads

ADVANCE
PREPARATION
The salad can be as-
sembled without the
dressing hours ahead
of time. Toss with the
dressing shortly before
serving.

Quinoa and Black Bean Salad with Lime Dressing

Quinoa is a nutrient-dense and delicately flavored grain.

FOR THE SALAD
- 1 cup quinoa
- 2 cups water or vegetable or chicken stock
- 1/4 teaspoon salt, plus more to taste
- 3 scallions, white and green parts, thinly sliced (optional)
- 1–2 serrano peppers (to taste), minced (optional)
- 1 medium red or green bell pepper, seeded and diced
- 1 medium tomato, diced
- 1/4 cup chopped fresh cilantro
- 1 15-ounce can black beans, drained and rinsed

FOR THE DRESSING
- 6 tablespoons fresh lime juice
- Salt to taste
- 1 small garlic clove, minced or pressed (optional)
- 1/4 cup plain yogurt or buttermilk
- 3 tablespoons extra-virgin olive oil

KEY NUTRIENTS
Protein
Beta Carotene
Vitamin A (red bell pep-
  pers)
Vitamin B$_6$
Folacin
Niacin
Riboflavin
Thiamin
Vitamin C
Copper
Iron
Magnesium
Manganese
Phosphorus
Potassium
Zinc

1. FOR THE SALAD: Rinse the quinoa thoroughly in several changes of cold water, draining it through a fine sieve each time. Bring the water or stock to a boil in a 2-quart saucepan. Add the quinoa and 1/2 teaspoon salt. Reduce the heat, cover, and simmer for 12 to 15 minutes, until the liquid is absorbed. Remove from the heat and let sit, covered, for 5 minutes. Uncover and transfer to a salad bowl. Let cool, then taste and adjust the salt. Toss with the remaining salad ingredients.

2. FOR THE DRESSING: Mix together the lime juice, salt, and garlic (if using) in a medium bowl. Whisk in the yogurt or buttermilk and oil.

3. Add the dressing to the salad, toss, and serve.

Broccoli and Chickpea Salad with Egg

ADVANCE PREPARATION

You can steam the broccoli and make the dressing a few hours ahead of time.

You can serve this quick, high-protein salad warm or cold. If your pantry is well stocked and you buy broccoli every week, dinner will always be on hand in the form of this dish.

1 pound broccoli, broken into florets, stems peeled and diced
1–2 15-ounce cans chickpeas (to taste), drained and rinsed
2 large eggs
Salt and freshly ground pepper to taste
Classic Vinaigrette (page 164), Lemon Vinaigrette (page 164), or Yogurt or Buttermilk Vinaigrette (page 165)
1 ounce Parmesan cheese, cut into slivers or grated

1. Place the broccoli in a steamer basket set in a saucepan with 1 inch of simmering water. Cover and steam for 4 to 5 minutes, until tender but not soft and still bright green. Transfer to a colander and run it under cold water, or transfer to a bowl of ice water, then drain. Transfer to a salad bowl and add the chickpeas.

2. Meanwhile, in another pot, soft-boil the eggs for 4 minutes. Drain and run under cold water for a couple of minutes.

3. Carefully peel the eggs, then cut them in half over the broccoli and chickpeas so the yolks run out over the mixture. Chop and add the egg whites. Sprinkle lightly with salt and pepper. Toss the salad with the dressing and Parmesan, then serve.

KEY NUTRIENTS
Protein
Beta Carotene
Vitamin A
Vitamin B$_6$
Folacin
Thiamin
Vitamin C
Copper
Iron
Magnesium
Manganese
Phosphorus
Potassium
Zinc
Monounsaturates

Salads

ADVANCE
PREPARATION
The salad, undressed,
will hold for a day in
the refrigerator.
Dressed, it will hold for
a couple of hours.

Curried Mixed-Grain Salad

I've been making one version or another of this hearty, protein-rich salad for years. The textures are marvelous, and it keeps very well.

^{1}/$_4$ cup pine nuts
1 cup canned chickpeas, drained and rinsed
^{1}/$_2$ cup brown rice, cooked (see page 266)
^{1}/$_2$ cup wheat berries, cooked (see page 267)
^{1}/$_2$ cup quinoa, cooked (see page 265)
1 bunch scallions, white and green parts, thinly sliced (optional)
^{1}/$_2$ pound broccoli florets, steamed for 4–5 minutes
1 tart apple, such as Granny Smith, peeled, cored, and diced, then tossed with 1 tablespoon fresh lemon or lime juice
^{1}/$_4$ cup dark or golden raisins

FOR THE DRESSING
^{1}/$_2$ cup plain yogurt or buttermilk
2 tablespoons Hellmann's or Best Foods mayonnaise
2 tablespoons fresh lime juice
1 tablespoon sherry vinegar
1 teaspoon Dijon mustard
1 teaspoon curry powder
Pinch of cayenne pepper
Salt to taste

^{1}/$_2$ head leaf lettuce, washed and dried

KEY NUTRIENTS
Protein
Beta Carotene
Vitamin A
Vitamin B$_6$
Folacin
Niacin
Riboflavin
Thiamin
Vitamin C
Copper
Iron
Magnesium
Manganese
Phosphorus
Potassium
Zinc

1. Toast the pine nuts in a small frying pan over medium heat. Shake them in the pan until they are lightly browned, then transfer immediately to a large bowl. Add all the remaining salad ingredients, except the lettuce, and toss together.

2. FOR THE DRESSING: Mix together all the ingredients in a small bowl.

3. Add the dressing to the salad and toss. Taste and adjust the seasonings.

4. Line a serving platter or wide bowl with the lettuce. Top with the salad and serve.

ADVANCE
PREPARATION

You can prepare every-
thing hours or even a
day in advance, but
don't toss the green
vegetable with the rice
and dressing too far
ahead of time, or the
color will fade. The
salad can hold with the
dressing for about an
hour in or out of the
refrigerator.

Wild Rice Salad

Wild rice makes a nutty, satisfying salad. Broccoli is the green
vegetable I usually choose for this, but you can also use green
beans or peas.

FOR THE SALAD

3 cups water or chicken or vegetable stock

1 cup wild rice, rinsed

$1/4$–$3/4$ teaspoon salt (depending on whether you're using water
      or salted or unsalted stock), plus more to taste

1 pound broccoli crowns, broken into florets; 1 pound
      peas, shelled; or $1/2$ pound green beans, trimmed and
      broken in half

$1/3$ cup walnut or pecan pieces

1 red bell pepper, seeded and diced

Up to $1/3$ cup chopped fresh herbs, such as parsley,
      thyme, tarragon, or chives, to taste (optional)

FOR THE DRESSING

2 tablespoons fresh lemon juice

1 tablespoon red wine vinegar or sherry vinegar

1 garlic clove, minced or pressed (optional)

Salt to taste

$1/3$ cup plain yogurt or buttermilk

3 tablespoons walnut oil

Freshly ground pepper to taste

1. **FOR THE SALAD:** Bring the water or stock to a boil in a
medium saucepan. Add the rice and salt. When the water comes
back to a boil, reduce the heat, cover, and simmer for 40 to 45 minutes, until the rice is tender. Spoon out a few grains and rinse them
with cold water. They should be splayed and tender to the bite,
with no hardness in the shells. Drain off any remaining liquid.

2. While the rice is cooking, place the broccoli, peas, or
beans in a steamer basket set in a saucepan with 1 inch of simmer-

KEY NUTRIENTS
Protein
Beta Carotene
Vitamin A
Vitamin B$_6$
Folacin
Niacin
Vitamin C
Manganese
Potassium
Omega-3s

ing water. Cover and steam until just tender, about 5 minutes. Transfer to a colander and run it under cold water, or transfer to a bowl of ice water, then drain.

3. Combine the rice, green vegetable, nuts, bell pepper, and herbs (if using) in a salad bowl.

4. FOR THE DRESSING: Mix together the lemon juice, vinegar, and garlic (if using) in a small bowl. Add salt to taste. Stir in the yogurt or buttermilk, walnut oil, and pepper. Combine well and taste; adjust the salt.

5. Add the dressing to the salad, toss, and serve.

ADVANCE
PREPARATION
The salad will keep for
a few days in the
refrigerator, but the
herbs will lose their
color.

Egg Salad

Most egg salads are simple, rather high-fat mixtures of seasoned hard-cooked eggs and mayonnaise, with celery or onion
mixed in. I make a lower-fat dressing of mayonnaise and yogurt and use lots of fresh herbs to give my egg salad a vibrant
flavor.

8 hard-cooked eggs (see page 155), finely chopped
   Salt and freshly ground pepper to taste
¼ cup chopped fresh herbs, such as parsley, tarragon,
      basil, or dill, or more to taste
2 celery stalks, finely chopped
1 small red onion, finely chopped and rinsed in cold water
      (optional)
¼ cup plain yogurt
4 teaspoons Hellmann's or Best Foods mayonnaise
1 tablespoon red wine vinegar
1 teaspoon Dijon mustard
½–1 teaspoon curry powder (optional)

1. Place the chopped eggs in a medium bowl and sprinkle
with salt and pepper. Add the herbs, celery, and onion (if using).

2. Stir together the yogurt, mayonnaise, vinegar, and mustard in a small bowl. Add salt and pepper to taste. Add the curry
powder, if using. Toss with the egg mixture. Taste and adjust the
seasonings. Refrigerate until ready to serve.

KEY NUTRIENTS
Protein
Vitamin A
Vitamin B$_{12}$
Folacin
Riboflavin
Iron
Phosphorus

Beef and Arugula Salad

ADVANCE
PREPARATION
The meat and dressing
will keep for a couple
of days in the refriger-
ator. Toss together
ahead of time for the
best flavor.

Make this salad when you have leftover beef from a roast or steak. Serve it as a lunch or supper main dish or as a starter.

4–5 cups arugula, trimmed, washed, and dried
1 ounce Parmesan cheese, shaved (optional)
2–4 tablespoons chopped fresh herbs, such as parsley,
    tarragon, chives, or chervil, to taste (optional)
    Salt and freshly ground pepper to taste

FOR THE DRESSING
2 tablespoons red or white wine vinegar or sherry vinegar,
    or 1 tablespoon vinegar and 1 tablespoon fresh lemon
    juice
2 teaspoons balsamic vinegar
1 tablespoon Dijon mustard
1 small garlic clove, minced or pressed
    Salt and freshly ground pepper to taste
1/4 cup plain yogurt or buttermilk
1/4 cup extra-virgin olive oil, or a mixture of olive oil and
    canola oil

2 cups cooked beef or steak, cubed or cut into thin strips

1. In a salad bowl, toss together the arugula, Parmesan (if using), herbs (if using), and salt and pepper.

2. FOR THE DRESSING: Mix together the vinegars and mustard in a medium bowl. Add the garlic and salt and pepper. Whisk in the yogurt or buttermilk and oil or oils.

3. In a separate medium bowl, combine half of the dressing and the beef; toss. If possible, let sit for 30 to 60 minutes.

4. Add the remaining dressing and the beef with its marinade to the salad. Toss well and serve.

KEY NUTRIENTS
Protein
Beta Carotene
Vitamin A
Vitamin B_6
Vitamin B_{12}
Folacin
Niacin
Riboflavin
Vitamin C
Vitamin E
Calcium
Copper
Iron
Magnesium
Manganese
Phosphorus
Potassium
Zinc
Monounsaturates
Omega-3s

Salads

ADVANCE
PREPARATION

The dressing and
toasted bread cubes
can be made several
hours before tossing
with the salad.

Frisée, Poached Egg, and Bacon Salad

This substantial salad is quite sufficient as a main dish and makes a great lunch or light supper. It can also be the opener to a meal.

FOR THE SALAD

2 small heads frisée or 1 large head curly endive
3 ounces slab bacon, rind removed and cut into $1/2$-inch dice, or 3 ounces regular bacon, cut into $1/2$ inch pieces, both cooked until crisp
2 thick slices crusty country bread or 8 slices baguette, toasted and cubed (about 2 cups)
4 large eggs
1 tablespoon vinegar (any kind)
Pinch of salt

FOR THE DRESSING

2–3 tablespoons red wine vinegar or sherry vinegar, to taste
1–2 tablespoons Dijon mustard, to taste
Salt and freshly ground pepper to taste
$1/2$ cup canola or peanut oil, or a combination of canola or peanut oil and extra-virgin olive oil

KEY NUTRIENTS
Protein
Beta Carotene
Vitamin A
Vitamin B$_{12}$
Folacin
Riboflavin
Vitamin C
Iron
Manganese
Phosphorus
Monounsaturates
Omega-3s

1. **FOR THE SALAD:** Remove the tough outer leaves from the frisée or endive. Separate the remaining leaves, wash well, dry, and break into smallish pieces. You should have about 6 cups. Place in a salad bowl. Add the bacon and bread cubes and toss to combine.

2. Poach the eggs. Fill a small or medium nonstick skillet with water to within $1/2$ inch of the rim. Bring to a boil. Meanwhile, break 1 egg into a teacup. Add the vinegar and salt to the boiling water. Reduce the heat to medium, lower the bottom of the cup gently into the water, taking care not to touch the water with your fingers, then tip the egg in. Repeat with another egg. Cover the pan

and remove from the heat. Poach for 4 minutes. Using a spatula or slotted spoon, carefully scoop up 1 egg at a time and transfer to a bowl of cold water. Bring the water back to a boil and cook the remaining 2 eggs as instructed. To serve, lift the eggs from the cold water, using the slotted spoon or gently in the palm of your hand, and drain briefly on a folded kitchen towel.

3. FOR THE DRESSING: In a small bowl, mix together the vinegar, mustard, and salt and pepper. Whisk in the oil, whisking well to amalgamate. The dressing will be quite thick.

4. Add the dressing to the salad and toss. Serve on individual plates or in wide bowls, placing a poached egg on each serving.

ADVANCE
PREPARATION
The dressing and all of
the salad ingredients
can be prepared sev-
eral hours ahead. The
potatoes can be
cooked and tossed with
the 2 tablespoons of
the dressing several
hours before serving.

Niçoise Salad

I like a salad that can be a main dish, as this one can. Everything in a niçoise salad appealed to me when I was pregnant —
tuna fish and eggs, lettuce and tomatoes, potatoes and green
beans, all in a tart dressing.

FOR THE DRESSING

3 tablespoons red wine vinegar or sherry vinegar, or more
 to taste

2 teaspoons Dijon mustard

1 garlic clove, minced or pressed
 Salt and freshly ground pepper to taste

$^2/_3$ cup extra-virgin olive oil, or $^1/_3$ cup oil and $^1/_3$ cup plain
 yogurt

FOR THE SALAD

1 pound new potatoes, scrubbed and quartered
 Salt and freshly ground pepper to taste

1 6-ounce can water-packed tuna, drained and flaked with
 a fork

1 small head Bibb lettuce, washed, dried, and leaves torn
 into large pieces, or 1 package (about 5 cups) baby
 salad greens, rinsed and dried

1 pound tomatoes, cut into wedges

$^1/_2$ pound green beans, trimmed, or broccoli florets, cut
 into bite-size pieces, steamed for 5 minutes

3 hard-cooked eggs (see page 155), quartered

OPTIONAL ADDITIONS

1 small cucumber, peeled and sliced

1 green or red bell pepper, seeded and thinly sliced

2–3 anchovy fillets (to taste), rinsed and chopped

$^1/_4$ cup chopped or slivered fresh herbs, such as basil,
 tarragon, chervil, chives, or parsley

KEY NUTRIENTS
Protein
Beta Carotene
Vitamin A
Vitamin B$_6$
Vitamin B$_{12}$
Folacin
Niacin
Riboflavin
Vitamin C
Vitamin E
Copper
Iron
Magnesium
Manganese
Phosphorus
Potassium
Monounsaturates

1. **FOR THE DRESSING:** Mix together the vinegar, mustard,
garlic, and salt and pepper in a medium bowl. Whisk in the olive
oil or the oil and yogurt.

2. FOR THE SALAD: Place the potatoes in a steamer basket set in a saucepan with 1 inch of simmering water. Cover and steam until just tender, 10 to 15 minutes. Remove from the heat, transfer to a large salad bowl, and toss at once with the salt and pepper and 2 tablespoons of the dressing. Add the tuna and toss with another 4 tablespoons of the dressing. Add the lettuce, tomatoes, beans or broccoli, eggs, and any of the additions of your choice. Toss with the remaining dressing and serve.

Makes 2 main-dish
servings or 4 starters
or side dishes

Tuna and Bean Salad

This dish proves how important a well-stocked pantry is. The whole thing can be pulled out of your cabinet — something I do often.

1 small white or red onion, very thinly sliced (optional)
¼ cup water (if using the onion)
1 tablespoon red or white wine vinegar (if using the onion)
1 6-ounce can water-packed tuna, drained
2 tablespoons chopped fresh parsley or other fresh herbs, such as chives, tarragon, dill, or sage
1 15-ounce can white beans, chickpeas, or borlotti beans, drained and rinsed

FOR THE DRESSING
2 tablespoons fresh lemon juice
2 tablespoons red or white wine vinegar
Salt and freshly ground pepper to taste
1 large garlic clove, minced or pressed (optional)
1 heaped teaspoon Dijon mustard
¼ cup plain yogurt or buttermilk
2–3 tablespoons extra-virgin olive oil (to taste)
Water for thinning (optional)

2 cups baby salad greens, rinsed and dried, for serving (optional)
Red and yellow cherry tomatoes for garnish (optional)

1. If using the onion, place in a small bowl with the water and vinegar. Set aside.

2. Drain the tuna and scrape into a large bowl, breaking it up with a fork. Add the parsley or other herbs. Drain the onion and add half to the tuna. Add the beans.

3. FOR THE DRESSING: Mix together the lemon juice, vinegar, and salt and pepper in a medium bowl. Add the garlic (if using) and mustard, then whisk in the yogurt or buttermilk and olive oil. Thin with a tablespoon or two of water, if desired.

4. Add the dressing to the tuna mixture and toss. Taste and adjust the seasonings.

5. If you wish, line a bowl or platter with the salad greens. Top with the salad. Scatter the remaining onions over the top. Garnish with the cherry tomatoes, if using. Serve immediately, or refrigerate and serve cold.

VARIATION

Tuna and Green Bean Salad

Substitute ½ pound fresh green beans for the canned beans, or use both. Trim the beans and break them in half. Place in a steamer basket set in a saucepan with 1 inch of simmering water. Steam the beans for 5 to 8 minutes, until crisp-tender but still bright green. Transfer to a bowl of cold water, drain, and toss with the tuna mixture. Continue with the recipe as instructed.

KEY NUTRIENTS
GREEN BEANS
Vitamin A
Folacin
Vitamin C
Iron
Manganese

ADVANCE
PREPARATION

All the elements, including the dressing, can be prepared hours ahead of assembling the salad.

Cobb Salad

Cobb salad, a California classic, makes a nutritious meal that combines chicken, egg, cheese, and vegetables.

FOR THE DRESSING

$1/4$ cup red wine vinegar or sherry vinegar, or more to taste

$1/4$ teaspoon sugar

1 tablespoon fresh lemon juice

1 teaspoon Worcestershire sauce

$1/4$ teaspoon dry English mustard

1 small garlic clove, minced or pressed

Salt and freshly ground pepper to taste

$1/2$ cup extra-virgin olive oil

$1/4$ cup canola oil

FOR THE SALAD

1 small head Bibb or romaine lettuce, leaves washed, dried, and coarsely chopped

1 bunch watercress, trimmed, washed, dried, and coarsely chopped

6 slices bacon, cooked until crisp and crumbled

3 hard-cooked eggs (see note), diced

2 medium tomatoes, seeded, and diced

2 boneless, skinless chicken breasts, poached (see page 156) and diced

1 ripe but firm avocado, preferably Hass, peeled, pitted, and diced

$1/2$ cup crumbled Roquefort cheese (about 2 ounces)

2 tablespoons snipped fresh chives

KEY NUTRIENTS
Protein
Beta Carotene
Vitamin A
Vitamin B_6
Vitamin B_{12}
Folacin
Niacin
Riboflavin
Vitamin C
Vitamin E
Calcium
Copper
Iron
Magnesium
Manganese
Phosphorus
Potassium
Monounsaturates
Omega-3s

1. **FOR THE DRESSING:** Mix together the vinegar and sugar in a small bowl or Pyrex measuring cup. Add the lemon juice, Worcestershire sauce, mustard, garlic, and salt and pepper. Whisk in the oils and set aside.

EVERY WOMAN'S

GUIDE TO EATING

DURING PREGNANCY

2. **FOR THE SALAD:** Toss the lettuce with the watercress in a salad bowl or deep serving platter. Arrange the other ingredients, except the chives, in bands over the lettuce. Sprinkle the chives over the top.

3. Pour as much of the dressing over the salad as you like and toss at the table. Serve with more dressing, if desired.

NOTE: To make hard-cooked eggs, place the eggs in a saucepan large enough to fit them in a single layer. Cover with cold water by about 1 inch. Place the pan over medium-high heat and bring to a boil. Turn the heat down to a simmer or a very slow boil and cook for 10 minutes. Drain the eggs and run under cold water for 2 to 4 minutes, then peel.

ADVANCE
PREPARATION
These salads will keep
for a couple of days in
the refrigerator. The
cilantro will lose its
color, so you might
want to add more be-
fore serving.

Three Chicken Salads

You can make a meal of chicken salad, and there are many different ways to season it. Begin with poached chicken breasts — or use leftover chicken from another dish — and make an Asian salad, a Mexican salad, or a curry.

Poached Chicken Breasts

    10 cups water
     1 onion, quartered
     2 garlic cloves, crushed
     2 whole chicken breasts, skinned and split
    $^1/_2$ teaspoon dried thyme or oregano, or a combination
1–1$^1/_2$ teaspoons salt, to taste

1. Combine the water, onion, and garlic in a medium saucepan and bring to a boil. Add the chicken breasts, reduce the heat, and bring to a simmer. Skim off any foam that rises to the top, then add the thyme and/or oregano. Cover partially, reduce the heat to low, and simmer for 15 minutes, until the chicken is cooked through. Add salt to taste. Let the chicken cool in the broth if there is time.

2. Remove the chicken from the broth when cool enough to handle. Strain the broth and set aside for another use. Remove the meat from the bones and shred. Do this by pulling strips of chicken away from the bone, then pulling larger pieces apart. It will pull apart naturally into shreds. You should have 3 to 3$^1/_2$ cups shredded chicken.

Curried Chicken Salad

     2 whole chicken breasts, skinned, poached and shredded
        (3–3$^1/_2$ cups; see above)
     1 bunch scallions, white and green parts, thinly sliced, or 1
        small red onion, finely chopped and rinsed

KEY NUTRIENTS
(FOR ALL VERSIONS)
Protein
Vitamin A
Vitamin B$_6$
Vitamin B$_{12}$
Folacin
Niacin
Vitamin C
Iron
Magnesium
Phosphorus
Monounsaturates (Mexican
    Chicken Salad)

¼ cup walnut pieces

1 tart apple, such as Granny Smith, peeled (if desired), cored, and chopped

2–4 tablespoons chopped fresh cilantro, to taste

FOR THE DRESSING

¼ cup plain yogurt

2 tablespoons peanut or canola oil

2 tablespoons fresh lime juice

4 teaspoons Hellmann's or Best Foods mayonnaise

1 tablespoon red wine vinegar

1 teaspoon Dijon mustard

1 teaspoon curry powder

1 teaspoon ground cumin

¼–½ teaspoon salt, to taste

Freshly ground pepper to taste

Broth from the poached chicken breasts or water for moistening (optional)

Lettuce leaves for serving (optional)

1. Combine the chicken, scallions or red onion, walnuts, apple, and cilantro in a medium bowl.

2. FOR THE DRESSING: Mix together all the ingredients in a medium bowl.

3. Add the dressing to the chicken mixture and toss. Taste and adjust the seasonings. If you'd like a moister salad, add a few tablespoons of broth or water.

4. If you wish, line a salad bowl or platter with the lettuce leaves. Top with the salad and serve.

Asian Chicken Salad

2 whole skinned chicken breasts, poached and shredded (3–3¹/₂ cups; see page 156)

1 jalapeño or 2 serrano peppers, seeded (if desired) and chopped (optional)

1 bunch scallions, white and green parts, thinly sliced separately (reserve the green parts for garnish)

1 small cucumber, peeled (if desired), seeded, and diced, or ¹/₂ European cucumber, diced

¹/₄ cup chopped fresh cilantro

FOR THE DRESSING

4–5 tablespoons buttermilk or plain yogurt, as desired

2 tablespoons dark sesame oil

1 tablespoon fresh lime juice

1 tablespoon seasoned rice wine vinegar or balsamic vinegar

1 tablespoon soy sauce

1 small garlic clove, minced or pressed

1–2 teaspoons (to taste) minced fresh ginger

Salt and freshly ground pepper to taste

Broth from the poached chicken breasts or water for moistening (optional)

Lettuce leaves for serving (optional)

1 tablespoon toasted sesame seeds or ground flax seeds

1. Combine the chicken, peppers, white parts of the scallions, cucumber, and cilantro in a large bowl.

2. FOR THE DRESSING: Combine all the ingredients in a medium bowl and mix well.

3. Add the dressing to the chicken mixture and toss. Taste and adjust the seasonings. If you'd like a moister salad, add a few tablespoons broth or water. If you wish, line a salad bowl or platter with the lettuce leaves. Top with the salad. Sprinkle with the reserved green parts of the scallions and the sesame or flax seeds, then serve.

Mexican Chicken Salad

2 whole skinned chicken breasts, poached and shredded
  (3–3½ cups; see page 156)
1 jalapeño or 2 serrano peppers, seeded (if desired) and
  chopped
1 bunch scallions, white and green parts, thinly sliced
3 medium tomatoes, chopped
1 ripe but firm avocado, preferably Hass, peeled, pitted,
  and diced
¼ cup chopped fresh cilantro

FOR THE DRESSING
⅓ cup extra-virgin olive oil
2 tablespoons fresh lime juice
2 tablespoons cider vinegar
1 garlic clove, minced or pressed (optional)
½ teaspoon crushed cumin seeds or ground cumin
¼ teaspoon salt, or more to taste
  Freshly ground pepper to taste

  Lettuce leaves for serving (optional)

1. Combine the chicken with the peppers, scallions, tomatoes, avocado, and cilantro in a large bowl.

2. FOR THE DRESSING: Mix together all the ingredients in a medium bowl.

3. Add the dressing to the salad and toss.

4. If you wish, line a salad bowl or platter with the lettuce leaves. Top with the salad and serve.

Asian Noodle Salad

I recommend Japanese buckwheat noodles, or soba, for this salad. Buckwheat is a high-protein grain and has a wonderful nutty flavor. You can find the noodles wherever Asian ingredients are sold. Enjoy this salad for lunch or dinner. It also makes a great leftover.

FOR THE SALAD

Salt

1/2 pound soba or udon

1/2 pound snow peas or sugar-snap peas, trimmed

1 tablespoon dark sesame oil

1 bunch scallions, white and green parts, thinly sliced separately (reserve the green parts for garnish)

1 red bell pepper, seeded and cut into slivers

1 whole boneless, skinless chicken breast, poached and shredded (see page 156), or 1/2 pound firm tofu, sliced and tossed with 1 tablespoon soy sauce

1/4 cup chopped fresh cilantro

FOR THE DRESSING

5 tablespoons buttermilk or plain yogurt

2 tablespoons seasoned rice wine vinegar

1 tablespoon soy sauce

1 tablespoon dark sesame oil

1/2 teaspoon hot chile oil or a pinch of cayenne pepper (optional)

1 small garlic clove, minced or pressed (optional)

1–2 teaspoons minced fresh ginger, to taste

Salt and freshly ground pepper to taste

Water for thinning (optional)

1. FOR THE SALAD: Bring a large pot of water to a rolling boil. Add a generous amount of salt and the noodles and cook for 3 minutes. Add the peas and cook for 3 minutes more. Remove a noodle using tongs. If it is still hard, cook for a few minutes more.

Some soba noodles are thinner than others, so you'll have to check the noodles to determine the cooking time.

2. When the soba is cooked al dente and the snow peas are bright green, drain, rinse with cold water, and transfer to a salad bowl. Add the sesame oil, white parts of the scallions, bell pepper, chicken or tofu, and cilantro.

3. FOR THE DRESSING: Mix together all the ingredients, except the water, in a small bowl. Thin with a little water, if desired.

4. Add the dressing to the noodles and toss. Sprinkle the green parts of the scallions on the salad. Serve warm, at room temperature, or chilled.

ADVANCE
PREPARATION

All the ingredients for
this salad can be pre-
pared hours ahead of
time. The fried tempeh
will keep for a few days
in the refrigerator.

Tempeh and
Sesame Salad

Tempeh is made from fermented soybeans. It's an excellent
protein source and has a meaty texture. Seasoned tempeh is
usually found in the dairy or tofu case in natural food stores
and some supermarkets.

FOR THE SALAD

1–2 tablespoons peanut or canola oil, as needed

^{1}/2 pound seasoned tempeh, cut into 4 pieces

3–4 scallions (to taste), thinly sliced (optional)

2 hearts of romaine lettuce (the inner leaves), washed,
dried, and coarsely chopped (4–5 cups)

1 small red or green bell pepper, seeded and diced

^{1}/3 cup chopped fresh cilantro

1 tablespoon sesame seeds

Soy sauce to taste

FOR THE DRESSING

2 tablespoons rice wine vinegar

1 tablespoon fresh lime juice

1 tablespoon soy sauce

^{1}/2 teaspoon hot chile paste (sambal oelek; optional)

^{1}/2 teaspoon sugar, or more to taste

1 small garlic clove, minced or pressed (optional)

^{1}/4 cup plain yogurt

2 tablespoons dark sesame oil

1–2 tablespoons peanut oil or water, to taste

1. FOR THE SALAD: Heat 1 tablespoon of the oil in a large frying
pan over medium-high heat. Add the tempeh in one layer. Cook
until browned on one side, about 2 minutes. Turn over, add more
oil if necessary, and cook until browned on the other side, about 2
minutes. Remove from the heat.

KEY NUTRIENTS
Protein
Beta Carotene
Vitamin A (red bell pep-
per)
Vitamin B$_6$
Folacin
Vitamin C
Iron
Magnesium
Manganese
Zinc

2. Combine the remaining salad ingredients in a large bowl. Slice the tempeh 1/4 inch thick and add to the salad.

3. FOR THE DRESSING: Stir together the vinegar, lime juice, soy sauce, chile paste (if using), sugar, and garlic (if using) in a small bowl. Whisk in the yogurt and sesame oil. Thin with the peanut oil or water.

4. Add the dressing to the salad, toss, and serve.

Vinaigrettes

Classic Vinaigrette
Makes about 1¹/₃ cups

ADVANCE
PREPARATION
This will keep for a
week in the refrigera-
tor.

If you have dressing on hand, you'll be much more likely to throw together a salad. This makes enough dressing for two or three big salads and many small ones. The garlic slices should not go into the salad; they are meant just to infuse the dressing.

KEY NUTRIENTS
Monounsaturates
Omega-3s (canola oil)

5 tablespoons sherry vinegar or red wine vinegar
1 tablespoon balsamic vinegar
1 tablespoon Dijon mustard
Salt, preferably coarse sea salt, to taste
1 cup extra-virgin olive oil, or ½ cup olive oil and ½ cup canola oil
2 garlic cloves, sliced lengthwise

1. Whisk together the vinegars, mustard, and salt in a small bowl. Whisk in the oil. If you are going to keep the dressing in a container without a squirter top, run a toothpick through the garlic slices, keeping them separated on the toothpick so that the surfaces are exposed to the dressing. Add the garlic to the dressing. Transfer to a container, preferably one with a squirter top. Refrigerate until ready to serve.

2. If the olive oil solidifies, remove the dressing from the refrigerator about 15 minutes before using. Shake or whisk well before tossing the salad.

NOTE: For a lower-fat or nonfat version, substitute nonfat plain yogurt or low-fat buttermilk for half or all of the oil.

Lemon Vinaigrette
Makes about ¹/₂ cup

ADVANCE
PREPARATION
This is best served no
more than 1 to 2 hours
after it's made.

Lemon juice is sometimes preferable to vinegar in a salad dressing. This one goes nicely with any green salad made with romaine lettuce, leaf lettuce, Boston lettuce, or spinach.

2 tablespoons fresh lemon juice, or 1 tablespoon fresh
    lemon juice and 1 tablespoon wine or sherry vinegar
1 teaspoon Dijon mustard or ¼ teaspoon dry English
    mustard
Salt to taste
1 small garlic clove, minced or pressed (optional)
6 tablespoons extra-virgin olive oil

Mix together the lemon juice or lemon juice and vinegar, mustard, salt, and garlic (if using) in a small bowl. Whisk in the oil.

ADVANCE
PREPARATION
This is best served no
more than 1 to 2 hours
after it's made.

KEY NUTRIENTS
Vitamin C
Monounsaturates

Yogurt or Buttermilk Vinaigrette
Makes about ½ cup

ADVANCE
PREPARATION
You can make this a few
hours ahead.

This low-fat vinaigrette can replace traditional vinaigrettes.

2 tablespoons red wine vinegar, sherry vinegar, or
    champagne vinegar, or 1 tablespoon fresh lemon juice
    and 1 tablespoon vinegar
1 teaspoon Dijon mustard
1 small garlic clove, minced or pressed
⅛–¼ teaspoon salt, to taste
¼ cup nonfat or low-fat plain yogurt or 5 tablespoons
    buttermilk
1 tablespoon extra-virgin olive oil
1 tablespoon water, if using yogurt, or more to taste
Freshly ground pepper to taste

Using a fork or small whisk, mix together the vinegar or vinegar and lemon juice, mustard, garlic, and salt in a small bowl. Stir in the yogurt or buttermilk, olive oil, and water (if using). Add the pepper and stir. Thin with more water, if desired.

VARIATION

Lemon Yogurt
or Buttermilk Vinaigrette

Omit the vinegar and use 2 tablespoons fresh lemon juice.

KEY NUTRIENTS
Vitamin B_{12}
Riboflavin
Calcium
Phosphorus

MAIN DISHES

Chicken Breasts Three Ways 169

Roast Chicken 171

Mediterranean Chicken Stew 172

Chicken, Lemon, and Olive Stew with
    Couscous 174

Stir-Fried Chicken and Broccoli 176

Turkey or Beef Burgers 178

Grilled or Pan-Seared Porterhouse Steak 179

Pan-Seared or Grilled London Broil 180

Steak or Chicken Fajitas 182

Roast Pork Loin with Fennel-Pepper Rub 184

Stir-Fried Pork and Greens 185

Roast Turkey 186

Wild Rice Stuffing 187

Halibut Cooked in the Microwave 189

Salmon Fillets Cooked in the Microwave 190

Red Snapper Fillets Baked in Foil 191

Whole Trout Baked in Foil 192

Sole with Olive Oil, Lemon, and Scallions 193

Snapper or Sole with Lemon, Capers, Oregano,
    and Olive Oil 194

Grilled or Broiled Fish Steaks with
    Asian Flavors 195

Grilled Tuna with Tomato-Balsamic Salsa 196

Creamy Pasta with Broccoli 197

Creamy Pasta with Greens 198

Pasta with Pesto and Green Beans 199

Summer Pasta with Tomatoes and Green Beans
    or Peas 200

Pasta with Tomato Sauce 201

Tortellini with Broccoli and Sage 203

Pasta with Tomato Mushroom Sauce 204

Zucchini "Pasta" 205

Quick Spinach and Tomato Lasagna 206

Greek Spinach Pie (Spanakopita) 208

Simple Homemade Pizza 210

Soft Tacos with Tofu and Tomatoes 211

Couscous with Chickpeas and Greens 212

Winter Vegetable Couscous 214

Quesadillas 216

Strata with Tomatoes and Greens 218

Hot or Cold Spinach Frittata 220

Fried Brown Rice and Vegetables 222

Pan-Cooked Tofu 223

Broiled or Grilled Tofu 224

Stir-Fried Tofu with Red Chard 225

Stir-Fried Tofu with Broccoli and
    Mushrooms 226

Spinach, Broccoli, or Asparagus Flan 228

Simmered Black Beans or Pinto Beans with
    Cilantro 229

Main Dishes

Refried Beans 230

Quick Black Bean Tacos 232

Soft Tacos or Tostadas with Chicken, Corn, and Avocado 233

Black Bean Tostadas (Chalupas) 234

Egg and Bean Tacos 235

Chicken Breasts Three Ways

ADVANCE PREPARATION
The marinades can be put together a few hours before you marinate the chicken.

There are many ways to cook a chicken breast. So rest assured, if that's all you feel like eating, you can go a long way before becoming bored with this versatile meat. Here are three different approaches.

With Asian Flavors

2 tablespoons water
1 tablespoon soy sauce
1 tablespoon peanut oil
1 garlic clove, minced or pressed (optional)
1 teaspoon grated or minced fresh ginger
$1/2$ teaspoon sugar
4 boneless, skinless chicken breast halves
Chopped scallions, chives, or fresh cilantro for serving (optional)

1. Stir together all the ingredients except the chicken breasts in a large bowl. Toss with the chicken breasts and let marinate for 15 minutes, turning at least once.

2. Heat a nonstick skillet or grill pan over medium-high heat. Drop a bit of water on the pan, and if it sizzles away at once, the pan is hot enough. Toss the chicken breasts with the marinade one more time so that they're well coated, then add them to the pan. Cook for 5–7 minutes per side, until golden on the outside and with no trace of pink on the inside, basting the tops with the marinade before you flip them over. Discard the remaining marinade.

3. Serve hot, with the scallions, chives, or cilantro sprinkled on the top, if desired.

KEY NUTRIENTS
Protein
Vitamin B_6
Vitamin B_{12}
Niacin
Iron
Magnesium
Phosphorus

Main Dishes

With Mediterranean Flavors

 3 tablespoons fresh lemon juice
 1 tablespoon olive oil
 2 garlic cloves, minced or pressed
 1 teaspoon chopped fresh rosemary and/or thyme or
      ¹/₂ teaspoon dried
   Salt and freshly ground pepper to taste
 4 boneless, skinless chicken breast halves

Proceed as directed in the previous recipe. Serve hot.

With Indian Flavors

 ¹/₂ cup plain yogurt
   Juice of 1 large lime
 1 tablespoon olive or canola oil
 1 garlic clove, minced or pressed (optional)
 ¹/₂ teaspoon ground cumin, or more to taste
 ¹/₂ teaspoon curry powder, or more to taste
   Salt to taste
 4 boneless, skinless chicken breast halves

1. Mix together the yogurt, lime juice, oil, garlic (if using), cumin, curry powder, and salt in a large bowl. Taste and adjust the seasonings. Toss with the chicken breasts and let marinate for 15 to 30 minutes, turning at least once.

2. Cook as directed on page 169. Serve hot.

Roast Chicken

ADVANCE PREPARATION
If you don't care about having the chicken hot, this can be roasted hours ahead of serving. It will keep in the refrigerator for 3 days. Carve all the meat off the carcass, place on a plate, and cover tightly with foil or plastic wrap.

Roast chicken is a great meal to make when you're tired and don't feel like dealing with food. The preparation is minimal, you throw it in the oven, turn it once, and have a meal for four in an hour. Leftovers are great for sandwiches.

1 $3^1/_2$- to 4-pound chicken, preferably free-range and
    hormone-free
1 tablespoon plus 1 teaspoon olive oil
  Salt and freshly ground pepper to taste
3 garlic cloves, crushed (optional)
5 sprigs fresh rosemary or tarragon (optional)

1. Preheat the oven to 450°F. Rinse the chicken inside and out under cold water, and blot dry with paper towels. Oil a baking dish with 1 teaspoon of the olive oil and place the chicken in it. Drizzle the remaining 1 tablespoon oil over the chicken and rub it into the skin with your hands. Sprinkle with salt and pepper. Place the garlic and 3 of the rosemary or tarragon sprigs, if using, in the cavity. Tuck the remaining herb sprigs into the wings, close to the body of the chicken. Turn the chicken breast side down.

2. Roast the chicken for 10 minutes. Reduce the oven temperature to 350°F. Roast for 30 minutes, then turn the bird onto its back. Roast for 30 minutes more, until the skin is golden brown. To test for doneness, stick a meat thermometer into the thickest part of the thigh. It should read 165°F. If you don't have a meat thermometer, pierce in the same place with a sharp knife. If the juices are clear, the chicken is done. If they are slightly pink, roast for 10 minutes more and check again.

3. Transfer the chicken to a cutting board, preferably one with indentations for the juices to run into, and let sit for 10 to 15 minutes before carving and serving.

KEY NUTRIENTS
Protein
Vitamin B_6
Vitamin B_{12}
Niacin
Riboflavin
Iron
Magnesium
Phosphorus
Zinc

Main Dishes

Mediterranean Chicken Stew

This delicious stew can be cooked ahead so that when you get home from work, hungry and exhausted, all you have to do is heat it up. Don't worry about the wine here; the alcohol evaporates as the stew simmers. You can use chicken stock instead, if you wish. Serve with rice, potatoes, or noodles.

- 1 3½- to 4-pound chicken, preferably free-range and hormone-free, skinned and cut into 6–8 pieces; or 3–3½ pounds chicken pieces (breasts, thighs, and legs) on the bone, skinned
- 1 tablespoon olive oil
- 1 medium onion, cut in half and thinly sliced
- 1 large red bell pepper, seeded and cut into ½-inch squares
- 3–4 garlic cloves (to taste), minced or pressed
- 1 28-ounce can whole tomatoes, drained and chopped, or one 28-ounce can recipe-ready chopped tomatoes, drained
  Salt to taste
- ½ cup chicken stock or dry white wine
- 2 teaspoons chopped fresh thyme or 1 teaspoon dried
- 1 bay leaf
  Freshly ground pepper to taste
- 3 tablespoons chopped fresh parsley

KEY NUTRIENTS
Protein
Beta Carotene
Vitamin A
Vitamin B$_6$
Vitamin B$_{12}$
Folacin
Niacin
Riboflavin
Vitamin C
Vitamin E
Iron
Magnesium
Phosphorus
Zinc

1. Rinse the chicken pieces and pat dry.

2. Heat 1 tablespoon of the oil in a large, heavy-bottomed casserole or Dutch oven over medium-low heat. Add the onion and cook, stirring, until tender, about 5 minutes. Add the bell pepper and cook, stirring, until soft, about 5 minutes. Add the garlic and stir together for about 30 seconds, until the garlic smells fragrant. Add the tomatoes and about $1/2$ teaspoon salt. Increase the heat to medium and cook, stirring often, for about 10 minutes, until the tomatoes have cooked down somewhat and the mixture smells very fragrant. Add the chicken and stock or wine and stir together. Bring to a simmer. If there is foam on the surface, skim it off.

3. Add the thyme and bay leaf to the chicken mixture and reduce the heat to low. Cover partially and simmer for 40 to 50 minutes, stirring and moving the chicken pieces around often, until the chicken is just about falling off the bone. Taste and season with salt and pepper.

4. Remove from the heat and stir in the parsley. Serve hot.

ADVANCE
PREPARATION

The dish can be made
through step 3 up to a
day ahead, but steam
the couscous again for
15 minutes when you
reheat the chicken.

Chicken, Lemon, and Olive Stew with Couscous

In this North African stew, the chicken is marinated with garlic
and a number of spices, then cooked with leeks. Just before
serving, the stew is completed with lemon juice, fresh herbs,
and green olives.

    1 3$\frac{1}{2}$- to 4-pound chicken, preferably free-range and
        hormone-free, skinned and cut into 6–8 pieces
    2 tablespoons olive oil
    2 large garlic cloves, minced or pressed
    1 teaspoon cracked coriander seeds
$\frac{1}{2}$ teaspoon ground ginger
$\frac{1}{2}$ teaspoon freshly ground pepper
$\frac{1}{2}$ teaspoon ground cumin
$\frac{1}{2}$ teaspoon paprika
$\frac{1}{2}$ teaspoon salt, or more to taste
    3 cups water
    1 large or 2 medium leeks, white and light green parts
        only, washed thoroughly and thinly sliced
      A few sprigs each fresh parsley and cilantro
    2 cups couscous
2$\frac{1}{2}$ cups salted water or chicken stock
$\frac{1}{4}$ cup imported green olives, pitted and cut in half
      Juice of 1–2 lemons (about $\frac{1}{4}$ cup), or more to taste
$\frac{1}{4}$ cup chopped fresh parsley or cilantro

1. Rinse the chicken pieces and pat dry.

2. Combine 1 tablespoon of the olive oil, the garlic, spices,
and salt in a large, flameproof casserole. Add the chicken and toss.
Cover and refrigerate for 30 to 60 minutes, stirring from time to
time.

KEY NUTRIENTS
Protein
Vitamin B$_6$
Vitamin B$_{12}$
Niacin
Riboflavin
Thiamin
Iron
Magnesium
Manganese
Phosphorus
Zinc

3. Add the water to the pot and bring to a boil. Using a slotted spoon, skim off any foam that rises to the top. When there is no longer any foam, add the leeks and parsley and cilantro sprigs to the pot. Reduce the heat, cover, and simmer gently for 30 minutes, until the chicken is just about tender.

4. While the chicken is simmering, combine the couscous and salted water or stock in a medium bowl. Soak for about 20 minutes, until tender, stirring every once in a while with a wooden spoon. Drain in a colander or strainer, then set the colander above the simmering chicken. Cover and steam for 15 minutes.

5. Add the olives to the chicken. Continue to simmer for 10 to 15 minutes more, until the chicken is falling off the bone.

6. Transfer the couscous to a large bowl or serving dish and toss with the remaining 1 tablespoon olive oil. Arrange the chicken pieces and olives on top. Bring the liquid in the casserole to a boil and reduce by half. Stir in the lemon juice and chopped parsley or cilantro. Taste and adjust the seasonings, adding more lemon juice or salt, if desired. Pour the sauce over the chicken and serve.

ADVANCE
PREPARATION
The broccoli can be
steamed and the glaze
assembled hours before
making the dish.

Stir-Fried Chicken and Broccoli

Although the list of ingredients looks long, stir-fries are incredibly easy to make. Once you've assembled the ingredients, the dish cooks in minutes.

FOR THE GLAZE

1/2 cup unsalted chicken or vegetable stock or water

2 tablespoons soy sauce

1 tablespoon rice wine vinegar, white vinegar, or cider vinegar

1/2 teaspoon sugar

FOR THE CHICKEN AND VEGETABLES

1 1/2 pounds broccoli, broken into florets

2 tablespoons canola or peanut oil

3/4 pound boneless, skinless chicken breasts, cut into 1/4-by-2-inch strips

1 tablespoon minced fresh ginger

1 tablespoon minced garlic

3/4 pound mushrooms, trimmed and thickly sliced

1 bunch scallions, white parts and some of the green parts, thinly sliced separately

1 tablespoon arrowroot or cornstarch dissolved in 1 1/2 tablespoons water

1 cup rice (white or brown) or bulgur, cooked (see page 266 or 263), for serving

KEY NUTRIENTS
Beta Carotene
Vitamin A
Vitamin B$_6$
Vitamin B$_{12}$
Folacin
Niacin
Vitamin C
Iron
Magnesium
Manganese
Phosphorus
Potassium

EVERY WOMAN'S

GUIDE TO EATING

DURING PREGNANCY

1. FOR THE GLAZE: Stir together all the ingredients in a small bowl.

2. FOR THE CHICKEN AND VEGETABLES: Place the broccoli in a steamer basket set in a saucepan with 1 inch of simmering water. Cover and steam just until crisp-tender, about 3 minutes. Transfer immediately to a bowl of ice water, then drain and pat dry.

3. Heat a wok or heavy-bottomed nonstick skillet over high heat until hot enough to evaporate a drop of water on contact. Add 1 tablespoon of the oil, swirl to coat the pan, and reduce the heat to medium-high. Add the chicken and cook, stirring, for 2 to 3 minutes, until the meat is cooked through. Remove the chicken from the pan and set aside. Add the remaining 1 tablespoon oil and the ginger and garlic to the pan. Cook, stirring with a wooden paddle or spoon, until fragrant and beginning to color, 20 to 30 seconds. Add the mushrooms and the white parts of the scallions and cook, stirring gently, for 2 minutes. Add the broccoli and cook, stirring constantly but gently, for 1 minute. Return the chicken to the pan.

4. Stir the glaze and add to the pan. Bring to a simmer and cook, stirring, for 1 minute, until the vegetables are just cooked through but still crisp. Give the cornstarch mixture a stir and add to the pan. Cook, stirring, until the sauce thickens and glazes the vegetables. Remove from the heat and sprinkle with the green parts of the scallions.

5. Serve at once over the rice or bulgur.

Turkey or Beef Burgers

ADVANCE
PREPARATION

You can make the un-
cooked burgers up to 1
day ahead. Just cover
and refrigerate until
you're ready to cook
them.

Ground turkey is lower in fat than beef. The trick to making it tasty is in the seasonings. Onion, garlic, ketchup, and Worcestershire sauce are great flavor enhancers.

    1 pound ground turkey or lean ground beef
    1/2 small white onion, finely chopped (about 1/3 cup)
    1-2 large garlic cloves (to taste), minced or pressed
        (optional)
    2 tablespoons Worcestershire sauce
    1-2 tablespoons ketchup, to taste
    1 tablespoon cold water
        Salt (about 1/2 teaspoon) and freshly ground pepper to
        taste
    4 whole wheat hamburger buns or pita breads for serving
        (optional)

OPTIONAL CONDIMENTS

Ketchup

Mustard

Hoisin or plum sauce

Salsa

Onion, bell pepper, and/or tomato slices

KEY NUTRIENTS
TURKEY (WHITE MEAT)
Vitamin B$_6$
Vitamin B$_{12}$
Niacin
Iron
Magnesium
Phosphorus
Zinc

TURKEY (DARK MEAT)
Vitamin B$_6$
Vitamin B$_{12}$
Niacin
Riboflavin
Iron
Phosphorus
Zinc

KEY NUTRIENTS
BEEF
Protein
Vitamin B$_6$
Vitamin B$_{12}$
Niacin
Riboflavin
Iron
Magnesium
Phosphorus
Potassium
Zinc

1. Rinse the onion with cold water. In a medium bowl, combine the ground turkey or beef, chopped onion, garlic (if using), Worcestershire sauce, ketchup, water, and salt and pepper. Shape into 4 patties. Press them into 3/4-inch-thick rounds.

2. Prepare a grill or heat a grill pan or nonstick skillet over medium-high heat until a drop of water evaporates immediately on contact. Cook the burgers for 4 to 5 minutes per side. They should be just cooked through and not at all pink.

3. Serve at once on hamburger buns or pita breads, if you wish, with the condiments of your choice.

Grilled or Pan-Seared Porterhouse Steak

ADVANCE PREPARATION
This is a cook-to-order dish.

When I crave red meat, this is what I want. The secret to this dish, known to food lovers as Steak a la Fiorentina, is very high heat. You need nothing else but a searingly hot fire, a dab of olive oil, and some salt and pepper for the steak. But do get the best-quality steak you can buy.

1 ³/₄- to 1-pound porterhouse steak, 1–1¹/₂ inches thick, trimmed
Salt and freshly ground pepper to taste
Olive oil for brushing

1. Let the steak sit at room temperature while you prepare the grill. Make a blazing hot fire in the grill; when the coals are white, with no black showing, the fire is ready. If you wish to cook the steak on the stove, heat a cast-iron skillet for 15 to 20 minutes over high heat.

2. Sprinkle the steak with salt and pepper and brush lightly with olive oil. Place the steak on the grill or in the pan. Cook for 7 minutes per side for rare, 9 minutes for medium-rare, and 10 minutes for well-done. Remove from the heat and serve.

KEY NUTRIENTS
Protein
Vitamin B$_6$
Vitamin B$_{12}$
Niacin
Riboflavin
Iron
Magnesium
Phosphorus
Potassium
Zinc

Main Dishes

Pan-Seared or
Grilled London Broil

Although red meat is not appealing to many pregnant
women, for some it provides a welcome shot of protein and
iron. Steak that is quickly pan-seared, then thinly sliced
across the grain, is called London broil. It is traditionally
made with leaner, tougher cuts of steak, such as flank steak,
top round, or shoulder, which will dry out if cooked too
long. Buy 1½- to 2-pound steaks, as they are thick, and if
you don't need that much meat, cut them into two or three
pieces and freeze what you don't cook. The steaks can be
thawed in the microwave as needed for quick, high-protein,
iron-rich dinners.

1 1½- to 2-pound top round steak, 1½ inches thick
1 large garlic clove, cut in half (if not marinating)
   Salt and freshly ground pepper to taste (if not
      marinating)

FOR THE MARINADE (OPTIONAL)
2 tablespoons olive oil
2 teaspoons soy sauce
1 teaspoon balsamic vinegar
1 garlic clove, minced
½ teaspoon minced fresh ginger

2 sprigs fresh tarragon, minced

1. If you are not marinating the steak, rub it with the garlic
and sprinkle generously with salt and pepper.

2. FOR THE MARINADE, IF USING: Mix together all the ingredients in a large bowl. Place the steak in the bowl and turn it over to
coat both sides. Cover tightly with plastic wrap or transfer to a zipper-lock bag and seal. Refrigerate for 1 to 2 hours.

3. Heat a heavy, preferably cast-iron pan or skillet over high heat until very hot. Remove the steak from the marinade, if using. Touch an edge of the steak to the pan; if the pan is hot enough, the steak should respond with an immediate brisk sizzle. Sear the steak for about 6 minutes per side. Check for doneness by making an incision in the center. The meat should be rare; do not overcook, or it will be tough. Alternatively, grill the meat over hot coals or a gas grill for 5 to 6 minutes per side.

4. Remove from the heat and let sit for 10 minutes. Sprinkle with the tarragon. Slice very thinly (no thicker than $1/4$ inch) on the diagonal (across the grain of the meat) and serve.

ADVANCE
PREPARATION
The salsa will hold for a
few hours in the refrig-
erator. The meat must
be marinated for sev-
eral hours.

Steak or Chicken Fajitas

Classic fajitas are grilled strips of marinated skirt steak
wrapped in warm flour tortillas and served with salsa and
other Mexican or Tex-Mex condiments, such as guacamole.
Now chicken fajitas are just as popular.

Juice of 3 limes
1 tablespoon vegetable or olive oil
2–3 garlic cloves (to taste), minced or pressed
2 scallions, white and green parts, minced, or $1/2$ red onion,
    minced and briefly rinsed in cold water
1 serrano pepper, minced
3 tablespoons minced fresh cilantro
1 1-pound skirt steak, cut into 3-inch-long strips, or 4
    boneless, skinless chicken breast halves, cut on the
    diagonal into 1-inch-long strips
Salt to taste
4 flour tortillas
Fresh Tomato Salsa (page 63)
$1/2$ head Bibb lettuce, leaves washed, dried, and shredded or
    torn into pieces

1. Mix together the lime juice, oil, garlic, scallions or onion,
pepper, and cilantro in a small bowl. Place the meat in a single
layer in a baking dish and pour on the marinade. Cover and refrigerate the steak for 12 to 24 hours or the chicken for 1 to 3 hours,
turning the meat from time to time.

2. Preheat the broiler. Remove the meat from the marinade
and season lightly with salt. Discard the marinade. Broil the steak
for 2 to 3 minutes per side for medium-rare, longer if you like it
well-done. Broil the chicken until firm to the touch and cooked
through, about 5 minutes per side.

KEY NUTRIENTS
STEAK
Protein
Vitamin B$_6$
Vitamin B$_{12}$
Niacin
Riboflavin
Iron
Magnesium
Phosphorus
Potassium
Zinc

CHICKEN
Protein
Vitamin B$_6$
Vitamin B$_{12}$
Niacin
Iron
Magnesium
Phosphorus

3. While the meat is cooking, wrap the tortillas in foil and warm on the grill, in a 350°F oven, or under the broiler.

4. When the meat is done, divide it among the tortillas. Add a spoonful of salsa and a handful of shredded lettuce to each tortilla. Roll up loosely and serve.

ADVANCE
PREPARATION

The pork loin can mari-
nate all day in the
refrigerator. Once
cooked, it will keep for
3 or 4 days and can be
served cold.

Roast Pork Loin
with Fennel-Pepper Rub

This recipe was given to me by my friend and colleague Russ
Parsons, food editor of the *Los Angeles Times*. This is a fragrant
pork roast, and the leftovers make great sandwiches.

1 3- to 3$^{1}/_{2}$-pound pork loin, preferably with the bone
1 garlic clove, cut in half
1 tablespoon peppercorns
2 teaspoons fennel seeds
2 teaspoons kosher salt
2 tablespoons olive oil

1. Place the pork loin on a wide plate and rub with the garlic. Grind together the peppercorns, fennel seeds, and salt, or crush
with the bottom of a heavy skillet. Cover the pork with the spice
mixture, rubbing it into the pork in a thick layer. Drizzle on the
olive oil and continue to massage the spice rub into the meat. Keep
picking up the rub that falls onto the plate and gradually work it
all into the meat. Cover with plastic and refrigerate for 2 hours.

2. Remove from the refrigerator and let sit at room temperature for 30 minutes. Preheat the oven to 325°F.

3. Place the roast on a rack in a roasting pan and roast for
1$^{1}/_{2}$ to 2 hours, until an instant-read meat thermometer reads 155°F
when the loin is pierced in several places. Do not touch the bone
when taking the temperature, as it will be hotter than the meat.

4. Let stand at room temperature for 20 to 30 minutes to
reabsorb the juices, then serve.

KEY NUTRIENTS
Protein
Vitamin B$_6$
Vitamin B$_{12}$
Niacin
Riboflavin
Thiamin
Iron
Phosphorus
Potassium
Zinc

Stir-Fried Pork and Greens

ADVANCE
PREPARATION
The greens can be
blanched up to a day
ahead and held in the
refrigerator in a plas-
tic bag, then cooked as
instructed just before
serving.

Many Asian dishes have the advantage of being one-dish meals that include protein, vegetable, and grain. Once you've prepared the ingredients, the cooking goes very quickly.

- 2 large bunches (1½–2 pounds) greens, such as Swiss chard, spinach, beet greens, turnip greens, or kale, stemmed and washed thoroughly.
- 1 tablespoon salt
- 2 tablespoons canola or peanut oil
- ¾ pound lean pork loin, cut into ¼-by-2-inch strips
- 2 large garlic cloves, minced or pressed (optional)
- 1 tablespoon grated or minced fresh ginger
- 2 tablespoons soy sauce, or more to taste
- 1 cup rice (white or brown) or bulgur, cooked (see page 266 or 263), or ½ pound Asian noodles, such as soba or somen, cooked (see page 262), for serving

1. Bring a large pot of water to a boil. Add the greens and salt. Cook for 2 to 5 minutes (depending on the type of greens), until tender. Drain and rinse with cold water. Gently squeeze out the water (you don't have to squeeze them completely dry) and coarsely chop.

2. Heat a wok or heavy-bottomed nonstick skillet over high heat until hot enough to evaporate a drop of water on contact. Add 1 tablespoon of the oil, swirl to coat the pan, and reduce the heat to medium-high. Add the pork and cook, stirring, for 2 to 3 minutes, until the meat is cooked through and there is no longer any trace of pink. Add the remaining 1 tablespoon oil, the garlic (if using), and ginger and cook, stirring with a wooden paddle or spoon, until fragrant and beginning to color, 20 to 30 seconds. Stir in the greens and soy sauce and heat through, stirring.

3. Serve with the rice, bulgur, or noodles.

KEY NUTRIENTS
Protein
Beta Carotene
Vitamin A
Vitamin B$_6$
Vitamin B$_{12}$
Folacin
Niacin
Riboflavin
Thiamin
Vitamin C
Vitamin E
Calcium
Copper (except spinach)
Iron
Magnesium
Manganese
Phosphorus
Potassium
Zinc

Main Dishes

Roast Turkey

We rarely think about cooking a great big turkey on days other than Thanksgiving or Christmas. Yet the birds are available year-round. A roast turkey weighing 10 to 12 pounds can feed you and your family for days. The recipe here is very straightforward; the bird bakes at 375°F, and you never have to turn it. You don't have to make a stuffing every time you roast a turkey, but the one here is quite good if you do.

1 10- to 12-pound turkey, preferably free-range and
    hormone-free
Wild Rice Stuffing (recipe follows; optional)
Salt and freshly ground pepper to taste
2 tablespoons olive oil

1. Preheat the oven to 375°F. Lightly oil a large roasting pan. Set your oven rack low enough so the turkey will fit in the oven.

2. Pull the giblets and neck out of the turkey cavity; discard or save for another purpose such as stock. Rinse the bird inside and out with cold water and blot dry with paper towels.

3. If you're stuffing the turkey, fill the large cavity with the stuffing. Sprinkle the turkey with salt and pepper and rub with the olive oil. Tuck the wings under the thighs and tie the legs together with kitchen twine. Place breast side up in the roasting pan. Roast for 11 to 15 minutes per pound. Baste the turkey, if you wish, brushing every 20 minutes with the drippings in the pan. The turkey is done when it reaches an internal temperature of 165°F. Take the temperature with a meat thermometer, sticking it into the thickest part of the thigh. The bird should be browned all over, and the flesh should feel firm and resilient when you press on it.

4. Remove from the oven and let rest for 20 minutes before carving and serving

Wild Rice Stuffing

This makes a great pilaf as well as a wonderful stuffing.

Makes 8–10 servings
as a stuffing, 6 as a
main-dish pilaf

ADVANCE
PREPARATION
The stuffing will hold
for a day in the refrig-
erator.

      4 cups chicken or vegetable stock
 1¹/₂ cups wild rice, rinsed
      Salt to taste
 ³/₄ cup whole almonds
      1 tablespoon olive oil
      1 medium onion or 3 shallots, chopped
 ¹/₂ pound mushrooms, trimmed and sliced
      2 garlic cloves, minced or pressed
      1 tablespoon butter
 ¹/₂ teaspoon dried thyme
 ¹/₂ cup chopped fresh parsley
      3 tablespoons chopped fresh sage
      Freshly ground pepper to taste

1. Bring the stock to a boil in a large saucepan. Add the wild rice and salt (if the stock isn't salted). Bring back to a boil, re-duce the heat, cover, and simmer for 40 minutes, until the rice is tender and splayed. Drain and set aside.

2. Preheat the oven to 375°F. Place the almonds on an un-greased baking sheet. Place in the oven and toast until golden brown, about 10 minutes. Transfer to a small bowl and coarsely chop.

3. Heat the oil in a large, heavy nonstick skillet over medium heat. Add the onion or shallots and cook gently, stirring, for 5 to 10 minutes, until tender and just beginning to color. Add the mushrooms, sprinkle with salt, and add the garlic and butter. Increase the heat to medium-high and cook, stirring, until the mushrooms begin to release their liquid, 3 to 5 minutes. Add the chopped almonds and thyme and continue to cook, stirring often, until the mushrooms are tender, 5 to 10 minutes. Stir in the rice,

KEY NUTRIENTS
Vitamin B₆
Folacin
Niacin
Riboflavin
Vitamin E
Calcium
Copper
Iron
Magnesium
Manganese
Phosphorus
Potassium
Zinc

Main Dishes

parsley, and sage and heat through. Sprinkle with pepper, then taste and adjust the salt.

4. Remove from the heat and let cool before stuffing the turkey.

NOTE: To reheat this stuffing, preheat the oven to 350°F. Place the stuffing in an oiled baking dish, cover, and bake for 20 minutes.

Halibut
Cooked in the Microwave

ADVANCE
PREPARATION
The fish can be mari-
nated in the refrigera-
tor for up to 1 day, but
it must be cooked at
the last minute.

Fish may or may not be appealing during the first months of pregnancy. The milder, the better, though, which is why I like halibut: it's meaty, but the flavor isn't as strong as other meaty fish such as salmon and tuna. Whatever the fish, the less you have to deal with it, the better, so the microwave is perfect. The fish will be done in minutes, and there's no lingering cooking odor. This recipe has Asian flavors, but you can just as easily substitute Mediterranean flavors — garlic and olive oil — or make it even simpler: a squeeze of lemon is all you need for a really fresh piece of fish.

  2 halibut fillets or steaks (about 6 ounces each)
  1 tablespoon fresh lime juice
  1 tablespoon soy sauce
  1 teaspoon dark sesame oil
  1 garlic clove, minced or pressed (optional)
  1 teaspoon grated or minced fresh ginger
$1/4$ teaspoon sugar

1. Rinse the fish steaks and pat dry. Stir together the remaining ingredients in a large bowl and toss with the fish. Let sit for 15 to 30 minutes, in or out of the refrigerator, turning the fish over halfway through.

2. Transfer to a microwave-safe plate or baking dish and drizzle some of the marinade over the fish. Cover with plastic wrap, pierce in a few places with the tip of a knife to vent, and cook at 100% power, or high, for 2 to 3 minutes. Let sit for 1 minute, then carefully uncover. If the fish does not pull apart easily with a fork, cook for 30 to 60 seconds more, then serve.

NOTE: Leave your mcirowave door open for an hour after cooking, so that odors don't linger inside.

KEY NUTRIENTS
Protein
Vitamin B_6
Vitamin B_{12}
Niacin
Vitamin E
Iron
Magnesium
Phosphorus
Potassium

Main Dishes

ADVANCE
PREPARATION

The fish can be pre-
pared on the plate with
its topping, covered,
and refrigerated for 1
hour before you mi-
crowave it.

Salmon Fillets
Cooked in the Microwave

Salmon cooks beautifully in the microwave. These fillets are
succulent, with little need for embellishment.

2 salmon fillets (about 6 ounces each)
Salt and freshly ground pepper to taste
Juice of $\frac{1}{2}$ lemon (optional)
A sprinkling of chopped fresh herbs, such as basil, dill,
    or tarragon (optional)
Herbed Yogurt Cheese (page 65), Tofu Green Goddess
    (page 67), or lemon wedges for serving

1. Rinse the salmon fillets and pat dry. Place side by side on
a microwave-safe plate or baking dish. Sprinkle with the salt and
pepper and lemon juice (if using). Sprinkle with the herbs, if
using, and cover the dish tightly with plastic wrap. Pierce the plastic in a few places with the tip of a knife to vent and cook at 100%
power, or high, for 2 to 3 minutes, until the salmon is opaque all
the way through. Let sit for 1 to 2 minutes, then check to see if the
salmon is done. Return to the microwave for 30 to 60 seconds
more, if necessary.

2. Divide the salmon between 2 plates. Pour any juices that
have collected on the cooking plate over the fish. Serve with the
Herbed Yogurt Cheese, Tofu Green Goddess, or lemon wedges.

NOTE: Leave your microwave door open for an hour after
cooking, so that odors don't linger inside.

KEY NUTRIENTS
Protein
Vitamin B_6
Vitamin B_{12}
Niacin
Riboflavin
Thiamin
Iron
Magnesium
Phosphorus
Potassium
Omega-3s

Red Snapper Fillets Baked in Foil

ADVANCE
PREPARATION
The packets can be assembled hours before cooking and held in the refrigerator. Remove from the refrigerator 15 to 30 minutes before cooking.

One of the easiest and neatest ways to prepare fish is to bake it in a foil packet. The fish steams in the packet, and the juices it releases make a nice sauce.

2 teaspoons olive oil, plus more for brushing
4 red snapper fillets (5–6 ounces each)
   Salt and freshly ground pepper to taste
1 lemon, sliced
4 sprigs fresh rosemary, or 1 teaspoon dried, crumbled
   rosemary
   Lemon wedges for serving

1. Preheat the oven to 450°F. Cut 4 sheets of heavy-duty aluminum foil (or 8 sheets of lighter foil for double thickness) into squares that are at least 2 inches longer than your fillets. Brush the dull side of the foil with olive oil.

2. Measure the snapper at the thickest point to determine the cooking time, which will be 5 minutes per $1/2$ inch of thickness. Lay each fillet on a square of foil. Sprinkle lightly with salt and pepper, then drizzle with $1/2$ teaspoon olive oil. Lay a few slices of lemon on top, then top with a sprig of rosemary or sprinkle with $1/4$ teaspoon dried rosemary. Fold the foil up loosely over the snapper and crimp the edges together tightly. Place the packets on a baking sheet and bake for 5 to 10 minutes, depending on the thickness of the fillets. The fish is done when the flesh is opaque and pulls apart easily when tested with a fork.

3. Cut the packets across the top. Serve in the foil packets on a plate, or transfer the fish to plates and pour the juices from the packets over the fish. Accompany with lemon wedges.

KEY NUTRIENTS
Protein
Vitamin B_6
Vitamin B_{12}

Main Dishes

ADVANCE
PREPARATION
The packets can be as-
sembled hours before
cooking and held in the
refrigerator. Remove
from the refrigerator
15 to 30 minutes be-
fore cooking.

Whole Trout Baked in Foil

One of the easiest types of fish to find these days is farmed trout. The small fish are sold whole, and they're often already boned. They're rich in omega-3s and have white or light pink flesh, depending on the type. Pink-fleshed trout are often called salmon trout. They are mild-tasting fish, much like salmon but a bit drier. One easy way to cook them is to bake them in a foil packet. Serve the trout with rice, other grains or potatoes, and a steamed green vegetable.

1 tablespoon olive oil, plus more for brushing
4 small trout or salmon trout, cleaned (with or without the
    bones), rinsed, and patted dry
Salt and freshly ground pepper to taste
4 sprigs fresh tarragon, fennel, or dill, or 1 teaspoon
    crushed fennel seeds
1 lemon, sliced

1. Preheat the oven to 450°F. Cut 2 sheets of heavy-duty aluminum foil (or 4 sheets of lighter foil for double thickness) into rectangles that are at least 2 inches longer than the fish. Brush the dull side of the foil with olive oil.

2. Measure the fish at the thickest point to determine the cooking time, which will be 5 minutes per ½ inch of thickness. Rub the fish inside and out with the oil, then sprinkle with salt and pepper. Place half the herb sprigs or fennel seeds inside the cavities and the rest on top of the fish. Lay each fish on a piece of foil and cover with lemon slices. Fold the foil up loosely over the trout and crimp the edges together tightly. Place the packets on a baking sheet and bake for 10 to 15 minutes, depending on the thickness of the fish. The fish is done when the flesh is opaque and pulls apart easily when tested with a fork.

3. Cut the packets across the top. Serve in the foil packets on a plate, or transfer the fish to plates and pour the juices from the packets over the fish.

KEY NUTRIENTS
Protein
Vitamin B$_6$
Vitamin B$_{12}$
Niacin
Riboflavin
Calcium
Iron
Magnesium
Phosphorus
Potassium
Omega-3s

Sole with Olive Oil, Lemon, and Scallions

Makes 3 or 4
servings

ADVANCE
PREPARATION
The dish can be assembled hours before cooking and held in the refrigerator. Remove from the refrigerator 15 to 30 minutes before cooking.

Sole is delicate and light — very easy to stomach at any time during pregnancy. The fillets are so thin that they cook in 5 to 8 minutes.

1 tablespoon plus 1 teaspoon olive oil
1 pound sole (or petrale sole) fillets
Salt and freshly ground pepper to taste
1 bunch scallions, white and green parts, sliced
Fresh lemon juice to taste

1. Preheat the oven to 425°F. Use 1 teaspoon of the olive oil to coat a baking dish large enough to accommodate all the fish in one layer. Lay the fillets in the dish, sprinkle with salt and pepper, and cover the dish tightly with aluminum foil. Bake for 5 to 8 minutes, until opaque and fork tender.

2. While the fish is baking, heat the remaining 1 tablespoon olive oil in a small frying pan and add the scallions. Cook, stirring, until they just begin to wilt, about 3 minutes. Set aside.

3. When the fish is done, remove from the oven and sprinkle with the lemon juice. Spoon the scallions over the top and serve.

KEY NUTRIENTS
Protein
Vitamin B$_{12}$
Riboflavin
Phosphorus

Main Dishes

ADVANCE
PREPARATION
The fish needs to
marinate for 15 to 30
minutes before
cooking.

Snapper or Sole with Lemon, Capers, Oregano, and Olive Oil

Lemon juice and capers make lively seasonings for this Mediterranean dish, and they're often particularly appealing to pregnant women. This is easy to make, even if you're not an experienced fish cook.

1/4 cup fresh lemon juice
1 tablespoon olive oil
1 tablespoon chopped fresh oregano or 1 teaspoon dried
2 garlic cloves, minced or pressed (optional)
   Salt to taste
1 1/2–2 pounds red snapper or sole fillets
1 tablespoon capers, drained, rinsed, and chopped

1. Mix together the lemon juice, olive oil, oregano, and garlic (if using) in a large bowl. Add the salt and fish and toss. Let sit for 15 to 30 minutes. Preheat the oven to 425°F.

2. Measure the fish at the thickest point. Place in a baking dish with the marinade, cover tightly, and bake for 4 to 5 minutes per 1/2 inch of thickness. When cooked, the fish should be opaque and pull apart easily when tested with a fork. Top with the capers and serve.

KEY NUTRIENTS
Protein
Vitamin B_6
Vitamin B_{12}
Niacin
Vitamin C
Iron
Magnesium
Phosphorus
Potassium

Grilled or Broiled Fish Steaks with Asian Flavors

Makes 4 servings

ADVANCE PREPARATION
The marinade can be made up to a day ahead of time.

Tuna, halibut, and salmon all work well in this recipe, and these fish are easy to find in supermarkets that sell fresh fish.

- 4 1-inch-thick tuna, salmon, or halibut steaks (6–8 ounces each)
- 1 tablespoon fresh lime juice
- 1 tablespoon rice wine vinegar
- 2 teaspoons dark sesame oil
- 1–2 garlic cloves (to taste), minced or pressed
- 2 teaspoons grated or minced fresh ginger
- 1/2 teaspoon sugar (optional)
- Lime wedges and/or plum sauce or hoisin sauce for serving (optional)

1. Rinse the fish steaks and pat dry. Place in a shallow baking dish. In a small bowl, mix together all the remaining ingredients, except the lime wedges and plum or hoisin sauce. Pour over the fish. Turn the steaks over so that they are coated on both sides. Cover the dish with plastic wrap. If you are going to cook the fish within 30 minutes, let sit at room temperature. If you are marinating the steaks for longer, place in the refrigerator. They can marinate for up to a few hours.

2. Prepare the grill (medium heat for a gas grill) or preheat the broiler, with the rack about 4 inches from the heat. Place the steaks on the grill or on a broiler pan and cook for 4 to 5 minutes (3 to 4 minutes for rare). Brush with marinade and carefully turn over, using a wide spatula or tongs. Brush with marinade again, then discard the remaining marinade. Cook for 4 to 5 minutes more (3 to 4 minutes for rare). Be careful not to overcook. Serve with lime wedges and/or plum or hoisin sauce, if desired.

KEY NUTRIENTS
Protein
Vitamin B$_6$
Vitamin B$_{12}$
Niacin
Vitamin E
Iron
Magnesium
Phosphorus
Potassium

Main Dishes

ADVANCE
PREPARATION
The sauce will hold for
several hours, at room
temperature or in the
refrigerator.

Grilled Tuna with Tomato-Balsamic Salsa

This is the same uncooked tomato sauce that I use with pasta during those summer months when the tomatoes are so good. It's not just great with pasta; it makes a terrific accompaniment to any grilled fish.

2 pounds (8 medium or 4 large) ripe tomatoes, peeled,
    seeded, and finely chopped
1¹/₂ tablespoons olive oil
2–3 teaspoons balsamic vinegar, to taste
3 tablespoons slivered fresh basil leaves
2 large garlic cloves, minced or pressed
    Salt to taste
6 ³/₄- to 1-inch-thick tuna steaks (6–8 ounces each)
    Freshly ground pepper to taste
    Fresh basil sprigs for garnish

1. Mix together the tomatoes, 1 tablespoon of the olive oil, the vinegar, slivered basil, garlic, and salt. Taste and adjust the salt.

2. Prepare a medium-hot grill or heat a nonstick grill pan over medium-high heat. Brush the tuna steaks with the remaining ¹/₂ tablespoon oil and season lightly with salt and pepper. Cook over high heat for 3 to 4 minutes per side (longer if desired).

3. Transfer to a platter or individual plates. Serve with the tomato salsa spooned partly over the fish, partly on the side. Garnish with the basil sprigs.

KEY NUTRIENTS
Protein
Vitamin A
Vitamin B$_6$
Vitamin B$_{12}$
Niacin
Vitamin C
Vitamin E
Iron
Magnesium
Phosphorus
Potassium

Creamy Pasta with Broccoli

ADVANCE
PREPARATION

The cottage cheese mixture will keep in the refrigerator until the expiration date on the cottage cheese container.

Cottage cheese blended with milk makes a creamy, low-fat pasta sauce. You can prepare the sauce while waiting for the water to boil.

1–2 garlic cloves, to taste (optional)
$1/2$ cup cottage cheese
$1/4$ cup milk
   Salt and freshly ground pepper to taste
2 tablespoons chopped fresh chives or parsley, or a combination (optional)
$3/4$ pound dried pasta, such as fusilli, penne, or farfalle
1 pound broccoli, broken into florets
1 ounce Parmesan cheese, grated (about $1/4$ cup)

1. Bring a large pot of water to a boil.

2. Meanwhile, chop the garlic, if using, in a mini-processor or food processor. When it adheres to the sides, stop the machine and scrape down the sides. Add the cottage cheese and blend until smooth. Scrape down the sides again. Add the milk and blend again until there is no trace of graininess. Add the salt and pepper. Transfer to a wide pasta bowl and stir in the chives and/or parsley, if using.

3. When the water comes to a boil, add 1 tablespoon salt and the pasta. Stir once to make sure the pasta doesn't stick to the bottom of the pot and cook until al dente. Add the broccoli to the pasta cooking water 3 to 4 minutes before the end of the estimated cooking time.

4. Meanwhile, stir 2 to 4 tablespoons of the cooking water into the cottage cheese mixture to thin it to your taste. Drain the pasta and broccoli and transfer to the bowl with the sauce. Add the Parmesan, toss together, and serve.

KEY NUTRIENTS
Beta Carotene
Vitamin A
Vitamin B_6
Vitamin B_{12}
Folacin
Niacin
Riboflavin
Thiamin
Vitamin C
Iron
Manganese
Phosphorus
Potassium

Main Dishes

ADVANCE
PREPARATION

The cottage cheese
mixture will keep in the
refrigerator until the
expiration date on the
cottage cheese con-
tainer.

Creamy Pasta with Greens

The cottage cheese–based "cream" sauce here and in the previous recipe can be used in combination with any pasta and any vegetable. If you use red chard or beet greens, the pasta sauce will be tinged pink.

2 bunches (about 1¹/₂ pounds) greens, such as Swiss chard,
    beet greens, kale, or spinach
1–2 garlic cloves, to taste (optional)
1 cup cottage cheese
¹/₄ cup milk
  Salt and freshly ground pepper to taste
³/₄ pound dried pasta, any shape
1 ounce Parmesan cheese, grated (about ¹/₄ cup)

1. Stem the greens and wash thoroughly, rinsing twice to make sure all the sand is removed. Coarsely chop. Bring a large pot of water to a boil.

2. Meanwhile, chop the garlic, if using, in a mini-processor or food processor. When it adheres to the sides, stop the machine and scrape down the sides. Add the cottage cheese and blend until smooth. Scrape down the sides again. Add the milk and blend again until there is no trace of graininess. Add the salt and pepper. Transfer to a wide pasta bowl.

3. When the water comes to a boil, add 1 tablespoon salt and the pasta. Stir once to make sure the pasta doesn't stick to the bottom of the pot and cook until al dente. Add the greens to the pasta cooking water 3 to 5 minutes before the end of the estimated cooking time.

KEY NUTRIENTS
Beta Carotene
Vitamin A
Vitamin B₆
Vitamin B₁₂
Folacin
Niacin
Riboflavin
Thiamin
Vitamin C
Vitamin E
Calcium
Copper (except spinach)
Iron
Magnesium
Manganese
Phosphorus
Potassium

4. Meanwhile, stir about 2 tablespoons of the cooking water into the cottage cheese mixture to thin it to your taste. Drain the pasta and greens and transfer to the bowl with the sauce. Add the Parmesan, toss together, and serve.

Pasta with Pesto and Green Beans

Makes 4 servings

ADVANCE PREPARATION
The beans can be trimmed and broken ahead of time, but this is a last-minute dish.

This is a quick meal, now that high-quality, commercially made pesto is so easy to find. Add green beans (or broccoli or peas), and you have a one-dish meal.

1/4–1/2 cup store-bought pesto, to taste
   1 tablespoon salt
 3/4 pound dried pasta, such as fettuccine, spaghetti, or
        fusilli
 1/2 pound green beans, trimmed and broken in half
 1/3 cup freshly grated Parmesan cheese for serving

1. Bring a large pot of water to a bowl. Place the pesto in a large bowl or heatproof serving dish.

2. When the water comes to a boil, add the salt and gradually add the pasta. Stir once to make sure the pasta doesn't stick to the bottom of the pot, then boil for 5 minutes. Add the green beans. Continue cooking until the pasta is cooked al dente.

3. Meanwhile, stir 1 to 2 tablespoons of the cooking water into the pesto and thin it to your taste. Drain the pasta and beans, toss with the pesto, and serve, passing the Parmesan at the table.

KEY NUTRIENTS
Vitamin A
Folacin
Niacin
Thiamin
Vitamin C
Iron
Manganese

Main Dishes

ADVANCE
PREPARATION
The tomato mixture,
without the herbs, can
be made several hours
ahead of serving. The
tomatoes will have
more flavor if you do
not refrigerate them.
Add the herbs shortly
before serving.

Summer Pasta with Tomatoes and Green Beans or Peas

You can make this easy one-dish pasta right through the end of tomato season.

1 1/2 pounds ripe tomatoes, seeded and diced
1–2 garlic cloves (to taste), minced or pressed (optional)
  Salt and freshly ground pepper to taste
1–2 tablespoons olive oil, to taste
1–2 teaspoons balsamic vinegar, to taste (optional)
  1 tablespoon slivered or chopped fresh basil or parsley
3/4 pound dried pasta, such as fusilli, rigatoni, farfalle, or penne
1/2 pound green beans, trimmed and broken in half, or 1 cup fresh or thawed frozen peas
  1 ounce Parmesan cheese, grated (about 1/4 cup)

1. In a large bowl, toss together the tomatoes, garlic (if using), salt and pepper, olive oil, vinegar (if using), and basil or parsley. Let sit at room temperature for 15 minutes or longer so the flavors can blend. Taste and adjust the seasonings.

2. Bring a large pot of water to a boil. Add 1 tablespoon of salt and the pasta. Cook for 5 minutes, then add the green beans or *fresh* peas (if using) and continue to cook until the pasta is al dente. If using thawed frozen peas, add them now.

3. Drain the pasta and vegetables and transfer to the bowl with the tomato mixture. Add the Parmesan, toss together, and serve.

KEY NUTRIENTS
Vitamin A
Niacin
Thiamin
Vitamin C
Vitamin E
Iron
Manganese

GREEN BEANS
Folacin

PEAS
Vitamin B_6
Copper
Magnesium
Phosphorus

Pasta with Tomato Sauce

ADVANCE
PREPARATION
The sauce will keep for
3 to 5 days in the
refrigerator and can be
frozen.

This is my basic tomato sauce, for which I use canned tomatoes. Use recipe-ready chopped tomatoes to save yourself the task of seeding and chopping. Practically any shape of pasta is suitable here. The ones I keep on hand include penne, fusilli, spaghetti, farfalle, and linguine. For variations, see the following page.

1 tablespoon olive oil
2–3 large garlic cloves (to taste), minced or pressed
1 28-ounce can tomatoes, drained (reserve 1/2 cup of the juice), seeded, and crushed (not pureed) in a food processor with the reserved juice, or finely chopped
1/2–3/4 teaspoon salt (to taste), plus 1 tablespoon for the pasta water
1/8 teaspoon sugar
2 tablespoons slivered fresh basil leaves or 3/4 teaspoon dried oregano or thyme, or a combination
Freshly ground pepper to taste
3/4 pound dried pasta, any shape
1/3 cup freshly grated Parmesan cheese

1. Heat the oil in a large, heavy nonstick skillet over medium heat and add the garlic. When the garlic begins to color, about 30 seconds, add the tomatoes and their juice, the salt, sugar, and dried herbs (if using). Cook, stirring often, for 15 to 25 minutes, until the tomatoes are cooked down, fragrant, and just beginning to stick to the pan but not dry. Stir in the fresh basil (if using) and add the pepper. Taste, adjust the seasonings, and turn off the heat.

2. Bring a large pot of water to a rolling boil. Add the remaining 1 tablespoon salt and the pasta. Cook until the pasta is al dente and drain. Toss at once with the sauce and serve, passing the Parmesan at the table.

KEY NUTRIENTS
Vitamin A
Niacin
Thiamin
Vitamin C
Vitamin E
Iron
Manganese

Main Dishes

KEY NUTRIENTS
CHICKPEAS
Protein
Thiamin
Folacin
Copper
Iron
Magnesium
Manganese
Phosphorus
Potassium
Zinc

KEY NUTRIENTS
GOAT CHEESE
Calcium

KEY NUTRIENTS
TUNA
Protein
Vitamin B$_6$
Vitamin B$_{12}$
Niacin
Iron
Magnesium
Phosphorus
Potassium

KEY NUTRIENTS
BROCCOLI
Beta Carotene
Vitamin A
Vitamin B$_6$
Folacin
Vitamin C
Manganese
Potassium

KEY NUTRIENTS
GREENS
Beta Carotene
Vitamin A
Vitamin B$_6$
Folacin
Riboflavin (spinach)
Vitamin C
Vitamin E
Calcium
Copper (except spinach)
Iron
Magnesium
Manganese
Potassium

ADDITIONS

Chickpeas

Make the tomato sauce as directed. Drain and rinse a 15-ounce can of chickpeas and add to the sauce. Heat through.

Goat Cheese

Make the tomato sauce as directed. Stir $^1/_2$ cup crumbled goat cheese into the warm sauce.

Tuna

Make the tomato sauce as directed. Drain a 6-ounce can of water-packed tuna and break it up with a fork. Stir it into the warm sauce. Add hot red pepper flakes to taste, if you wish.

Broccoli

Make the tomato sauce as directed. Trim the stems from $^3/_4$ to 1 pound broccoli and break the tops into small florets. Peel the stems, quarter lengthwise, and slice. Cook the pasta as directed, but after the pasta has boiled for 5 minutes, add the broccoli to the cooking water.

Greens

Make the tomato sauce as directed. Wash and stem 1 large bunch (about 1 pound) spinach, chard, beet greens, or kale. Bring the pasta water to a boil. Add the salt and greens. Cook for 1 to 4 minutes, depending on how tough the greens are. Remove from the water with a slotted spoon and transfer to a bowl of cold water. Drain, squeeze dry, and coarsely chop. Stir into the warm sauce. Bring the water back to a boil and cook the pasta as directed.

Tortellini with Broccoli and Sage

ADVANCE PREPARATION
This is a last-minute operation.

This is another quick dinner that you can pull together using a combination of fresh and prepared foods.

1 tablespoon salt
3 cups fresh, frozen, or dried cheese tortellini
1 pound broccoli, broken into florets
1 tablespoon olive oil
6 fresh sage leaves, cut into slivers (optional)
Freshly ground pepper to taste
1 ounce Parmesan cheese, grated (about $1/4$ cup)

1. Bring a large pot of water to a boil. Add the salt and tortellini. Reduce the heat so that the water is at a gentle rather than a fast boil. Cook according to the package directions, usually 6 to 8 minutes for fresh or frozen tortellini, 15 minutes for dried.

2. Add the broccoli to the pot 3 to 4 minutes before the end of the estimated cooking time. Warm a serving dish.

3. When the tortellini is cooked al dente and the broccoli is tender, drain. Transfer to the warm serving dish. Add the oil, sage (if using), pepper, and Parmesan; toss. Serve at once.

KEY NUTRIENTS
Beta Carotene
Vitamin A
Vitamin B_6
Vitamin B_{12}
Folacin
Niacin
Riboflavin
Thiamin
Vitamin C
Iron
Manganese
Phosphorus
Potassium

Main Dishes

ADVANCE
PREPARATION
The sauce will keep for
3 to 5 days in the
refrigerator and can be
frozen.

Pasta with Tomato
Mushroom Sauce

Cooked sliced mushrooms contribute a meaty texture and
deep savory flavors to the basic tomato sauce for pasta. This
sauce also makes a great topping for polenta (see page 260).

$^3/_4$ pound mushrooms, trimmed and sliced
   Salt to taste
1 tablespoon olive oil
2–3 large garlic cloves (to taste), minced or pressed
$^1/_4$–$^1/_2$ teaspoon chopped fresh or dried thyme or rosemary
1 28-ounce can whole or chopped tomatoes (reserve $^1/_2$
   cup of the juice), seeded, and crushed (not pureed) in
   a food processor with the reserved juice, or finely
   chopped
$^1/_2$–$^3/_4$ teaspoon salt (to taste), plus 1 tablespoon for the pasta
   water
$^1/_8$ teaspoon sugar
2 tablespoons slivered fresh basil leaves or $^3/_4$ teaspoon
   dried oregano, or a combination
   Freshly ground pepper to taste
$^3/_4$ pound dried pasta, any shape
$^1/_3$ cup freshly grated Parmesan cheese for serving

KEY NUTRIENTS
Vitamin A
Folacin
Niacin
Riboflavin
Thiamin
Vitamin C
Vitamin E
Copper
Iron
Manganese
Phosphorus
Potassium

1. Heat a large, heavy nonstick skillet over medium heat
and add the mushrooms. Sprinkle with salt and cook, stirring,
until they begin to release their liquid, 3 to 5 minutes. Add the oil
and continue to cook until the mushrooms have softened, 5 to 10
minutes. Stir in the garlic and dried thyme or rosemary, if using.
When the garlic begins to color, 30 to 60 seconds, add the tomatoes
and their juice, the salt, and the sugar. Cook, stirring often, for 15 to
20 minutes, until the tomatoes are cooked down, fragrant, and just
beginning to stick to the pan but not dry. Stir in the fresh thyme or
rosemary (if using) and the pepper. Taste, adjust the seasonings,
and turn off the heat.

2. Bring a large pot of water to a rolling boil. Add the remaining 1 tablespoon salt and the pasta. Cook until the pasta is al dente and drain. Toss at once with the sauce and serve, passing the Parmesan at the table.

VARIATION

Pasta with Quick Tomato Mushroom Sauce

Substitute commercial tomato sauce for homemade. Cook the mushrooms with the garlic and herbs as directed above and stir into the commercial sauce. Use 1 to 1½ cups for ¾ pound pasta.

Zucchini "Pasta"

Makes 4 servings

If you are concerned about carbohydrates but love pasta, try this dish. It's crucial that you don't overcook the zucchini. It should be al dente, like al dente fettuccine.

ADVANCE PREPARATION
You can make the ribbons hours ahead of time, but the actual cooking should be done right before serving.

8 small or 3 or 4 large zucchini (about 2 pounds)
2 tablespoons olive oil
Salt and freshly ground pepper to taste
Tomato sauce for pasta (cooked or uncooked; homemade or commercial) or pesto (homemade or commercial)
½ cup freshly grated Parmesan cheese for serving

1. Using a vegetable peeler, cut the zucchini into thin ribbons. Turn the squash as you make the ribbons.

2. Heat the oil in a large nonstick skillet over medium-high heat. Add the zucchini ribbons and stir for 3 to 5 minutes, until translucent and softened. Add the salt and pepper, top with the sauce, and serve. Pass the cheese at the table.

KEY NUTRIENTS
TOMATO SAUCE
Vitamin A
Folacin
Vitamin C
Vitamin E

Main Dishes

ADVANCE
PREPARATION
The lasagna can be as-
sembled a day ahead of
time, covered in plas-
tic, and refrigerated
overnight. Add 5 min-
utes to the covered
baking time if chilled.
The assembled lasagna
also can be wrapped in
plastic, then foil, and
frozen for a month.

Quick Spinach and Tomato Lasagna

This lasagna, from my *Light Basics Cookbook* (William Morrow, 1999) is a no-fuss dish. Thanks to no-boil lasagna noodles
and commercial tomato sauce, it can be assembled in 10 to 15
minutes.

1½ cups cottage cheese
  1 26-ounce jar tomato sauce for pasta
  1 10-ounce package frozen spinach, thawed and squeezed
    dry
  ½ pound no-boil lasagna noodles
  ⅔ cup freshly grated Parmesan cheese
  3 tablespoons fresh or dry bread crumbs
  2 tablespoons olive oil, plus more for brushing

1. Oil or butter a 3-quart gratin or baking dish. Preheat the
oven to 375°F.

2. In a food processor, blend the cottage cheese until fairly
smooth. Add ½ cup of the tomato sauce and blend until smooth.
Add the spinach and briefly blend until the spinach is mixed in (do
not puree).

KEY NUTRIENTS
Protein
Beta Carotene
Vitamin A
Vitamin B₆
Vitamin B₁₂
Folacin
Niacin
Riboflavin
Thiamin
Vitamin C
Vitamin E
Calcium
Iron
Magnesium
Manganese
Phosphorus
Potassium
Zinc

3. To assemble the lasagna, have all the ingredients within
reach. Spoon about ½ cup of the sauce into the baking dish and
spread over the bottom of the dish. Arrange a layer of lasagna noodles over the sauce. Break the noodles, if necessary, to make a layer
that covers the entire surface of the dish. Dot the noodles with
spoonfuls of the cottage cheese mixture and gently spread over the
noodles. Top with a layer of sauce and a sprinkling of Parmesan
(about 1½ tablespoons). Repeat the layers — pasta, cottage cheese
mixture, sauce, and Parmesan — two or three more times, depending on the shape of your dish. Make sure you end up with a

layer of tomato sauce topped with Parmesan. Sprinkle on the bread crumbs, then drizzle on the oil.

4. Cut a piece of foil large enough to cover the dish. Brush the dull side with oil. Place it over the lasagna, oiled side down. Bake for 25 minutes, uncover, and bake for 15 minutes more, until the top is beginning to brown. Let sit for 5 to 10 minutes before serving. Serve hot or warm, cut in squares.

ADVANCE
PREPARATION
The spinach and leeks
can be prepared and
cooked up to 1 day be-
fore assembling the
tart. The tart can be
assembled 1 day ahead
as well. Keep in the re-
frigerator.

Greek Spinach Pie
(Spanakopita)

Bursting with spinach, this nutritious vegetarian main dish is
protein-rich and a real crowd pleaser.

2¼ pounds fresh spinach, stemmed and washed thoroughly
 1 tablespoon olive oil, plus more for brushing
 3 large leeks, white and light green parts only, washed
    thoroughly and thinly sliced
 3 large eggs, beaten
 ¼ cup chopped fresh dill (optional)
 6 ounces feta cheese, crumbled (about 1½ cups)
    Salt and freshly ground pepper to taste
 9 sheets phyllo dough
 1 egg white, lightly beaten

1. Place the wet spinach in a large nonstick skillet over
medium-high heat and wilt. Transfer to a colander and press out
as much water as possible. When the spinach is cool enough to
handle, wrap in a towel and squeeze out more water. Finely chop
and set aside.

KEY NUTRIENTS
Protein
Beta Carotene
Vitamin A
Vitamin B$_6$
Vitamin B$_{12}$
Folacin
Riboflavin
Vitamin C
Vitamin E
Calcium
Iron
Magnesium
Manganese
Phosphorus
Potassium

2. Preheat the oven to 375°F. Heat the oil in a large skillet
over medium-low heat and add the leeks. Cook for about 10 minutes, stirring often, until softened and just beginning to brown.
Add the spinach and stir together. Remove from the heat.

3. Beat the eggs in a large bowl. Stir in the spinach and
leeks, dill (if using), feta, and salt and pepper. Taste and adjust the
seasonings.

4. Brush a 10½- to 12-inch tart pan with olive oil and layer
in 4 sheets of phyllo, placing them not quite evenly on top of each

other so that the edges overlap the sides of the pan all the way around. Brush each sheet, including the edges, lightly with oil before adding the next sheet. Top with the spinach mixture. Fold the edges of the dough over the spinach mixture and brush them with oil. Layer the remaining 5 sheets of dough over the top, brushing each sheet lightly with oil, and tuck the edges of the dough into the sides of the pan. Brush the top with the beaten egg white. Pierce the top in several places with a sharp knife. Bake for 45 to 50 minutes, until the top is golden brown. Serve hot or at room temperature.

Simple Homemade Pizza

Use a prepared crust, such as Boboli, for this easy pizza. You
can add any number of toppings to the basic pie.

1 12- or 14-inch prepared pizza crust
2 tablespoons olive oil
1–1½ pounds ripe tomatoes, peeled, seeded, and chopped, or
      one 14-ounce can tomatoes, drained and chopped
2–3 large garlic cloves (to taste), minced or pressed
1 tablespoon slivered fresh basil leaves or 1 teaspoon
      dried oregano
Salt, to taste
Freshly ground pepper to taste

OPTIONAL ADDITIONS

2 red, yellow, or green bell peppers, thinly sliced, or more
    to taste
1–2 onions, thinly sliced, to taste
½ pound mushrooms, trimmed and thinly sliced
¼ cup imported black olives, pitted
2–4 tablespoons capers (to taste), drained and rinsed
4 canned artichoke hearts, drained, rinsed, and thinly
    sliced

¼ cup freshly grated Parmesan cheese

1. Preheat the oven to 450° F for at least 30 minutes, preferably with a baking stone on the middle rack.

2. Brush the pizza crust with 1 tablespoon of the oil. In a
medium bowl, mix together the tomatoes, garlic, basil or oregano,
salt, and pepper. Spread over the crust. Top with any of the additions of your choice. Drizzle on the remaining 1 tablespoon oil.
Transfer to the baking stone, if using, or to a baking sheet and bake
for 15 to 30 minutes, until the crust is browned. Sprinkle on the
Parmesan and serve.

Soft Tacos
with Tofu and Tomatoes

Makes 4 servings

ADVANCE
PREPARATION
The filling will keep for
2 or 3 days in the
refrigerator.

This dish is definitely one of my favorite tofu dishes. Silken tofu has a great eggy texture, and it absorbs the flavors of the tomato mixture beautifully, resulting in a filling that is much like Mexican scrambled eggs: spicy and wonderful. I also like the contrasting texture of the onion.

1 28-ounce can tomatoes, drained
2 garlic cloves, coarsely chopped
1 serrano or jalapeño pepper, coarsely chopped, or more
  to taste
1 tablespoon canola oil
1 small or medium onion, chopped
1 teaspoon ground cumin
  Salt to taste
1 pound medium or firm silken tofu
2–3 teaspoons soy sauce, to taste
3 tablespoons chopped fresh cilantro
8 corn tortillas, warmed (see page 40)
  Salsa, homemade (page 63) or commercial (optional)

1. Combine the tomatoes, garlic, and pepper in a blender and blend until fairly smooth.

2. Heat the oil in a large nonstick skillet over medium heat and add the onion. Cook, stirring, until tender, 3 to 5 minutes. Increase the heat to medium-high, add the cumin, stir once, and add the tomato puree. It should sizzle immediately. Cook, stirring, until the mixture is thick, 5 to 10 minutes. Season with salt. Add the tofu, mashing it into the sauce with the back of a spoon. Add the soy sauce and continue to cook for 5 minutes more, until the tofu is heated through. Stir in the cilantro. Taste and adjust the seasonings.

3. Place 2 tortillas on each plate and top with the tofu mixture. Serve, passing salsa to spoon over the top, if desired.

KEY NUTRIENTS
Protein
Vitamin A
Folacin
Thiamin
Vitamin C
Vitamin E
Calcium
Iron
Magnesium
Phosphorus

Main Dishes

ADVANCE
PREPARATION

The stew and the cous-
cous will keep for 3 to
4 days in the refrigera-
tor. You can reheat the
couscous in the mi-
crowave or a 350°F
oven, or steam it again
over the stew or water.

Couscous with Chickpeas and Greens

This hearty meal will probably fill you up, so you may want to eat smaller portions over a couple of days. It's a delicious vege-tarian main dish. You can find *harissa* in gourmet shops and some Middle Eastern groceries.

1 pound (2 heaped cups) dried chickpeas, washed, picked over, and soaked in 2 quarts water for 6 hours or overnight

8 cups water

4 large garlic cloves, minced or pressed (optional)

2 leeks, white parts only, washed thoroughly and sliced

1 medium onion, chopped

2 tablespoons *harissa* (Tunisian chile paste) or $1/4$–$1/2$ teaspoon cayenne pepper (to taste), plus more for serving (optional, especially if you have heartburn)

2 tablespoons tomato paste

2–3 teaspoons salt (to taste), plus 1 teaspoon for the couscous

1 teaspoon coriander seeds, ground (optional)

1 teaspoon caraway seeds, ground (optional)

2 large bunches ($1^{1}/_{2}$–2 pounds) greens, such as Swiss chard, spinach, or turnip greens, stemmed, washed thoroughly, and coarsely chopped

3 cups couscous

$2^{1}/_{2}$ cups hot water

KEY NUTRIENTS
Protein
Beta Carotene
Vitamin A
Vitamin B$_6$
Folacin
Niacin
Riboflavin (spinach)
Thiamin
Vitamin C
Vitamin E
Calcium
Copper
Iron
Magnesium
Manganese
Phosphorus
Potassium
Zinc

1. Drain the chickpeas and transfer to a large pot. Add the 8 cups water and bring to a boil. Reduce the heat and simmer for 1 hour.

2. After 1 hour, add the garlic (if using), leeks, onion, *harissa* or cayenne (if using), tomato paste, salt, coriander, and caraway (if using) to the pot. Bring back to a simmer, cover, and cook for 30 to 60 minutes, until the chickpeas and vegetables are thoroughly tender and the broth is fragrant. Stir in the greens, a handful at a time, allowing each handful to cook down a bit before adding the next. Simmer for 10 to 15 minutes, until the greens are tender. Remove from the heat. Taste and adjust the seasonings, then strain off 1 cup of the cooking liquid.

3. Place the couscous in a medium bowl with 1 teaspoon salt. Combine the hot water and cooking liquid in a large measuring cup or small bowl and pour over the couscous. The couscous should be completely submerged, with about 1/2 inch water on top. Let sit for 20 minutes, until the water is absorbed. Stir every 5 minutes with a wooden spoon or rub the grains between your thumbs and fingers, so that the couscous doesn't form clumps. Fluff it with a fork or your hands. Taste and add more salt, if necessary. Drain in a colander or strainer.

4. Place the couscous in the colander or strainer above the simmering stew or over a small amount of water in a large pot if you don't want to keep cooking the greens. Cover and steam for 10 to 15 minutes.

5. Place a generous spoonful of couscous in each of 6 wide soup bowls or plates, top with the stew, and serve. If you wish, pass additional *harissa* or cayenne at the table.

ADVANCE
PREPARATION
The vegetable mixture
and the couscous will
keep for 3 to 4 days in
the refrigerator. Do
not stir in the parsley
or cilantro until you
reheat the stew. You
can reheat the cous-
cous in the microwave
or in a covered casse-
role in a 350°F oven,
or steam it again over
the vegetable mixture.

KEY NUTRIENTS
Protein
Beta Carotene
Vitamin A
Vitamin B$_6$
Folacin
Niacin
Riboflavin (spinach)
Thiamin
Vitamin C
Vitamin E
Calcium
Copper
Iron
Magnesium
Manganese
Phosphorus
Potassium
Zinc

Winter Vegetable Couscous

This dish is filling but very low in fat, with lots of healthy root vegetables, such as turnips and leeks, and vitamin-rich vegetables, such as winter squash. You can find *harissa* in gourmet shops and some Middle Eastern groceries.

1 cup dried chickpeas, washed and picked over

11 cups water

4 large garlic cloves, minced or pressed

2 onions, sliced

2 large carrots, peeled and thickly sliced

2 medium turnips, peeled and cut into wedges

1 leek, white part only, washed thoroughly and sliced

1 bay leaf

2–3 teaspoons salt, to taste

1 teaspoon dried thyme

1/2 teaspoon ground cinnamon

Pinch of saffron threads (optional)

1 pound winter squash, such as butternut or hubbard, peeled and cut into 3/4-inch dice

1 teaspoon *harissa* (Tunisian chile paste) or 1/4 teaspoon cayenne pepper, plus more for serving (optional, especially if you have heartburn)

Freshly ground pepper to taste

1 bunch (about 3/4 pound) Swiss chard or spinach, stemmed, washed thoroughly, and coarsely chopped

2 cups couscous

1/4 cup chopped fresh cilantro or parsley

1. Soak the chickpeas in 3 cups of the water for several hours or overnight; drain.

2. Combine the drained chickpeas, remaining 8 cups water, half the garlic, the onions, carrots, turnips, leek, and bay leaf in a stockpot or Dutch oven. Bring to a boil, reduce the heat, cover, and simmer for 1 hour. Add 2 teaspoons of the salt, the remaining garlic, the thyme, cinnamon, saffron (if using), squash, and *harissa* or cayenne (if using). Simmer for 30 to 60 minutes more, until the chickpeas are tender. Taste and adjust the salt and *harissa* or cayenne. Add a generous amount of pepper, then stir in the chard or spinach.

3. Place the couscous in a medium bowl. Strain off 2½ cups of the cooking liquid from the chickpeas and vegetables and pour over the couscous. Let sit for 20 minutes, until the water is absorbed. Stir every 5 minutes with a wooden spoon or rub the grains between your thumbs and fingers, so that the couscous doesn't form clumps. Fluff it with a fork or your hands. Taste and add salt, if necessary. Drain in a colander or strainer.

4. Place the couscous in the colander or strainer above the vegetable mixture, making sure the bottom of the colander does not touch the liquid (remove some of the liquid if it does). Cover and steam for 15 minutes. (Alternatively, warm the couscous in a covered casserole in a 350°F oven for 20 minutes.) Transfer the couscous to a serving bowl. Stir the cilantro or parsley into the vegetable mixture.

5. To serve, divide the couscous among 4 wide soup bowls and ladle on a generous helping of the vegetable mixture. If you wish, pass additional *harissa* or cayenne at the table.

Quesadillas

Making nutritious meals and snacks quickly is all-important during the exhausting first and last months of pregnancy. Corn tortillas have more nutrients and less fat than flour tortillas. If you are making a meal of these quesadillas, serve with beans or Refried Beans (page 230) and/or rice. Follow with a salad.

Classic Quesadilla
Makes 1 quesadilla

1 corn tortilla
2 heaped tablespoons grated cheddar or Monterey jack
    cheese
Salsa, homemade (page 63) or commercial for serving

Heat the tortilla in a nonstick skillet over medium-high heat until flexible. Turn over and sprinkle the cheese over the surface. When the cheese begins to melt, fold the tortilla over with a spatula. Heat for about 30 seconds, then turn it over and continue to heat until the tortilla is lightly browned in places on both sides. Transfer to a plate and serve hot, accompanied by the salsa.

Low-Fat, High-Protein Quesadillas
Makes 8 quesadillas, serving 4

Keep a batch of this low-fat filling in the refrigerator so that you can make these quesadillas for a quick snack or meal.

1 cup nonfat cottage cheese
1/3 cup grated Monterey jack cheese
8 corn tortillas
Salsa, homemade (page 63) or commercial for serving

1. Blend together the cottage cheese and Monterey jack cheese in a food processor until completely smooth.

2. Heat 1 to 3 of the tortillas in a large nonstick skillet over medium-high heat until flexible. Turn over and top each tortilla with 2 tablespoons of the cheese mixture. Fold the tortilla over with a spatula. Heat through, turning the folded tortilla over from time to time, until the cheese melts and the tortilla is browned in places on both sides. Don't worry if some of the cheese runs out onto the pan (it probably will). Transfer to plates and serve hot, passing the salsa to spoon over the top.

VARIATIONS

Quesadillas with Black Beans

Add 2 tablespoons cooked black beans (page 229) or Refried Beans (page 230) to each Classic Quesadilla (or Low-Fat, High-Protein Quesadilla). Top the cheese with the beans and proceed with the recipe.

Quesadillas with Greens

For 8 Classic Quesadillas or Low-Fat, High-Protein Quesadillas, stem and thoroughly wash 2 large bunches (1½ to 2 pounds) Swiss chard, spinach, or other greens. Bring a large pot of water to a boil. Add about 2 teaspoons salt and the greens. Blanch for 1 to 4 minutes (depending on the type of greens), until tender. Transfer to a bowl of cold water, drain, and squeeze out the water. Coarsely chop. Top the cheese on each tortilla with 3 tablespoons chopped greens and proceed with the recipe.

WITH BLACK BEANS
ADVANCE
PREPARATION

The beans will keep for a few days in a covered bowl in the refrigerator and can be frozen.

KEY NUTRIENTS
Protein
Vitamin B$_6$
Folacin
Thiamin
Copper
Iron
Magnesium
Manganese
Phosphorus
Potassium

WITH GREENS
ADVANCE
PREPARATION

The cooked greens will keep for a few days in a covered bowl in the refrigerator and can be frozen.

KEY NUTRIENTS
Beta Carotene
Vitamin A
Vitamin B$_6$
Folacin
Riboflavin (spinach)
Vitamin C
Vitamin E
Calcium
Copper (except spinach)
Iron
Magnesium
Manganese
Potassium

Main Dishes

217

ADVANCE
PREPARATION

The bread and tomato
layers can be assem-
bled hours before
beating together the
eggs and milk and com-
pleting the casserole.

Strata with Tomatoes and Greens

A strata is like a savory bread pudding and is a comforting and nutritious meal. Bread, tomatoes, and greens are layered and bound with eggs, milk, and cheese. This is a great way to use up bread that has gone or is going stale.

Salt

1 bunch (about $3/4$ pound) spinach or Swiss chard, stemmed and washed thoroughly

1 14-ounce can diced tomatoes, drained, or 4 medium fresh tomatoes, peeled, seeded, and chopped

2–3 large garlic cloves (to taste), 1 or 2 minced, 1 cut in half

$1/8$ teaspoon sugar

Freshly ground pepper to taste

$1/2$ pound slightly stale white or whole wheat bread, sliced about $1/2$ inch thick (see note)

2 ounces Gruyère cheese, grated (about $1/2$ cup)

4 large eggs

2 cups milk

$1/4$–$1/2$ teaspoon dried thyme, to taste (optional)

1. Preheat the oven to 350°F. Oil or butter a 2-quart baking or gratin dish.

2. Bring a large pot of water to a boil. Add 1 tablespoon of salt and the greens. Blanch for 2 to 4 minutes, until tender. Transfer immediately to a bowl of cold water. Drain, squeeze out the water, and coarsely chop. Place in a large bowl and add the tomatoes, minced garlic, and sugar. Season with salt and pepper and toss.

3. If the bread is soft, toast it lightly and rub all the slices, front and back, with the cut garlic. If the bread is stale, just rub it

KEY NUTRIENTS
Protein
Beta Carotene
Vitamin A
Vitamin B$_6$
Vitamin B$_{12}$
Folacin
Riboflavin
Vitamin C
Vitamin E
Calcium
Copper (except spinach)
Iron
Magnesium
Manganese
Potassium
Phosphorus
Zinc

with the garlic. Layer half of the slices in the baking dish. Top with half of the tomato-greens mixture. Sprinkle on half of the cheese. Repeat the layers.

4. Beat together the eggs and milk in a medium bowl. Add a scant $^1/_2$ teaspoon salt, a sprinkling of pepper, and the thyme (if using). Pour over the bread mixture. Bake for 40 to 50 minutes, until firm and browned. Serve hot or warm.

NOTE: If the bread is so stale that it's difficult to cut, soak it in 1 cup milk just until soft enough to slice, about 1 minute.

Hot or Cold
Spinach Frittata

Here's a delicious way to obtain a vitamin-packed serving of
greens with protein-rich eggs. Carry wedges of this to work for
lunch, or eat it for dinner. If garlic doesn't agree with you at
this time, leave it out.

2 bunches (about 1½ pounds) spinach, stemmed and
     washed thoroughly, or two 10-ounce packages frozen
     spinach
Salt
8 large eggs
Freshly ground pepper to taste
2–4 garlic cloves (to taste), minced or pressed (optional)
3 tablespoons milk
1 tablespoon olive oil

1. If using fresh spinach, bring a large pot of water to a
rolling boil. Add about 1 teaspoon salt and the spinach. Cook for 1
minute and drain. Rinse with cold water, gently squeeze dry, and
coarsely chop. Alternatively, you can wilt the spinach in a large
nonstick skillet over high heat in the water left on the leaves after
washing. For frozen chopped spinach, thaw in the microwave,
squeeze out the water, and coarsely chop.

KEY NUTRIENTS
Protein
Beta Carotene
Vitamin A
Vitamin B_6
Vitamin B_{12}
Folacin
Riboflavin
Vitamin C
Vitamin E
Calcium
Iron
Magnesium
Manganese
Phosphorus
Potassium

2. Beat the eggs in a large bowl. Season with salt and pepper, then add the garlic (if using), milk, and spinach.

3. Heat the oil in a 10- or 12-inch, heavy-bottomed nonstick skillet over medium-high heat. Hold your hand above the
pan; it should feel hot. Drop a bit of egg into the pan, and if it sizzles and cooks at once, the pan is ready. Pour in the egg mixture.
Swirl the pan to distribute the mixture evenly over the surface.
During the first few minutes of cooking, shake the pan gently, tilt-

ing it slightly with one hand, while lifting up the edges of the omelet with a wooden or plastic spatula in the other hand to let the eggs run underneath. Reduce the heat to low, cover (use a pizza pan if you don't have a lid that fits your skillet), and cook for 10 minutes, shaking the pan gently every once in a while. From time to time, remove the lid and loosen the bottom of the omelet with the spatula, tilting the pan so that the bottom doesn't burn. It will, however, turn a deep golden brown; this is fine. The eggs should be just about set; if they're not, cook for a few minutes longer. Preheat the broiler.

4. Finish the omelet under the broiler for 2 to 3 minutes, watching very carefully to make sure the top doesn't burn. It should brown slightly, and it will puff up. Remove from the heat, shake the pan to make sure the omelet isn't sticking, and let cool for 5 to 15 minutes.

5. Loosen the edges of the omelet with the spatula, then carefully slide it from the pan onto a large, round platter. Serve immediately, or let cool to room temperature, cover, and refrigerate. Serve cold or reheat gently.

VARIATION: You can make this with other greens, such as Swiss chard, beet greens, or kale. Boil tougher greens for 2 to 4 minutes, drain, and proceed as instructed.

ADVANCE
PREPARATION

You can prepare the
ingredients and steam
the broccoli hours be-
fore cooking the dish.
The stir-frying is a
last-minute operation.

Fried Brown Rice and Vegetables

Fried rice is a great dish for using up leftovers — meat, tofu, vegetables, and, of course, rice. It can be simple or elaborate. If you have nothing in the fridge but a carrot or a bunch of broccoli — fine, as long as you have garlic, ginger, soy sauce, and eggs.

1 bunch broccoli, broken into florets, stems peeled and chopped
2 tablespoons peanut or canola oil
1 bunch scallions, white and green parts, sliced separately
2 teaspoons grated or minced fresh ginger
2 large garlic cloves, minced or pressed
2 large eggs, lightly beaten
3 cups cooked brown rice (1 cup uncooked)
1–2 tablespoons soy sauce, to taste
2–3 tablespoons chopped fresh cilantro, to taste

1. Place the broccoli in a steamer basket set in a saucepan with 1 inch of simmering water. Cover and steam for 3 to 5 minutes, until crisp-tender. Transfer to a bowl of ice water, drain, and set aside.

2. Heat the oil in a wok or large nonstick skillet over high heat until a drop of water evaporates on contact. Reduce the heat to medium-high and add the white parts of the scallions. Cook, stirring, for about 2 to 3 minutes, until translucent. Add the ginger and garlic. Cook, stirring, for about 30 seconds, until fragrant and beginning to color. Add the broccoli and stir together for 1 minute, then add the eggs. As soon as they begin to set, stir in the rice and soy sauce. Toss together for a couple of minutes, until the rice is heated through and the eggs are dispersed throughout the rice. Remove from the heat and stir in the cilantro. Taste and adjust the soy sauce, then serve.

KEY NUTRIENTS
Beta Carotene
Vitamin A
Vitamin B$_6$
Folacin
Niacin
Vitamin C
Iron
Magnesium
Manganese
Phosphorus
Potassium

Pan-Cooked Tofu

Tofu browns very nicely in a nonstick skillet, taking on a firm, almost meaty texture. You can marinate it first or season it with a dipping sauce (see pages 60–61) or with soy sauce after browning. Use this tofu in other stir-fried dishes or add it to salads. It's great to have on hand in the refrigerator.

1 pound firm tofu
1–2 tablespoons canola or peanut oil, as needed

1. Drain the tofu, blot dry with paper towels, and cut into ¼-inch-thick slices (thicker if desired) or dice it. Marinate, if desired, in a dipping sauce for 15 minutes or longer.

2. Heat 1 tablespoon of the oil in a large nonstick skillet over medium-high heat. Add the tofu slices in one layer and cook for 2 to 4 minutes, until lightly browned. Turn the tofu over and brown the other side. Alternatively, stir-fry the diced tofu, moving it around and flipping it constantly, for 3 to 5 minutes, until lightly browned on all sides. Add more oil, if necessary. Don't overcook, or the tofu will be hard.

3. Serve hot or at room temperature.

ADVANCE PREPARATION
The tofu can be marinated in the refrigerator for several days. Browned tofu can be kept, covered, in the refrigerator for a day or two.

KEY NUTRIENTS
Protein
Calcium
Iron

Main Dishes

ADVANCE
PREPARATION
The tofu can be mari-
nated for a few days.

Broiled or Grilled Tofu

Be careful not to overcook the tofu. It should be browned, but you need to remove it from the heat after 2 to 4 minutes per side, before the edges become blackened and hard. The tofu will definitely benefit from a marinade. It's best served hot, although leftovers can make a great sandwich (see page 79).

1 pound firm tofu
Dipping sauce of your choice for marinating (see pages
    60–61) or 1 tablespoon canola or peanut oil for
    brushing
Dipping sauce of your choice (see pages 60–61) or soy
    sauce for serving

1. Preheat the broiler or prepare a medium-hot grill. Oil a baking sheet or grill pan.

2. Drain the tofu and pat dry with paper towels. Cut into ¹/₂-inch-thick slices and blot each slice with paper towels. Marinate for at least 15 minutes or simply brush with oil. Broil or grill until just beginning to brown, about 2 to 4 minutes per side. Serve hot with the dipping sauce or soy sauce.

KEY NUTRIENTS
Protein
Calcium
Iron

Stir-Fried Tofu
with Red Chard

ADVANCE
PREPARATION
The greens can be
blanched a day ahead
of time and refriger-
ated. The tofu can mar-
inate for several days
in the refrigerator.

Red chard has a particularly nice way of coloring this savory tofu dish. If you can't find red chard, you can use regular Swiss chard, beet greens, or other greens. Serve this with rice, noodles, or other grains.

2 tablespoons soy sauce
2 tablespoons grated or minced fresh ginger
2 teaspoons sugar
3/4 pound firm tofu, cut into 1-by-1/2-inch pieces
1 tablespoon salt
2 bunches (1 1/2-2 pounds) red chard, stemmed and washed thoroughly
1 tablespoon canola or peanut oil
1-2 garlic cloves (to taste), minced or pressed (optional)

1. Mix together the soy sauce, 1 tablespoon of the ginger, and the sugar in a medium bowl. Add the tofu, toss, and set aside. Marinate for 15 minutes or longer. Refrigerate if not using right away.

2. Bring a large pot of water to a boil. Add the salt and chard. Blanch for 2 minutes, until tender to the bite. Transfer immediately to a bowl of ice water. Drain, squeeze out some of the water, and coarsely chop. If the stems are not too stringy, cut into thin slices.

3. Heat the oil in a large, heavy nonstick skillet or wok over medium-high heat. Add the chard stems, if using, and cook, stirring, for 1 minute. Using a slotted spoon, transfer the tofu to the pan and cook, stirring, until lightly browned, 2 to 4 minutes. Add the garlic, if using, and the remaining 1 tablespoon ginger and stir together for 1 minute. Stir in the chard leaves and cook, stirring, for 1 to 2 minutes more, until heated through and fragrant. Serve hot.

KEY NUTRIENTS
Protein
Beta Carotene
Vitamin A
Vitamin B$_6$
Folacin
Vitamin C
Vitamin E
Calcium
Copper
Iron
Magnesium
Manganese
Potassium

Main Dishes

ADVANCE
PREPARATION
The broccoli can be
steamed and the mari-
nade assembled up to a
day ahead. The tofu
can be marinated for
several days. Keep all
in the refrigerator.

Stir-Fried Tofu with Broccoli and Mushrooms

Tofu can be combined with just about any vegetable for a delicious vegetarian stir-fry. Broccoli works well because the little
flowers absorb the flavors of the marinade and sauce so nicely.

FOR THE MARINADE
1/4 cup soy sauce
1 tablespoon dark sesame oil
1 tablespoon rice wine vinegar
2 garlic cloves, minced
1 teaspoon sugar

FOR THE STIR-FRY
1 pound firm tofu, cut into slices about 1/4 inch thick and
    1 1/2–2 inches long
1 large bunch broccoli (about 1 1/2 pounds)
1/2 cup water or chicken or vegetable stock
2 tablespoons peanut or canola oil
1/2 pound mushrooms, trimmed and thickly sliced
1 tablespoon grated or minced fresh ginger
1 bunch scallions, white and green parts, trimmed and
    sliced
Salt to taste
2 teaspoons arrowroot or cornstarch dissolved in 3
    tablespoons water
1 cup rice, cooked (see page 265); or 6 ounces Asian
    noodles, such as soba or somen, cooked (see page
    262), for serving
Soy sauce for serving

KEY NUTRIENTS
Protein
Beta Carotene
Vitamin A
Vitamin B$_6$
Folacin
Niacin
Riboflavin
Vitamin C
Calcium
Copper
Iron
Manganese
Phosphorus
Potassium

1. FOR THE MARINADE: Mix together all the ingredients in a
large bowl.

2. FOR THE STIR-FRY: Toss the tofu with the marinade. Cover
and refrigerate for at least 15 minutes. Toss the tofu from time to
time to distribute the marinade evenly.

3. Trim the stems from the broccoli and break the tops into small florets. Peel the stems, quarter lengthwise, and slice. Place the broccoli in a steamer basket set in a saucepan with 1 inch of simmering water. Cover and steam for 3 to 4 minutes, until crisp-tender. Rinse abundantly with cold water, or transfer to a bowl of ice water, then drain. Set aside.

4. Using a slotted spoon, transfer the tofu from the marinade to a small bowl. (You can keep the marinade in the refrigerator and reuse with more tofu. Never reuse it if you have marinated fish or meat.) Mix 2 tablespoons of the marinade with the water or stock and set aside.

5. Heat a wok or large, heavy nonstick skillet over medium-high heat until a drop of water evaporates immediately on contact. Add the oil and swirl it around. Add the mushrooms and cook, stirring, until they begin to release their liquid, about 3 minutes. Add the tofu and cook, stirring and tossing, until the tofu is lightly browned, 3 to 5 minutes. Stir in the ginger and the scallions, add a pinch of salt, and cook, stirring, for about 1 minute, until the ginger colors slightly and the scallions are just tender. Add the broccoli and the water or stock mixture, bring to a simmer, and stir together for 1 to 2 minutes, until the broccoli is heated through and the stock simmering. Give the arrowroot or cornstarch mixture a stir and add to the pan. Cook, stirring, until the sauce glazes the tofu and vegetables, which will happen very quickly.

6. Serve at once with the rice or noodles, passing the soy sauce at the table.

Spinach, Broccoli, or Asparagus Flan

This vegetable flan is like a quiche without a crust. You don't have the hassle and the fat calories of a crust, but you still get the creamy, nutritious filling. It's a great vehicle for vegetables. If you're making a low-fat version, add some nonfat dry milk for a richer, creamier filling.

 1 tablespoon olive oil
 ½ medium onion, chopped
 4 large eggs, beaten
 1 cup milk
 2 tablespoons nonfat dry milk, if using 1% or nonfat milk
 ½ teaspoon salt
 Freshly ground pepper to taste
 1 cup chopped blanched spinach or other greens, or 2 cups cooked chopped broccoli or asparagus
 2 ounces Gruyère cheese, grated (about ½ cup)

1. Preheat the oven to 375°F. Oil a 9- or 10-inch pie plate, baking dish, or tart pan.

2. Heat the oil in a small, heavy nonstick skillet over medium heat. Add the onion and cook, stirring, until tender, about 5 minutes. Remove from the heat.

3. Beat together the eggs, milk, dry milk (if using), salt, and pepper in a medium bowl. Stir in the vegetables, cooked onion, and cheese. Turn into the baking dish and bake for 30 minutes, or until the top is browned and the flan is firm. Serve hot, warm, or at room temperature.

Simmered Black Beans or Pinto Beans with Cilantro

ADVANCE PREPARATION
The beans will keep for about 4 days in the refrigerator and freeze well. Cover first with plastic wrap or wax paper before covering with foil, so that the beans don't react with the aluminum. Remember to remove the plastic wrap or wax paper before reheating.

A bowl of brothy beans can make a very satisfying meal. I like to season mine with cilantro and serve them with warm corn tortillas. One pot of beans can make a few meals: a bowl of beans one night, Quesadillas with Black Beans (page 217) the next, and perhaps a main-dish salad, such as Bean Salad with Cumin Vinaigrette (see page 134) for lunch.

1 pound dried black beans or pinto beans, washed and picked over
7–8 cups water, as needed
1 medium onion, chopped
4 large garlic cloves, minced or pressed, or more to taste
Salt to taste (about 2 teaspoons)
2–4 tablespoons chopped fresh cilantro (to taste), plus more for garnish if desired

1. Soak the beans in 7 cups of the water for at least 6 hours. If the weather is hot, put them in the refrigerator.

2. Transfer the beans with their soaking liquid to a large, heavy bean pot, casserole, or Dutch oven. They should be covered by 1 inch of water. Add more water if they are not and bring to a boil. Reduce the heat and skim off any foam that rises to the top. Continue to skim off foam until there isn't any more. Add the onion and half the garlic. Reduce the heat to low, cover, and simmer for 1 hour.

3. Add the salt, remaining garlic, and cilantro. Continue to simmer for 1 hour more, until the beans are quite soft and the broth is thick and fragrant. Taste for salt and garlic and add more if needed.

4. Serve hot, or for the best flavor, let sit overnight in the refrigerator, reheat, and serve.

KEY NUTRIENTS
Protein
Vitamin B$_6$
Folacin
Thiamin
Calcium (pinto beans)
Copper
Iron
Magnesium
Manganese
Phosphorus
Potassium

Main Dishes

ADVANCE
PREPARATION
Refried beans will keep
for 3 days in the
refrigerator and for
several months in the
freezer. Cover first
with plastic wrap or
wax paper before cov-
ering with foil, so that
the beans don't react
with the aluminum. Re-
member to remove the
plastic wrap or wax
paper before
reheating. Keep the re-
served cooking liquid
in a covered container
in the refrigerator.

Refried Beans

A tasty pot of beans can be transformed into delicious refried beans without using lard or even very much oil. This is a boon for those of you who love Mexican food but have to shun fried foods because of calories, fats, and pregnancy-related heart-burn. These beans, which I have been making for many years, cook in their own broth. They're great for tostadas, tacos, and nachos.

Simmered Black Beans or Pinto Beans with Cilantro (page 229)
2 tablespoons canola oil
1 tablespoon ground cumin
2 teaspoons pure ground chili powder, mild or medium-hot
Salt to taste (optional)

1. Drain off about 1 cup of liquid from the cooked beans, and set aside. Mash half the beans coarsely in a food processor or with a bean or potato masher. Don't puree them; you want texture. Stir the mashed beans back into the pot.

2. Heat the oil in a large, heavy-bottomed nonstick skillet over medium heat. Add the cumin and chili powder and cook, stir-ring for about 1 minute, until the spices begin to sizzle and cook. Increase the heat to medium-high and add the beans. (This can be done in batches, in which case you should cook the spices in batches as well.) Fry the beans, stirring and mashing often, until they thicken and begin to get aromatic and crusty on the bottom. Stir up the crust each time it forms and mix it into the beans. Cook for about 20 minutes, stirring often and mashing the beans with the back of a wooden spoon or a bean masher. The beans should be thick but not dry. Add the reserved cooking liquid if they seem too dry, but if you will be reheating them later, save some of the liquid for moistening before you reheat them. Taste and adjust the salt, if necessary.

KEY NUTRIENTS
Protein
Vitamin B$_6$
Folacin
Thiamin
Copper
Iron
Magnesium
Manganese
Phosphorus
Potassium

3. Serve immediately, or set aside in the pan if you will be serving within a few hours; reheat in the pan. Otherwise, transfer the beans to a lightly oiled baking dish, cover with foil, and refrigerate. Reheat for 30 minutes in a 325°F oven. In either case, moisten with the reserved cooking liquid before reheating.

VARIATION
Quick Refried Beans

Although canned beans never taste as good as beans you cook with lots of onion, garlic, and spices, they are suitable for making refried beans in a hurry. For 2 cups refried beans, you will need two 15-ounce cans beans (4 cans yields the same amount as this recipe). Do not drain off the liquid or puree the beans. Heat the oil and spices as directed above. Pour in the beans with their liquid and mash with the back of a wooden spoon or a bean masher. Cook, stirring, as instructed. You will need to add water, as refried canned beans will dry out considerably.

ADVANCE
PREPARATION
Cooked black beans
will keep for about 4
days in the refrigera-
tor and freeze well.
Cover first with plastic
wrap or wax paper be-
fore covering with foil,
so that the beans don't
react with the alu-
minum. Remember to
remove the plastic
wrap or wax paper be-
fore reheating.

Quick Black Bean Tacos

You can use canned or homemade black beans for these easy,
nutritious tacos. The filling is a bit runny. If you wish, you can
mash the beans so that it's easier to eat the soft tacos with your
hands.

3 cups cooked black beans with some liquid (see page 229)
    or Refried Beans (page 230); or two 15-ounce cans
    black beans
8 corn tortillas, warmed (see page 40)
1 cup salsa, homemade (page 63) or commercial
2 ounces feta cheese or packaged queso fresco, crumbled
    (about 1/2 cup)

1. Heat the beans in a large saucepan over medium heat
until bubbling. If the bean broth is very liquid, boil the beans until
the liquid reduces somewhat. Mash the beans, if desired.

2. Spoon the beans with a bit of their liquid onto the tortillas. Top each with salsa and cheese, fold the tortillas over the filling, and serve.

KEY NUTRIENTS
Protein
Vitamin A
Vitamin B_6
Folacin
Thiamin
Vitamin C
Vitamin E
Copper
Iron
Magnesium
Manganese
Phosphorus
Potassium

Soft Tacos or Tostadas with Chicken, Corn, and Avocado

ADVANCE PREPARATION

The cooked chicken will keep for a couple of days in the refrigerator. The chicken mixture can be made several hours ahead of serving and refrigerated.

Here's another quick summer meal that combines protein, vegetables, and grain in one healthy package.

4 cups water
Salt to taste (about ½ teaspoon)
2 boneless, skinless chicken breast halves, preferably free-range and hormone-free
2 ears corn
1 ripe avocado, peeled, pitted, and diced
1 large tomato, finely chopped
1–3 serrano peppers or 1–2 jalapeño peppers (to taste), seeded for a milder dish and minced
5–6 tablespoons fresh lime juice, to taste
6 tablespoons chopped fresh cilantro
8 corn tortillas, warmed (see page 40)
Salsa, homemade (page 63) or commercial for serving

1. Bring the water to a boil in a large saucepan. Add the salt and chicken breasts. Reduce the heat and simmer for 10 to 13 minutes, until the breasts are cooked through. Remove the chicken from the pan and let cool. When cool enough to handle, shred the chicken. You should have about 2 cups shredded chicken.

2. Place the corn in a steamer basket set in a saucepan with 1 inch simmering water. Cover and steam for 5 minutes. Rinse with cold water, then cut the kernels from the cob.

3. In a medium bowl, toss together the chicken, corn, avocado, tomato, peppers, lime juice, and cilantro. Taste and adjust the seasonings.

4. Top the tortillas with the chicken mixture and serve, passing the salsa at the table.

KEY NUTRIENTS
Vitamin A
Vitamin B_6
Vitamin B_{12}
Folacin
Niacin
Thiamin
Vitamin C
Vitamin E
Copper
Iron
Magnesium
Phosphorus
Potassium

Main Dishes

ADVANCE
PREPARATION

The refried beans will
hold for 3 days in the
refrigerator and can be
frozen. Cover first with
plastic wrap or wax
paper before covering
with foil, so that the
beans don't react with
the aluminum. Remem-
ber to remove the
plastic wrap or wax
paper before
reheating. The tortilla
crisps will hold for sev-
eral hours. The ricotta
or cottage cheese can
be blended and mixed
with the yogurt 2 to 3
days ahead of time.
Stir before using. The
toasted almonds will
keep for weeks in the
refrigerator.

Black Bean Tostadas
(Chalupas)

This is my favorite Mexican meal: crisp corn tortillas slathered
with savory refried black beans and topped with fresh tomato
salsa and crumbled cheese. It makes a terrific, high-protein
vegetarian main dish.

12 corn tortillas
 1 cup ricotta or cottage cheese
 1/3 cup plain yogurt
    Refried Beans (page 230; use black beans)
 2 cups shredded lettuce
 1 1/2 cups salsa, homemade (page 63) or commercial
    Scant 1/2 cup whole almonds, toasted (see page 187) and
        coarsely chopped
 2 ounces feta cheese or packaged queso fresco, crumbled
    (about 1/2 cup)

1. Cut the tortillas in half for smaller portions or leave
whole. If you have a microwave, place 1 or 2 tortillas in the microwave and cook for 1 minute at 100% power, or high. Turn the
tortillas over and cook for 1 minute more. Repeat until the tortillas
are crisp and lightly browned. If you don't have a microwave, toast
in a 350°F oven until crisp. Set aside.

2. Blend the ricotta or cottage cheese in a food processor
until smooth. Add the yogurt and continue to blend until smooth.
Set aside.

3. Reheat the beans in the pan, adding the reserved cooking liquid if they seem dry. Or reheat the beans for 30 minutes in a
lightly oiled, covered baking dish in a 325°F oven. Spoon some of
the reserved liquid over the top if they seem dry.

KEY NUTRIENTS
Protein
Beta Carotene
Vitamin A
Vitamin B$_6$
Vitamin B$_{12}$
Folacin
Riboflavin
Thiamin
Vitamin C
Vitamin E
Copper
Iron
Magnesium
Manganese
Phosphorus
Potassium

4. Spread a generous spoonful of black beans over each crisp tortilla. Top with some of the ricotta or cottage cheese mixture, then a generous handful of lettuce. Spoon on some salsa and sprinkle with the almonds and crumbled cheese. Serve immediately.

Egg and Bean Tacos

Makes 4 servings

ADVANCE
PREPARATION
The Refried Beans can
be made 3 or 4 days
ahead and held in the
refrigerator.

You can cook and refry your beans for this dish, or use canned beans for a quicker dish. These tacos are great for breakfast, lunch, or dinner.

8 large eggs
$^3/_4$ cup Refried Beans (page 230; use black beans)
Salt to taste
1 tablespoon olive oil
$^1/_2$ small white onion, finely chopped (about $^1/_3$ cup; optional)
1–2 jalapeño peppers, seeded and minced (optional)
8 corn tortillas, warmed (see page 40)

1. Beat the eggs in a large bowl. Add the beans and beat together. Add the salt.

2. Heat the oil in a large, heavy-bottomed nonstick skillet over medium heat. Add the onion and peppers, if using. Cook, stirring, until the onion is tender, about 5 minutes. Add the egg-and-bean mixture and cook, stirring constantly, until the eggs are scrambled. Remove from the heat and serve on the warm tortillas.

KEY NUTRIENTS
Protein
Vitamin A
Vitamin B_6
Vitamin B_{12}
Folacin
Riboflavin
Thiamin
Calcium
Copper
Iron
Magnesium
Manganese
Phosphorus
Potassium

GRAIN AND VEGETABLE DISHES

Asian Greens 238

Mediterranean Greens 239

Wilted Spinach with Lemon Juice 240

Southern Italian–Style Broccoli Rabe 241

Broccoli with Garlic and Lemon 242

Roasted Beets and Beet Greens 243

Steamed Artichokes with Dips 244

Braised Red Cabbage 246

Pan-Cooked Summer Squash 247

Summer Vegetable Gratin 248

Zucchini and Rice Gratin 249

Corn Gratin 250

Tomato Gratin 251

Steamed New Potatoes or Fingerlings with
    Herbs 252

Baked Potatoes Two Ways 253

Baked Potato Skins 254

Potato Gratin 255

Baked Sweet Potatoes 256

Basmati Rice Pilaf with Chickpeas 257

Basmati Rice Pilaf with Peas 258

Easy Polenta 260

Polenta with Tomato Sauce and Beans 261

Asian Noodles 262

Basic Cooking Directions for Some Grains 263

    BULGUR 263

    COUSCOUS 263

    QUINOA 265

    RICE 265

    WILD RICE 267

    WHEAT BERRIES 267

ADVANCE
PREPARATION
The blanched greens
will keep for a couple
of days in the refriger-
ator.

Asian Greens

Ginger, garlic, and soy sauce are the seasonings for these healthy greens. You can omit the garlic if it doesn't sit well with you.

2 large bunches (1¹/₂–2 pounds) greens, such as Swiss
    chard, beet greens, turnip greens, or kale, stemmed
    and washed thoroughly
1 tablespoon salt, plus more to taste
1 tablespoon canola or peanut oil
2 large garlic cloves, minced or pressed (optional)
1 tablespoon grated or minced fresh ginger
1 tablespoon soy sauce, or more to taste

1. Bring a large pot of water to a boil. Add the 1 tablespoon salt and the greens. Cook for 2 to 4 minutes (depending on the type of greens), until tender. Drain and rinse with cold water. Gently squeeze out the water (you don't have to squeeze them completely dry) and coarsely chop.

2. Heat the oil in a large, heavy nonstick skillet over medium-high heat. Add the garlic, if using, and ginger. Cook, stirring, until fragrant and beginning to color, about 30 to 60 seconds. Stir in the greens and add the soy sauce and salt to taste. Heat through and serve immediately.

KEY NUTRIENTS
Beta Carotene
Vitamin A
Vitamin B₆
Folacin
Vitamin C
Vitamin E
Calcium
Copper (except
    spinach)
Iron
Magnesium
Manganese
Potassium

Mediterranean Greens

ADVANCE PREPARATION
The blanched greens will keep for a couple of days in the refrigerator.

A number of seasonings can add a Mediterranean dimension to greens: garlic and lemon, garlic and hot red pepper flakes, or just plain garlic and olive oil.

1 tablespoon salt, plus more to taste
2 large bunches (1¹/₂–2 pounds) greens, such as Swiss chard, beet greens, turnip greens, or kale, stemmed and washed thoroughly
1 tablespoon olive oil
1–2 garlic cloves (to taste), minced or pressed
   Juice of ¹/₂ lemon
   Hot red pepper flakes to taste (optional)

1. Bring a large pot of water to a boil and add the 1 tablespoon salt. Add the greens and cook for 2 to 4 minutes (depending on the greens), until tender. Drain and rinse with cold water. Gently squeeze dry and coarsely chop.

2. Heat the oil in a large, heavy nonstick skillet over medium heat. Add the garlic and cook for about 30 seconds, until it begins to color. Add the greens and cook, stirring, until heated through. Stir in the lemon juice, salt, and hot pepper. Serve hot or cold. If serving cold, add the lemon juice just before serving.

KEY NUTRIENTS
Beta Carotene
Vitamin A
Vitamin B₆
Folacin
Vitamin C
Vitamin E
Calcium
Copper (except spinach)
Iron
Magnesium
Manganese
Potassium

Grain and

Vegetable Dishes

ADVANCE
PREPARATION
Cooked spinach will
keep for 3 or 4 days in
the refrigerator. Cover
the bowl tightly with
plastic wrap.

Wilted Spinach
with Lemon Juice

Serve this fresh spinach — just wilted and doused with a bit of fresh lemon juice — as a side dish with fish, chicken, or meat, or with vegetarian dishes such as Basmati Rice Pilaf with Chickpeas (page 257) or Spinach, Broccoli, or Asparagus Flan (page 228).

1½ pounds fresh spinach, stemmed and washed thoroughly
Salt and freshly ground pepper to taste
Juice of 1 lemon or lemon wedges for serving

Heat a large nonstick skillet over high heat and add the spinach leaves in batches. As each batch begins to wilt, add another handful. Cook, stirring, until all the spinach is wilted. Season with salt and pepper and stir for 1 to 2 minutes, until the spinach is a deep, bright green. Squeeze on the lemon juice (if using) and serve. If not using the juice, serve with the lemon wedges.

KEY NUTRIENTS
Beta Carotene
Vitamin A
Vitamin B_6
Folacin
Riboflavin
Vitamin C
Vitamin E
Calcium
Iron
Magnesium
Manganese
Potassium

EVERY WOMAN'S

GUIDE TO EATING

DURING PREGNANCY

Southern Italian–Style Broccoli Rabe

Broccoli rabe, also called rapini and cima, is a thick-stemmed green with broccoli-like flowers. This is a classic southern Italian side dish, or you can toss it with pasta.

1½ pounds broccoli rabe
2 teaspoons salt, plus more to taste
2 tablespoons olive oil
2–3 garlic cloves (to taste), minced or pressed
1 dried hot chile pepper, seeded and crumbled, or
    ¼ teaspoon hot red pepper flakes

1. Bring a large pot of water to a boil while you prepare the ingredients.

2. Wash the broccoli rabe and break or cut off the tough stem ends. When the water comes to a boil, add the 2 teaspoons salt and broccoli rabe. Boil for 5 minutes, until the stems are tender. Remove ½ cup cooking water from the pot and reserve. Drain the broccoli rabe.

3. Heat the oil in a large, heavy-bottomed nonstick skillet over medium heat. Add the garlic and chile pepper or red pepper flakes. Cook, stirring, for about 30 seconds, until the garlic begins to color. Stir in the rabe and the reserved cooking water and cook, stirring, until the water evaporates. Season with salt and serve.

ADVANCE PREPARATION

This can be made several hours ahead of time and reheated gently. The broccoli rabe can be boiled and held in the refrigerator for a few days.

KEY NUTRIENTS
Beta Carotene
Vitamin A
Vitamin B$_6$
Folacin
Vitamin C
Vitamin E
Calcium
Copper
Iron
Magnesium
Manganese
Potassium

Grain and

Vegetable Dishes

ADVANCE
PREPARATION

This can be made hours
ahead and reheated,
but don't add the
lemon juice until just
before serving. If you
do, the broccoli will
discolor, and the fla-
vors will not be as
vivid.

Broccoli with Garlic and Lemon

Lemon and garlic, classic seasonings for Mediterranean-style greens, also work well with broccoli. If garlic doesn't appeal to you while you're pregnant, omit it.

- 1 large bunch broccoli (about 1½ pounds)
- 1 tablespoon olive oil
- 1–2 garlic cloves (to taste), minced or pressed (optional)
  Salt and freshly ground pepper to taste
- 1–3 tablespoons fresh lemon juice, to taste

1. Break or cut off the broccoli florets. Peel the stems, cut them into halves or quarters lengthwise, and slice about ½ inch thick. Place the broccoli in a steamer basket set in a saucepan with 1 inch of simmering water. Cover and steam for 5 minutes, or until tender. Transfer to a colander and run it under cold water, or transfer to a bowl of ice water, then drain.

2. Heat the oil in a large, heavy nonstick skillet over medium heat. Add the garlic, if using, and cook, stirring, until it just begins to color, 30 seconds to 1 minute. Add the broccoli and stir to heat through. Add the salt and pepper and lemon juice. Serve hot or warm.

KEY NUTRIENTS
Beta Carotene
Vitamin A
Vitamin B$_6$
Folacin
Vitamin C
Manganese
Potassium

Roasted Beets and Beet Greens

The easiest way to cook beets is to roast them in their skins. This method also results in particularly sweet, tender beets. While they are roasting, blanch the greens, then serve the two together.

1 bunch beets, with greens
2 teaspoons salt, plus more to taste
Freshly ground pepper to taste
1/2 lemon

1. Preheat the oven to 425°F. Cut away the greens from the beets, about 1/2 inch up from the base of the stems, and set aside. Scrub the beets under warm water with a vegetable brush. Place in a baking dish and add about 1/4 inch of water. Cover tightly with a lid or foil and bake for 30 to 60 minutes, depending on the size of the beets. Medium-size beets take about 40 minutes, large beets 50 to 60 minutes, and small beets about 30 minutes. Test for doneness by sticking a knife into a beet. It should slide in easily. Remove from the oven and let cool. If there is time, leave the lid on while the beets cool; they will continue to steam, and it will be even easier to slip off the skins.

2. While the beets are in the oven, prepare the greens. Stem and wash thoroughly in several changes of water. Bring a large pot of water to a boil. Add the 2 teaspoons salt and the greens. Boil for about 2 minutes, until tender. Transfer to a bowl of cold water, then drain. Gently squeeze out the water and coarsely chop. Place in a serving dish or on individual plates. Season with salt and pepper. Keep warm or let cool to room temperature.

3. When the beets are cool enough to handle, cut away the ends and slip off the skins. Cut into wedges or slices and place on top of the greens. Squeeze on some lemon juice and serve.

Makes 2 servings

ADVANCE PREPARATION
Roasted beets, peeled or unpeeled, and blanched greens, will keep for several days in the refrigerator. They can be reheated in the microwave or dipped in a pot of simmering water.

KEY NUTRIENTS
Beta Carotene
Vitamin A
Vitamin B$_6$
Folacin
Vitamin C
Vitamin E
Calcium
Copper
Iron
Magnesium

Grain and

Vegetable Dishes

ADVANCE
PREPARATION
Cooked artichokes will
keep, covered, for 3 to
5 days in the refriger-
ator.

Steamed Artichokes with Dips

A steamed artichoke, hot or cold, can start a meal or make one. Sometimes artichokes are so large that one will be sufficient for two people.

2 large or 4 medium artichokes
¹/₂ lemon

OPTIONAL DIPS
Classic Vinaigrette (page 164)
Low-Fat Mayonnaise (page 64)
Tofu Mayonnaise (page 66)
Yogurt Dip with Mint or Dill (recipe follows)
Creamy Garlic Dip (recipe follows)

1. Lay each artichoke on a cutting board and, using a sharp chef's knife, cut away the entire top quarter in one slice. Now cut away the thorny ends of the leaves with a scissors. This goes faster than you think. Cut off the stems so that the artichoke will stand upright. Rinse thoroughly under cold water. Rub the cut surfaces with the lemon.

2. Place the artichokes in a steamer basket set in a saucepan or wok with 1 inch of simmering water. Or place them right in the water. Cover and steam for 30 to 40 minutes, depending on the size. Check from time to time to make sure the water hasn't all evaporated. Test for doneness by pulling a leaf away; it should not resist.

3. Serve hot with any of the dips of your choice. Or rinse with cold water, let cool, and serve at room temperature. You also may serve the artichokes cold.

KEY NUTRIENTS
Folacin
Vitamin C
Copper
Iron
Magnesium
Manganese
Phosphorus
Potassium

Yogurt Dip with Mint or Dill

Makes about $^3/_4$ cup

$^3/_4$ cup plain yogurt or Yogurt Cheese (page 65)
1 tablespoon Hellmann's or Best Foods mayonnaise
1–2 garlic cloves (to taste), cut in half
$^1/_4$ teaspoon salt
$^1/_4$ cup chopped fresh mint or dill
Fresh lemon juice to taste

Stir the yogurt or Yogurt Cheese and mayonnaise together in a small bowl. Pound the garlic and salt to a paste with a mortar and pestle or mash on a cutting board with the back of a chef's knife. Stir into the yogurt, along with the mint or dill and lemon juice. Chill until ready to serve.

ADVANCE PREPARATION
These dips are best served the day they are made, as the garlic becomes quite pungent over time.

KEY NUTRIENTS
Vitamin B$_{12}$
Riboflavin
Calcium (yogurt dip)
Phosphorus

Creamy Garlic Dip

Makes about $^3/_4$ cup

1 garlic clove, cut in half
$^1/_4$ teaspoon salt, or more to taste
$^1/_2$ cup cottage cheese
3 tablespoons plain yogurt
2 tablespoons Hellmann's or Best Foods mayonnaise

Pound the garlic and salt to a paste with a mortar and pestle or mash on a cutting board with the back of a chef's knife. Blend the cottage cheese in a food processor or mini-processor until fairly smooth. Add the yogurt and mayonnaise and continue to blend until very smooth. Add the garlic-salt paste and combine well. Taste and adjust the salt. Chill until ready to serve.

ADVANCE PREPARATION
The dip can be made 1 to 2 days ahead.

KEY NUTRIENTS
Vitamin B$_{12}$
Riboflavin
Phosphorus

ADVANCE
PREPARATION
This is best made a day
ahead. It will keep for
4 to 5 days in the
refrigerator.

Braised Red Cabbage

Bacon or lard is used in traditional German braised red cabbage, which is often served with roast pork. So that vegetarians won't miss out on this dish, I give an alternative here.

1 medium head (2–2¹/₂ pounds) red cabbage, quartered, cored, and shredded crosswise
2 slices bacon, diced, or 2 tablespoons peanut oil
¹/₂ medium onion, minced
1 tablespoon sugar
1 large tart apple, such as Granny Smith, peeled, cored, and chopped
¹/₄ cup red wine vinegar
Salt to taste (¹/₄–¹/₂ teaspoon if using bacon; up to 1 teaspoon if using oil)
³/₄–1 cup water, as needed

1. Cover the cabbage with cold water in a large bowl while you prepare the remaining ingredients.

2. Heat the bacon in a large nonreactive skillet or Dutch oven over low heat until it renders its fat, or heat the oil. Add the onion and cook, stirring, until tender, about 5 minutes. Add the sugar and cook, stirring, until the mixture is golden, about 5 minutes. Stir in the apple, cover, and cook, stirring from time to time, for 3 to 4 minutes. Drain the cabbage and add to the skillet. Toss to coat thoroughly with fat, then stir in the vinegar and toss together. Cover the pot and braise for 10 minutes, or until the cabbage is bright pinkish purple. Add the salt and ³/₄ cup of the water. Increase the heat to medium-low and bring to a simmer. Cover and simmer for 1 to 1¹/₂ hours, stirring from time to time. Add more water, if necessary. The cabbage should be very tender. Taste and adjust the salt.

KEY NUTRIENTS
Folacin
Vitamin C

3. Serve immediately if you must, or transfer to a covered container and refrigerate overnight. Reheat gently and serve.

Pan-Cooked
Summer Squash

ADVANCE
PREPARATION
For best results, serve
at once.

This simple cooked squash makes a great side dish. It also can
be combined with black beans or pinto beans and crumbled
cheese on corn tortillas for quesadillas or soft tacos.

1 tablespoon olive oil
2 garlic cloves, minced or pressed (optional)
1–1¹/₂ pounds summer squash (a mixture of colors is nice),
     sliced about ¹/₄ inch thick (if very large, cut
     lengthwise into halves or quarters, then slice)
Salt to taste (about ¹/₄ teaspoon)
Freshly ground pepper to taste
Chopped fresh herbs, such as parsley, thyme, or chives,
     for garnish (optional)

Heat the oil in a large, heavy nonstick skillet over medium
heat. Add the garlic, if using, and cook for about 30 seconds, just
until it begins to smell fragrant. Add the squash and salt. Cook,
stirring often, for 5 to 10 minutes, until the squash is tender and
translucent. Add lots of pepper, then garnish with the herbs, if you
wish. Serve hot.

KEY NUTRIENTS
Folacin
Vitamin C

Grain and

Vegetable Dishes

ADVANCE
PREPARATION
This can be made several hours ahead of serving.

Summer Vegetable Gratin

This beautiful, bright, vegetable-studded summer gratin will provide you with high-quality protein and can be eaten as a main dish or side dish. For a lower-fat version, use 1% milk and enrich with nonfat dry milk.

- 1 tablespoon olive oil
- 1 small sweet onion, chopped
- 1 medium or large red bell pepper, seeded and diced
- 3 medium zucchini ($1^1/_4$–$1^1/_2$ pounds), diced
- 1–2 large garlic cloves (to taste), minced or pressed
  Salt to taste (about $^3/_4$ teaspoon)
- 1 ear corn, kernels cut from the cob
  Freshly ground pepper to taste
- 1 teaspoon chopped fresh thyme or $^1/_2$ teaspoon dried
- 3 large eggs
- $^3/_4$ cup milk
- 2 tablespoons nonfat dry milk, if using 1% milk
- 2 ounces Gruyère cheese, grated (about $^1/_2$ cup)

1. Preheat the oven to 375°F. Oil a 2-quart baking or gratin dish.

2. Heat the oil in a large, heavy nonstick skillet over medium heat. Add the onion and cook, stirring, until just tender, 3 to 5 minutes. Add the bell pepper and cook, stirring, until it begins to soften, about 3 minutes. Add the zucchini, garlic, and about $^1/_4$ teaspoon salt and continue to cook, stirring often, until the zucchini is translucent but still bright green. Stir in the corn, pepper, and thyme and cook, stirring, for a few minutes more, until the corn is barely tender. Transfer to the baking dish.

3. In a medium bowl, beat together the eggs, milk, and dry milk (if using). Add about $^1/_2$ teaspoon salt and season with pepper. Add the cheese and stir together. Pour over the zucchini mixture. Bake for 30 to 40 minutes, until firm and browned. Serve hot or at room temperature.

KEY NUTRIENTS
Protein
Beta Carotene
Vitamin A
Vitamin B_6
Vitamin B_{12}
Folacin
Riboflavin
Thiamin
Vitamin C
Calcium
Iron
Magnesium
Phosphorus

Zucchini and Rice Gratin

ADVANCE
PREPARATION
This can be made a day
ahead and held in the
refrigerator, tightly
wrapped.

Here's another nutritious main dish or side dish that is easy to pack for lunch. Eggs and rice are the binder for this Provençal gratin.

2 tablespoons olive oil
1 medium onion, minced
2 pounds zucchini or yellow summer squash (or a mixture), finely diced
2 garlic cloves, minced or pressed
Salt and freshly ground pepper to taste
2 large eggs
2 ounces Gruyère cheese, grated (about ½ cup)
½ cup uncooked long-grain or medium-grain rice (about 1½ cups cooked)
½ cup chopped fresh parsley
1 teaspoon chopped fresh thyme or ½ teaspoon dried
2 tablespoons fresh or dry bread crumbs

1. Preheat the oven to 375°F. Brush a 2-quart baking or gratin dish with olive oil.

2. Heat 1 tablespoon of the oil in a large, heavy nonstick skillet over medium heat. Add the onion and cook, stirring, until tender, about 5 minutes. Add the squash, garlic, and salt and pepper. Cook, stirring often, for 8 to 10 minutes, until the squash is tender but not mushy. Remove from the heat and let cool slightly.

3. Beat the eggs in a medium bowl. Stir in the squash and onion, cheese, rice, parsley, and thyme. Transfer to the baking dish, sprinkle with the bread crumbs, and drizzle with the remaining 1 tablespoon oil. Bake for 45 minutes, until firm and browned.

4. Let cool briefly on a rack and serve warm. Or refrigerate and serve cold.

KEY NUTRIENTS
Folacin
Vitamin C

Grain and

Vegetable Dishes

ADVANCE
PREPARATION
This can be made sev-
eral hours ahead and
reheated.

Corn Gratin

Corn, not cream, makes this marvelous gratin creamy. It can be eaten as a main dish or side dish.

- 3 large ears corn
- $2/3$ cup milk
- $3/4$ teaspoon salt
- $1/2$ teaspoon sugar
- 4 large eggs
- $1/2$ teaspoon crushed cumin seeds
  Freshly ground pepper to taste
- 2 ounces Gruyère cheese, grated (about $1/2$ cup)

1. Preheat the oven to 375°. Oil or butter a 2-quart baking or gratin dish.

2. Cut the kernels from 1 ear of corn and set aside. Cut the kernels from the other 2 ears and place in a blender with the milk, salt, and sugar. Blend until fairly smooth.

3. Beat the eggs in a large bowl. Stir in the corn mixture, reserved corn kernels, cumin, pepper, and cheese. Pour into the gratin dish and bake for 45 to 60 minutes, until firm and browned. Serve hot or warm.

KEY NUTRIENTS
Protein
Vitamin A
Vitamin B$_{12}$
Folacin
Riboflavin
Thiamin
Vitamin C
Calcium
Iron
Magnesium
Phosphorus
Zinc

Tomato Gratin

ADVANCE
PREPARATION
You can make this dish
hours ahead.

This is a dish to make at the height of tomato season, but also if you have some tomatoes lying around that are less than perfect. The long cooking brings out the sugars in the tomatoes. The gratin is as good at room temperature as it is hot. It makes a great side dish with grilled meat or fish.

2 pounds ripe but firm tomatoes, sliced ½ inch thick
  Salt to taste
1 teaspoon sugar
1 cup fresh or dry bread crumbs
2 tablespoons chopped fresh parsley
2–3 tablespoons olive oil, to taste

1. Preheat the oven to 400°F. Oil a 2-quart baking or gratin dish.

2. Layer the tomatoes in the dish, sprinkling each layer with salt and a little of the sugar. In a small bowl, toss together the bread crumbs, parsley, and olive oil. Spread over the tomatoes in an even layer. Bake for about 1½ hours, until the top is golden brown and the juices in the dish are quite thick. Serve warm, at room temperature (my preference), or cold.

KEY NUTRIENTS
Vitamin A
Vitamin C
Vitamin E

Grain and

Vegetable Dishes

Steamed New Potatoes or Fingerlings with Herbs

ADVANCE PREPARATION
You can steam the potatoes hours ahead and refrigerate. Reheat by steaming for another couple of minutes or by plunging into a pot of simmering water and draining.

New potatoes with herbs go well as a side dish with just about anything — meat, fish, chicken, or a savory vegetarian tart, omelet, or gratin.

1¹/₂ pounds small waxy potatoes, such as new potatoes or
      fingerlings, scrubbed, or larger potatoes, such as
      Yukon Gold, scrubbed and quartered
1 tablespoon olive oil
Coarse sea salt and freshly ground pepper to taste

OPTIONAL HERBS
6–12 fresh sage leaves (to taste), cut into slivers
1 tablespoon snipped fresh dill
1–2 tablespoons chopped fresh parsley and/or chives, to
      taste
1 tablespoon snipped fresh chervil

1. Place the potatoes in a steamer basket set in a saucepan with 1 inch of simmering water. Cover and steam for 10 to 20 minutes, until tender. Drain.

2. Transfer the potatoes to a warm serving bowl. Add the olive oil, salt and pepper, and any of the herbs of your choice. Serve hot.

KEY NUTRIENTS
Vitamin B$_6$
Niacin
Vitamin C
Copper
Iron
Magnesium
Manganese
Potassium

Baked Potatoes
Two Ways

Baked Russet Potatoes

Idaho russets are the best potatoes for baking. There's nothing to it.

4 Idaho russet potatoes, scrubbed
  Yogurt Cheese (page 65) or sour cream, plain or mixed
      with chopped fresh chives or other herbs, for serving

Preheat the oven to 425°F. Pierce the potatoes in a few places with a sharp knife or fork. Place directly on the middle oven rack and bake for about 1 hour, until tender. Remove from the oven and slice down the middle, then across. Serve with Yogurt Cheese or sour cream.

Dry-Roasted Waxy Potatoes

These hassle-free potatoes need no oil and taste so good that you won't want to reach for the butter or sour cream. Don't use russets — the normal baking potatoes — for these; they're too dry. Use a waxy or semiwaxy potato, such as Yukon Gold or White Rose. If you are sensitive to carbohydrates, this is a better baked potato for you than a russet.

1¹/₂–2 pounds medium waxy or semiwaxy potatoes, scrubbed
          and cut in half lengthwise
       Salt, preferably coarse sea salt, and freshly ground
          pepper to taste
       Dried thyme to taste (optional)

Preheat the oven to 400°F. Put the potatoes on a baking sheet, cut side up. Sprinkle with the salt and pepper and thyme, if using. Bake for 30 to 40 minutes, until tender and the tops are puffed and browned. Serve hot or warm.

ADVANCE
PREPARATION
You can make these an hour before serving and keep them warm in the oven. Just turn off the oven when they're done and leave them in there.

KEY NUTRIENTS
Vitamin B$_6$
Niacin
Vitamin C
Copper
Iron
Magnesium
Manganese
Potassium

Grain and

Vegetable Dishes

ADVANCE PREPARATION
The potatoes can be baked hours or even days ahead of hollowing out and crisping the shells.

Baked Potato Skins

Floury russet potatoes have quite a high glycemic index, so if you have to watch your carbs, they're best avoided. However, the skins are fine and taste great when baked until crisp. Seek out organic potatoes for this dish: potatoes absorb pesticides very easily, and much of the residue settles in the skins.

    2 large organic baking potatoes, scrubbed
    1 tablespoon butter, melted
      Salt and pepper to taste
  ³/₄ cup Herbed Yogurt Cheese (page 65)

1. Preheat the oven to 400°F. Pierce the potatoes in a few places with a sharp knife or fork. Place directly on the middle oven rack and bake for 1 hour, until tender on the inside and crisp on the outside. Remove from the oven and let cool until you can handle them.

2. Cut the potatoes in half lengthwise. Scoop out and set aside the flesh for another purpose; you can leave a little flesh lining the shells. Place the shells on a baking sheet. Brush with the butter, season with salt and pepper, and return to the oven. Bake for 10 to 15 minutes, until crisp. Fill with the cheese and serve.

KEY NUTRIENTS
Vitamin B₆
Vitamin B₁₂
Niacin
Riboflavin
Vitamin C
Calcium
Copper
Iron
Magnesium
Manganese
Phosphorus
Potassium

Potato Gratin

ADVANCE
PREPARATION
This should be baked as
soon as it is assembled,
but it can be made
ahead and reheated in
a 350°F oven for 20
minutes.

Serve a potato gratin with your meal, and you'll get lots of delicious, useful calories. You can use 1% milk, if you wish. This is a toned-down version of a classic French potato gratin, with virtually no butter or cream.

    2 large garlic cloves, cut in half lengthwise
    3 pounds baking or Yukon Gold potatoes, scrubbed and
        sliced about 1/4 inch thick
    2 large eggs
 3 1/2 cups milk
    1 teaspoon salt, or to taste
      Freshly ground pepper, to taste
    3 ounces Gruyère cheese, grated (about 3/4 cup)

1. Preheat the oven to 375°F. Rub the inside of a 3-quart baking or gratin dish with the garlic. Arrange the potatoes in an even layer in the dish.

2. Beat the eggs in a medium bowl. Add the milk, salt, pepper, and cheese. Pour over the potatoes. Bake for 1 to 1 1/2 hours, until the top is golden and crusty. During the first hour, remove the gratin from the oven every 15 minutes and break up the top layer with a large spoon or knife, then stir and fold it into the rest of the potatoes. Serve hot or warm.

KEY NUTRIENTS
Vitamin B$_6$
Vitamin B$_{12}$
Niacin
Riboflavin
Vitamin C
Calcium
Copper
Iron
Magnesium
Manganese
Potassium
Phosphorus

Grain and

Vegetable Dishes

ADVANCE
PREPARATION
Cooked sweet potatoes
actually benefit from
sitting in the refriger-
ator for several hours
or overnight, as they
continue to exude their
sweetness. Place in a
covered dish in the re-
frigerator and reheat
in the microwave or a
350°F oven.

Baked Sweet Potatoes

You can bake several sweet potatoes at once and keep them in the refrigerator. They make a great snack or lunch (one of my favorites is sliced sweet potato and cottage cheese) and become even sweeter as they sit.

4 medium or 2 large sweet potatoes, scrubbed
4 teaspoons butter or 2 limes, quartered (optional)

1. Preheat the oven to 425°F. Cover a baking sheet with foil.

2. Pierce the sweet potatoes in several places with a sharp knife or fork. If the ends are shriveled, cut them off. Place on the baking sheet. Bake 1 to 1^1/$_2$ hours for very large potatoes until soft and oozing, or about 40 minutes for smaller potatoes.

3. Cut large potatoes in half lengthwise and divide among individual plates. Slit smaller potatoes down the middle and place on the plates. Top each with 1 teaspoon butter or a squeeze of lime juice, if desired.

KEY NUTRIENTS
Beta Carotene
Vitamin A
Vitamin B$_6$
Vitamin C
Copper
Manganese

Basmati Rice Pilaf with Chickpeas

ADVANCE PREPARATION
You can make this a few hours in advance. Transfer the finished rice to a lightly oiled 2-quart baking dish. Spread it in an even layer and let cool completely. To reheat, cover with foil and bake in a 350°F oven for 20 minutes.

This pilaf makes a beautiful side dish, but it also packs substantial protein and as such can become an important component of a vegetarian meal.

- 1 cup basmati rice
- 1 tablespoon olive oil
- 1 small onion, chopped
- 1/2 teaspoon cumin seeds, crushed
- 1 cup cooked chickpeas, drained and rinsed
- 2 1/2 cups chicken or vegetable stock or water
- 1/2 teaspoon salt, or to taste
- Freshly ground pepper to taste

1. Wash the rice in several rinses of cold water until the water runs clear. Cover with water and let sit while you prepare the remaining ingredients, then drain.

2. Heat the oil in a heavy saucepan over medium heat. Add the onion and cumin and cook, stirring, until the onion is tender, about 5 minutes. Increase the heat and stir in the rice, chickpeas, and stock or water. Bring to a boil and add the salt and pepper. Reduce the heat to low, cover, and simmer for 15 to 20 minutes, until the liquid has just about been absorbed. Remove from the heat.

3. Place a clean, dry dishtowel over the pan and cover tightly with the lid. Let sit, covered, for 15 to 20 minutes. Serve hot.

KEY NUTRIENTS
Folacin
Niacin
Thiamin
Copper
Iron
Magnesium
Manganese
Phosphorus
Potassium
Zinc

Grain and

Vegetable Dishes

ADVANCE
PREPARATION
This can be made a few
hours ahead and re-
heated, although the
peas will shrivel. After
tossing the rice with
the peas and almonds,
transfer the rice to a
lightly oiled baking
dish, and let cool. To
reheat, cover with foil
and bake in a 350°F
oven for 20 minutes.

Basmati Rice Pilaf
with Peas

You can serve this subtly seasoned pilaf as a side dish or main
dish. Top it with thick yogurt or Yogurt Cheese if you're serving it as a main course.

     1 cup basmati rice
    ³/₄ teaspoon cumin seeds
     1 tablespoon olive or canola oil
    ¹/₂ medium onion, minced
     2 cups chicken or vegetable stock or water
¹/₂–³/₄ teaspoon salt, to taste (optional; depending on the
         stock)
     1 cup very sweet fresh or thawed frozen peas
    ¹/₄ cup slivered almonds
       Plain yogurt or Yogurt Cheese (page 65) for serving
         (optional)

KEY NUTRIENTS
Vitamin A
Vitamin B₆
Folacin
Niacin
Riboflavin
Thiamin
Vitamin C
Vitamin E
Calcium
Copper
Iron
Manganese
Magnesium
Phosphorus
Potassium
Zinc

1. Wash the rice in several rinses of cold water until the
water runs clear. Cover with water and let sit while you prepare the
remaining ingredients, then drain.

2. Toast the cumin seeds in a small skillet over medium
heat. Shake the pan constantly, and as soon as the seeds darken
slightly and smell toasty, transfer to a small bowl.

3. Heat the oil in a heavy 3- or 4-quart saucepan over
medium heat. Add the onion and cook, stirring, for about 3 minutes, until it begins to soften. Add the toasted cumin seeds and
cook, stirring, for another 2 to 3 minutes, until the onion is tender.
Stir in the rice and cook, stirring, for a couple of minutes, until the
grains are separate. Pour in the stock or water. Bring to a boil and
add salt, if necessary. Reduce the heat to low, cover, and simmer for
10 minutes, until steam holes cover the surface of the rice and

much of the liquid has evaporated. Add the peas and almonds to the surface of the rice (do not stir). Cover the pot and steam for 5 to 10 minutes more. Remove from the heat.

4. Place a clean, dry dishtowel over the pan and cover tightly with the lid. Let sit, covered, for 15 to 20 minutes. Transfer to a serving bowl and toss with the peas and almonds. Serve with yogurt or Yogurt Cheese, if desired.

ADVANCE
PREPARATION
The polenta will keep
for several days in the
refrigerator.

Easy Polenta

Polenta, the Italian cooked cornmeal mush, is very easy to make, although it does require more than an hour in the oven. Serve alone as a side dish, or serve as a main dish, topped with Tomato Sauce and Beans. Cold polenta can be sliced and reheated in the oven, toasted, or grilled.

    4 cups water
    1 cup polenta
 1¹/₄ teaspoons salt
    1 tablespoon butter

Preheat the oven to 350°F. Combine all the ingredients in a 2-quart baking dish. Stir together and bake for 1 hour. Remove from the oven, stir, and return to the oven for 10 minutes more. Remove from the oven and let sit for 5 minutes. Serve hot.

KEY NUTRIENTS
Thiamin
Magnesium
Phosphorus

Polenta with Tomato Sauce and Beans

Makes 4 servings

Easy Polenta (page 260)
1 tablespoon olive oil
2–3 large garlic cloves (to taste), minced or pressed
1 28-ounce can whole tomatoes, drained (reserve 1/2 cup of
the juice), seeded, and crushed (not pureed) in a food
processor with the reserved juice, or finely chopped
1 tablespoon slivered fresh basil or sage leaves or 3/4
teaspoon dried oregano or thyme, or a combination
1/2–3/4 teaspoon salt, to taste
1/8 teaspoon sugar
1 15-ounce can cannellini beans, drained and rinsed
Freshly ground pepper to taste
1/3 cup freshly grated Parmesan cheese for serving

1. While the polenta is baking, heat the oil in a large, heavy nonstick skillet over medium heat. Add the garlic and cook for about 30 seconds, until it begins to color. Stir in the tomatoes and their juice, dried oregano or thyme (if using), salt, and sugar. Add the beans and cook, stirring often, for 10 to 20 minutes, until the tomatoes are cooked down, fragrant, and just beginning to stick to the pan but not dry. Stir in the fresh basil or sage, if using. Add the pepper, then taste and adjust the seasonings. Turn off the heat.

2. Remove the polenta from the oven and let sit for 5 minutes. Spoon on the tomato and bean topping. Sprinkle on the Parmesan and serve. Alternatively, spoon the polenta onto 4 individual plates, top with the tomato mixture and Parmesan, and serve.

ADVANCE PREPARATION
The tomato and bean sauce will keep for 3 days in the refrigerator.

KEY NUTRIENTS
Vitamin A
Vitamin B$_6$
Folacin
Thiamin
Vitamin C
Vitamin E
Copper
Iron
Magnesium
Manganese
Phosphorus
Potassium

Grain and

Vegetable Dishes

ADVANCE
PREPARATION
The cooked noodles will
keep for 3 days in the
refrigerator.

Asian Noodles

The Asian noodles I use most often are Japanese buckwheat
noodles, called soba, or wheat noodles, called udon. Unlike
Italian semolina pasta, Asian pasta is usually not cooked in
salted water, and the noodles are softer when cooked. They can
be prepared ahead and reheated in a little oil, or eaten cold.

$1/2$–$3/4$ pound soba or udon
1–3 teaspoons dark sesame oil, as needed

1. Bring a large pot of water to a boil. Gradually add the
noodles, then stir with a long-handled spoon to make sure they
don't stick together. When the water comes back to a rolling boil,
add a cup of cold water. Bring back to a boil, then add another cup
of cold water. Bring back to a boil again and add a third cup of
cold water. By the time the water comes back to a boil, the noodles
should be cooked through. Drain and rinse with cold water.

2. Transfer the noodles to a serving bowl and toss with the
sesame oil. Serve immediately, or store in a tightly covered bowl in
the refrigerator.

KEY NUTRIENTS
SOBA
Manganese

UDON
Niacin
Thiamin
Iron
Manganese

Basic Cooking Directions for Some Grains

Bulgur
Makes about 3 cups

Bulgur is wheat that has been precooked, dried, and cracked. It needs only a soak in boiling water. It's a light grain with a nutty flavor.

1 cup fine or medium bulgur
¼–½ teaspoon salt, to taste
2½ cups boiling water
1–2 teaspoons butter or olive oil, to taste (optional)

1. Place the bulgur in a medium bowl and add the salt. Stir with a spoon or mix with your hands to distribute the salt evenly. Pour on the boiling water. Let sit for 15 to 20 minutes, until the bulgur is soft. Drain through a strainer, pressing the bulgur to extract all the water.

2. Reheat the bulgur in a medium saucepan over low heat or in the microwave at 100% power, or high, for about 30 seconds. If desired, add the butter or oil and serve.

Couscous
Makes about 5 cups

We think of couscous as a grain, but the grainlike particles are actually tiny pellets of semolina pasta. However, couscous isn't cooked like pasta. It's soaked, then steamed, so that the grains become fluffy and light. Like pasta, couscous is usually the centerpiece of a dish.

2 cups couscous
½–¾ teaspoon salt, to taste
2½ cups warm water or chicken or vegetable stock

ADVANCE PREPARATION
Cooked grains keep well in the refrigerator for a few days. You can reheat grains in the oven or microwave. Follow the alternative directions for steaming couscous in the oven or microwave (see page 264) for all grains.

KEY NUTRIENTS
BULGUR
Folacin
Iron
Magnesium
Manganese

KEY NUTRIENTS
COUSCOUS
Niacin
Thiamin
Iron
Manganese

Grain and

Vegetable Dishes

1. Place the couscous in a medium bowl and add the salt. Mix with your hands to distribute the salt evenly. Pour the water or stock over the couscous; the couscous should be completely submerged, with about ½ inch water on top. Let sit for 20 minutes, until the water is absorbed and the couscous is slightly al dente. Stir every 5 minutes with a wooden spoon or rub the couscous between your moistened thumbs and fingers, so that it doesn't form clumps. After 20 minutes, fluff it with a fork or with your hands. Taste and adjust the salt, if necessary.

2 Place the couscous in a colander or strainer and set it over boiling water (or over the dish you are serving it with), making sure that the bottom of the colander does not touch the liquid. Remove some of the liquid if it does. If there is a space between the edge of the colander and the rim of the pot, wrap a towel around the pot so that the steam doesn't escape. Steam, uncovered, for 20 minutes.

3. Transfer to a large bowl or platter. If you wish, you can steam the couscous twice for an even fluffier grain. Proceed as above — this can be done hours before you are ready to eat — and repeat just before eating.

VARIATION

Alternative Steaming Methods

To steam the couscous in the oven, preheat the oven to 350°F. Place the couscous in a lightly oiled baking dish and cover tightly with foil. Bake for 20 minutes, until heated through. To use the microwave, place the couscous in a microwave-safe bowl and cover tightly with plastic wrap. Pierce the plastic with a knife and cook at 100% power, or high, for 1 minute. Let sit for 1 minute, then carefully remove the plastic and fluff with a fork. Repeat, if desired.

Quinoa

Makes about 3 cups

This high-protein grain has its origins in Peru. It's a wonder grain that is high in iron, potassium, and magnesium. It has a delicate taste and cooks up in 15 minutes, making it a convenience food as well. Always rinse quinoa before cooking.

1 cup quinoa
2 cups water or chicken or vegetable stock
¹⁄₄ teaspoon salt, plus more to taste

Place the quinoa in a bowl and rinse thoroughly in several changes of cold water, draining it through a fine sieve each time. Bring the water or stock to a boil in a 2-quart saucepan. Add the quinoa and salt. Reduce the heat, cover, and simmer for 12 to 15 minutes, until the liquid is absorbed and little spirals appear in the grain. Remove from the heat and let sit, covered, for 5 minutes. Season with additional salt, if desired.

KEY NUTRIENTS
QUINOA
Protein
Vitamin B$_6$
Folacin
Niacin
Riboflavin
Thiamin
Copper
Iron
Magnesium
Manganese
Phosphorus
Potassium
Zinc

Rice

There are many types of rice, and each has its own particular cooking method. The types of rice used in this book are basmati, white, and brown. Wild rice is actually not a rice but a grass, although the cooking instructions are given in this section.

BASMATI OR WHITE RICE

Makes about 3 cups white rice, 3¹⁄₂ to 4 cups basmati

BASMATI RICE is the fragrant, delicate rice used in Indian cooking and in many Middle Eastern dishes. There is more than one way to cook it. You can use the same method you use for white rice, but rinse the rice in several changes of water before adding it to the boiling water. Or you can cook it following the instructions for pilafs on pages 257 and 258.

KEY NUTRIENTS
BASMATI OR
WHITE RICE
Niacin
Thiamin
Iron
Manganese

Grain and

Vegetable Dishes

WHITE RICE comes in long-grain and medium-grain varieties. This widely used rice has been hulled and the germ removed, and it is fairly quick-cooking.

    2 cups water
    1 cup basmati or white rice
$^1/_2$–$^3/_4$ teaspoon salt, to taste

Bring the water to a boil in a 1- or 2-quart saucepan. Add the rice and salt. When the water comes back to a boil, stir *once* (and only once). Reduce the heat to low, cover the pot tightly, and simmer for 15 minutes. Remove the cover and look and listen. There will be holes in the surface, into which you can peer to see if the water has evaporated. You will hear any remaining water simmering as well. If you're not sure whether all the water has been absorbed, stick a chopstick — not a spoon — into the rice to see if it is beginning to stick to the bottom of the pan. If there is still water simmering, return the lid to the pan and continue to cook, checking every 5 minutes. When the water has evaporated, remove from the heat. Place a clean, dry dishtowel over the pan, cover with the lid, and let the pan sit without touching it for at least 10 minutes. The rice will continue to steam and grow fluffy, and the towel will absorb the steam.

BROWN RICE
Makes about 3 cups
BROWN RICE has been husked, but it still contains all of its bran and germ, so it has more B vitamins, fiber, and trace minerals than white rice. It takes twice as long to cook and has a chewier, heartier texture. The method for cooking brown rice is exactly the same as that for white or basmati rice, except you use 2$^1/_4$ cups water or stock for 1 cup rice, and you cook the rice for 35 to 50 minutes. Check after 35 minutes, as instructed above.

KEY NUTRIENTS
BROWN RICE
Niacin
Magnesium
Manganese
Phosphorus

Wild Rice

Makes about 3 cups

KEY NUTRIENTS
WILD RICE
Vitamin B$_6$
Folacin
Niacin
Zinc

The dark brown grains of this wild grass have a marvelous nutty flavor.

    3 cups water or chicken or vegetable stock
    1 cup wild rice, rinsed
    $^1/_2$–$^3/_4$ teaspoon salt, to taste (optional; depending on the
        stock)

Bring the water or stock to a boil in a large saucepan. Add the rice and salt (if using). When the rice comes back to a boil, reduce the heat, cover, and simmer for 40 minutes, until the rice is tender and the kernels are splayed. Remove from the heat and drain off any liquid that remains.

Wheat Berries

Makes about 4 cups

KEY NUTRIENTS
WHEAT BERRIES
Folacin
Iron
Magnesium
Manganese

Wheat berries are the whole wheat kernels. They can be found in natural food stores. The grains are hearty and chewy and benefit from soaking before cooking. I think they lend themselves best to salads and soups. Cooked wheat berries freeze well.

    1 cup wheat berries
    3 cups water
    $^1/_2$ teaspoon salt, or to taste

Soak the wheat berries in water to cover by 1 inch for several hours, then drain. Transfer to a large saucepan. Add the water and bring to a boil. Reduce the heat, cover, and simmer for 1 hour. Add the salt and continue to simmer for 30 minutes more, until the grains are tender but still chewy. Remove from the heat and drain off any liquid that remains.

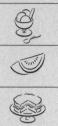

DESSERTS

Bread Pudding with Apples or Peaches 269

Chocolate Pudding 270

Berry Cream 271

Brownies 272

Flourless Orange Cake 273

Cherry Clafoutis 274

Pear Crumble or Crisp 275

Baked Apples 276

Dried Figs in Orange Juice 277

Melon with Mint and Lime 277

Pears Poached in Ginger Honey Syrup 278

Frozen Banana Yogurt 279

Rice Pudding 280

Orange and Mint Salad 281

Strawberries and Peaches with Mint 281

Strawberries with Mint and Citrus Juice 282

Strawberry Orange Soup 282

Bread Pudding
with Apples or Peaches

ADVANCE
PREPARATION
Bread pudding is best
freshly made, but you
can keep it for a few
days and reheat it in a
300°F oven.

This is a great way to use up bread that is getting stale, and it also makes a high-protein, comforting dessert, snack, or breakfast. Don't use sourdough bread for this. Whole wheat bread is good. An egg bread, such as challah, makes a great choice.

$1/2$ cup golden raisins
$1/2$ pound bread, thickly sliced (about 6 slices)
2 tablespoons unsalted butter, softened
2 apples, peeled, cored, and sliced, or 3 peaches, pitted
    and sliced
4 large eggs
$1/3$ cup packed light brown sugar
$2^1/4$–$2^1/2$ cups milk, as needed
1 teaspoon pure vanilla extract
$1/4$–$1/2$ teaspoon freshly grated nutmeg, to taste
Whipped cream or sour cream for serving (optional)

1. Preheat the oven to 350°F. Butter a 2-quart baking or gratin dish. Place the raisins in a small bowl, pour on boiling water to cover, and let sit for 1 minute. Drain and place the raisins on paper towels.

2. Spread both sides of the bread with the butter and cut into 2-inch cubes. Transfer to a medium bowl, add the apples or peaches and raisins, and toss. Arrange in the baking dish in an even layer.

3. Beat together the eggs and brown sugar in a medium bowl. Beat in $2^1/4$ cups of the milk, the vanilla, and nutmeg. Pour over the bread. If the bread isn't submerged, add a little more milk.

4. Bake for 45 to 60 minutes, until set. Serve warm, topped with a little whipped cream or sour cream, if you wish.

KEY NUTRIENTS
Protein
Vitamin A
Vitamin B_6
Vitamin B_{12}
Folacin
Niacin
Riboflavin
Thiamin
Vitamin C
Calcium
Copper
Iron
Magnesium
Manganese
Phosphorus
Potassium

Desserts

ADVANCE
PREPARATION
The pudding will keep
for 5 days in the
refrigerator.

Chocolate Pudding

There's not a more comforting dessert around than chocolate pudding, and it has the added value of being packed with protein and calcium. Although this one isn't quite as quick as opening a packet of the instant kind, it's very easy to make, and it yields a far tastier and more nutritious result.

$2^{1}/_{3}$ cups milk
$^{1}/_{2}$ cup plus 1 tablespoon sugar
Pinch of salt
5 tablespoons unsweetened cocoa powder
2 tablespoons cornstarch, sifted
1 large egg
2 large egg yolks
1 teaspoon pure vanilla extract
Lightly whipped cream or milk for serving

1. Place 2 cups of the milk, $^{1}/_{4}$ cup of the sugar, and the salt in a medium, heavy-bottomed saucepan and bring to a boil over medium heat.

2. Meanwhile, mix together the remaining $^{1}/_{4}$ cup plus 1 tablespoon sugar, the cocoa, and cornstarch in a medium bowl. Whisk in the remaining $^{1}/_{3}$ cup milk, and stir until smooth and free of lumps.

3. Carefully whisk the hot milk mixture into the bowl; return the mixture to the saucepan. Slowly bring to a boil over medium heat, stirring often. Boil gently, stirring constantly, until the mixture is thick, 2 to 5 minutes. Let cool slightly.

4. Whisk the egg and egg yolks together in a small bowl. Slowly whisk in 1 cup of the hot (not boiling) cocoa mixture, then whisk the mixture back into the saucepan. Whisk constantly over

KEY NUTRIENTS
Protein
Vitamin B$_{12}$
Riboflavin
Calcium
Phosphorus

medium-low heat, being careful not to boil (or the eggs will curdle), until it thickens a little more, 3 to 5 minutes. Stir in the vanilla and remove from the heat.

5. Pour into 4 ramekins, pudding dishes, or glass sundae dishes and cover with plastic wrap. If you don't want a skin to form on the surface, lay the plastic directly on the surface of the pudding. Chill for 2 to 3 hours or longer, then serve with whipped cream or milk.

Berry Cream

Makes 4 servings

This creamy mixture of frozen berries with their juice and blended cottage cheese makes a great dessert, breakfast, or snack. Keep frozen berries in the freezer so you can make it often. Raspberries are terrific in this dish, but mixed berries are great, too.

ADVANCE PREPARATION
This will keep for a few days in the refrigerator.

1 12-ounce package frozen raspberries or mixed berries
1 tablespoon fresh lemon juice
2 tablespoons sugar
1 cup cottage cheese
1/4 cup plain yogurt

1. Let the berries thaw in a medium bowl in the refrigerator. There should be a fair amount of juice. Add the lemon juice and sugar, stir together well, and let sit for 15 minutes or longer.

2. Blend the cottage cheese in a food processor until smooth. Add the yogurt and continue to blend until there is no trace of graininess. Stir into the berries. Chill in a covered bowl or serve right away.

KEY NUTRIENTS
Protein
Vitamin B$_{12}$
Folacin
Riboflavin
Calcium
Manganese
Phosphorus

Desserts

ADVANCE
PREPARATION

Brownies keep well for
about 5 days in the
pan. They can also be
frozen for a few
months.

Brownies

Brownies are the fulfillment of any chocolate craving. They're easy to make and even easier to eat. The better the quality of chocolate you use, the better they will be.

2 ounces unsweetened chocolate, broken into pieces
8 tablespoons (1 stick) unsalted butter, cut into pieces
$^2/_3$ cup all-purpose flour
Pinch of salt
2 large eggs
1 cup sugar
1 teaspoon pure vanilla extract
$^1/_2$ heaped cup walnuts or pecans, coarsely chopped
4 ounces bittersweet chocolate, cut into small pieces, or
$^2/_3$ cup bittersweet chocolate chips

1. Preheat the oven to 350°F. Butter an 8- or 9-inch square baking pan.

2. Combine the unsweetened chocolate and butter in a bowl set over a pan with 1 inch of simmering water and melt, stirring every 15 seconds. Remove from the heat just before fully melted and stir to complete the melting. Or melt in the microwave at 50% power for 2 to 3 minutes. Stir and let cool slightly.

3. Sift the flour and salt into a medium bowl.

4. Beat the eggs and sugar together in another medium bowl until thick and lemon-colored. Beat in the vanilla. Fold in the melted chocolate, then the flour mixture. Fold in the nuts and bittersweet chocolate. Do not overwork the batter.

5. Transfer the batter to the baking pan and bake for 25 to 30 minutes, until a toothpick inserted in the center comes out with just a little batter on it. The brownies should still be moist in the center when done. Let cool completely in the pan on a rack, then cut into squares.

Flourless Orange Cake

ADVANCE
PREPARATION
This cake is better the
day after you make it.
It will keep for about 5
days.

This is one of the easiest cakes imaginable, and you won't believe it will actually bake into a nice, moist, firm cake. There's no flour. Instead, ground almonds give the cake a wonderful texture. Grind them in the food processor; take care not to overprocess them or they will become too oily.

  2 medium thin-skinned oranges, preferably seedless
  6 large eggs
  1 cup sugar
1^1/$_2$ teaspoons baking powder
1^1/$_2$ cups ground almonds

1. Scrub the fruit well. Place in a medium saucepan and cover with water. Bring to a boil, then reduce the heat, cover, and simmer for 2 hours, checking every once in a while to make sure the water hasn't boiled off too much. Drain and let cool. When cool enough to handle, carefully cut the fruit in half and remove all the seeds, if any (otherwise the cake will be bitter).

2. Preheat the oven to 350°F. Grease and flour a 9^1/$_2$- or 10-inch springform pan and line it with parchment paper.

3. Put the fruit, skin and all, in a food processor and puree. Measure out 1^1/$_4$ cups.

4. In a large bowl, beat the eggs with the sugar and baking powder at medium-high speed until thick and lemon-colored. Add the ground almonds and mix well. Mix in the orange at low speed, in two or three additions, beating for 20 seconds after each addition. Pour into the pan.

5. Bake for 1 hour, until the cake is firm and a knife inserted in the center comes out clean. If the top begins to get too brown halfway through, cover loosely with foil. Let cool for 10 minutes in the pan, then remove the outer rim and let cool completely.

KEY NUTRIENTS
Vitamin A
Vitamin B$_{12}$
Folacin
Niacin
Riboflavin
Vitamin E
Calcium
Copper
Iron
Magnesium
Manganese
Phosphorus
Potassium
Zinc
Omega-3s

Desserts

ADVANCE
PREPARATION
The clafoutis will hold
for several hours. You
can reheat it in a
250°F oven if desired.
Leftovers make a great
breakfast.

Cherry Clafoutis

The clafoutis is a classic French dessert. A cross between a flan and a pancake, it can be made with any number of fruits. Cherry clafoutis is traditionally made without pitting the cherries, so make sure your diners know if you don't pit them.

1½ pounds fresh sweet cherries, such as Bing, stems removed and pitted (if desired)
3 tablespoons kirsch or other berry-flavored liqueur
6 tablespoons sugar
4 large eggs
Seeds from 1 vanilla bean or ½ teaspoon pure vanilla extract
⅔ cup sifted unbleached or all-purpose flour
¾ cup milk
½ cup plain yogurt
Pinch of salt
Powdered sugar for topping

1. Toss the cherries with the kirsch and 2 tablespoons of the sugar in a large bowl. Let sit for 30 minutes. Meanwhile, preheat the oven to 400°F. Butter a 10-inch ceramic tart pan or 1½- to 2-quart baking dish.

2. Drain the liquid from the cherries into a small bowl. Set the cherries aside. Transfer the liquid to the bowl of an electric mixer or a large bowl. Add the eggs, the seeds from the vanilla bean or vanilla extract, and the remaining 4 tablespoons sugar. Beat together. Slowly beat in the flour. Add the milk, yogurt, and salt. Mix together well. This can also be mixed at high speed in a blender.

3. Arrange the cherries in the baking dish. Pour in the batter. Bake for 35 to 45 minutes, or until the top is browned and puffed and the clafoutis is firm.

4. Remove from the oven and sprinkle with powdered sugar (place in a strainer and tap the strainer above the clafoutis). Let cool in the dish on a rack. Serve warm or at room temperature.

KEY NUTRIENTS
Protein
Vitamin A
Vitamin B₁₂
Folacin
Riboflavin
Vitamin C
Calcium
Iron
Phosphorus

Pear Crumble or Crisp

ADVANCE
PREPARATION
The crumble can be
made a few hours
ahead and reheated in
a 300°F oven

Crumbles are as enticing as good fruit pies, without the hassle of the piecrust. This one is pure indulgence.

FOR THE TOPPING
- 1 cup old-fashioned rolled oats
- 1/2 cup all purpose flour or whole wheat pastry flour
- 1/4 cup packed light brown sugar
- 1/4 teaspoon salt
- 1/4 teaspoon freshly grated nutmeg
- 6 tablespoons (3/4 stick) cold unsalted butter

- 2 tablespoons fresh lemon juice
- 2 tablespoons sugar
- 1 tablespoon cornstarch or 1 teaspoon arrowroot
- 1/2 teaspoon ground ginger
- 2 1/2 pounds ripe but firm pears
- Plain yogurt sweetened with honey, whipped cream, vanilla ice cream, or frozen yogurt for serving

1. FOR THE TOPPING: Mix together the oats, flour, brown sugar, salt, and nutmeg. Cut the butter into small pieces and work in, either by taking up the mixture in handfuls and rubbing briskly between your fingers and thumbs, or by using the pulse action in a food processor. The mixture should have a crumbly consistency.

2. Preheat the oven to 375° F. Butter a 2- to 2 1/2-quart baking or gratin dish.

3. Combine the lemon juice, sugar, cornstarch or arrowroot, and ginger in a large bowl. Peel, core, and slice the pears. Toss at once with the lemon juice mixture. Turn into the prepared baking dish. Sprinkle on the topping in an even layer. Bake for 45 minutes, until the top is crisp and browned. If you wish, finish browning the top briefly under the broiler, taking care not to burn it.

4. Serve warm with the yogurt, whipped cream, ice cream, or frozen yogurt.

KEY NUTRIENT
Vitamin C

Desserts

ADVANCE
PREPARATION

The apples can be
baked several hours
ahead and reheated for
15 minutes in a 325°F
oven.

Baked Apples

These easy baked apples can be moistened with the reduced
apple juice from the pan. You can season them with cinnamon
or ginger — or both! Gravenstein, Braeburn, Pink Ladies, and
Granny Smith apples are all suitable for this dish.

    4 firm tart apples (see headnote)
    1/2 lemon
    1 tablespoon dark or light brown sugar
    1/2 teaspoon ground ginger or 1 teaspoon ground cinnamon
    1/2 cup apple juice
    A few strips lemon zest
    Plain yogurt for serving (optional)

1. Preheat the oven to 350°F.

2. Peel the top quarter of each apple. Cut a cone out of the
stem end using a paring knife or the tip of your peeler, then pull
the cone out by the stem. Rub the peeled parts of the apples with
the lemon. Place in a buttered baking dish.

3. Mix together the brown sugar and ginger or cinnamon
in a cup. Sprinkle over the apples. Pour the apple juice over the apples and into the dish. Add the lemon zest to the juice in the dish.
Cover with aluminum foil and bake for 30 to 40 minutes, until the
apples are tender. Remove the foil, spoon some of the juice over
the apples, and bake for 5 to 10 minutes more, until the sugar has
dissolved.

4. Serve warm or at room temperature. Spoon some of the
juice from the dish over the apples and accompany with yogurt, if
desired.

KEY NUTRIENT
Vitamin C

Dried Figs
in Orange Juice

Dried figs are a terrific source of fiber and make a delicious snack or dessert. Here they are marinated in calcium-fortified orange juice.

1 pound dried figs, cut into quarters or halves, depending on the size
3 cups calcium-fortified orange juice
Plain yogurt for serving (optional)

Place the figs in a medium bowl and add the orange juice. Refrigerate for 8 to 12 hours. Serve with yogurt, if you wish.

Melon with
Mint and Lime

Melon can be particularly appealing when you have little taste for food because it's so thirst-quenching and refreshing. The natural sugar in the fruit will give you energy, and the lime juice may ease your nausea. Any ripe melon works here — cantaloupe, honeydew, crenshaw, and watermelon are all good.

1 ripe melon, seeded and cut into chunks
Juice of 1 lime
2 tablespoons fresh mint leaves, chopped or cut into slivers

Toss all the ingredients together in a medium bowl. Cover and refrigerate until ready to serve.

VARIATION
Pineapple with Mint

Substitute 1 pineapple, peeled, cored, quartered, and sliced, for melon, omitting the lime juice.

ADVANCE PREPARATION
This will keep for a week in the refrigerator, but the figs will give up their flavor into the juice.

KEY NUTRIENTS
Vitamin B$_6$
Vitamin C
Calcium
Copper
Iron
Magnesium
Manganese
Potassium

Makes 4 servings

ADVANCE PREPARATION
The cut-up melon will keep for several days in the refrigerator. The lime juice and mint will lose their fresh taste after a day, however, so you might want to keep the melon cut up and toss it with the other ingredients as you eat it.

KEY NUTRIENTS
Beta Carotene (orange-fleshed melons)
Vitamin A (orange-fleshed melons)
Potassium

KEY NUTRIENTS
PINEAPPLE
Vitamin C
Manganese

Desserts

Pears Poached in Ginger Honey Syrup

Ginger infusions are wonderful for poaching fruit, and they can also ease morning sickness and soothe colds and sore throats.

2 tablespoons grated or minced fresh ginger
3 cups boiling water
$1/4$ cup mild-flavored honey, such as clover or acacia, or $1/3$ cup sugar
4 pears, peeled, cored, and cut into thick wedges
1 tablespoon fresh lemon juice

1. Place the ginger in a bowl or Pyrex measuring cup and pour on the boiling water. Cover and let steep for 15 minutes. Strain into a $1^{1}/_{2}$- or 2-quart saucepan and add the honey or sugar. Bring to a boil and reduce by about a third. Reduce the heat to a simmer.

2. Toss the pears with the lemon juice and add to the ginger syrup. Simmer for 10 minutes, until translucent. Remove from the heat. Transfer the pears to an attractive serving bowl and return the ginger syrup to the heat. Increase the heat and boil until the syrup thickens slightly, 3 to 5 minutes. Pour over the pears and let cool. Serve at room temperature, or refrigerate and serve cold.

KEY NUTRIENT
Vitamin C

EVERY WOMAN'S

GUIDE TO EATING

DURING PREGNANCY

Frozen Banana Yogurt

ADVANCE
PREPARATION
This will keep for weeks
in the freezer but must
be softened in the
refrigerator before
serving. If you keep
frozen bananas on
hand it is quickly made
to order.

Sweet frozen foods are often the most appetizing foods during pregnancy. But ice cream can be a hazard for those who have to be careful about weight gain. This creamy frozen mixture is satisfying in the same way, and it's just fruit and yogurt. Keep frozen bananas on hand so you can satisfy the cravings you will inevitably have once you've tasted this treat the first time.

    4 large or 6 medium ripe or very ripe bananas
1½ cups plain yogurt
    1 tablespoon mild honey, such as clover
    1 teaspoon pure vanilla extract
       Freshly grated nutmeg to taste (optional)

1. Peel the bananas, cut into thick slices, and place in zipper-lock freezer bags. Freeze for 24 hours or longer, until frozen solid.

2. Place the yogurt, honey, and vanilla in a food processor and add the banana chunks. Using the pulse action, process several times until the mixture is almost smooth, with a few chunks. Then turn on the food processor and process until smooth. Add the nutmeg, if you wish.

3. Serve at once, or freeze for 2 to 3 hours. If the mixture freezes solid, soften in the refrigerator for 30 minutes before serving.

VARIATION

Frozen Strawberry Banana Yogurt

Add 1 pint fresh strawberries, hulled and frozen, to the food processor with the bananas.

KEY NUTRIENTS
Protein
Vitamin B$_6$
Folacin
Vitamin C
Calcium
Magnesium
Manganese
    (Strawberry-Banana
    Yogurt)
Potassium

Desserts

ADVANCE
PREPARATION

This can be made hours
ahead of serving, but
you should take it off
the heat 5 minutes
earlier. You will have to
thin the mixture with
hot milk when you are
ready to serve it.

Rice Pudding

Rice pudding can be particularly appealing during the early months of pregnancy, when you're tired and nauseous and just want something sweet and easy. This meets those criteria, and it also has a lot of food value.

2 cups water
1 cup white rice
$1/4$ teaspoon salt
1 2-inch cinnamon stick
4 cups milk
$1/2$ cup sugar, or $1/3$ cup sugar and 1 tablespoon mild-
  flavored honey, such as clover or acacia
$1/2$ cup dark or golden raisins (optional)
  Freshly grated nutmeg to taste

1. Bring the water to a boil in a medium, heavy-bottomed saucepan and add the rice, salt, and cinnamon stick. When the mixture comes back to a boil, stir the mixture once, cover, reduce the heat to medium-low, and simmer for 15 minutes, until the liquid is absorbed and the rice is tender. Increase the heat to medium and stir the milk, sugar or sugar and honey, and raisins (if using) into the rice. Bring back to a simmer, stirring. Reduce the heat to medium-low and continue to simmer, stirring often, until the mixture has thickened but is still soupy, 20 to 25 minutes.

2. Remove from the heat, sprinkle with the nutmeg, and serve hot or warm.

KEY NUTRIENTS
Vitamin B$_6$
Vitamin B$_{12}$
Niacin
Riboflavin
Thiamin
Calcium
Copper
Iron
Magnesium
Manganese
Phosphorus
Potassium

Orange and Mint Salad

There is always dessert on hand if you have oranges and mint. Oranges help with the absorption of iron from nonmeat sources.

5 navel oranges or 8 blood oranges
  Juice of $1/2$ orange or 1 blood orange
2 tablespoons slivered fresh mint leaves
  Fresh mint sprigs for garnish

1. Peel the oranges and remove the pith. Slice crosswise and transfer to an attractive bowl. Cover and refrigerate.

2. Just before serving, toss the oranges with the juice and mint. Serve, garnishing each dish with a mint sprig.

Makes 4 servings

ADVANCE PREPARATION
This will hold for a couple of hours in the refrigerator but is best made close to serving time, or the juice will become more acidic.

KEY NUTRIENTS
Folacin
Vitamin C

Strawberries and Peaches with Mint

Fresh fruit is the dessert I most often recommend to pregnant women. But there are many ways to embellish it. This is a great summer dish.

1 pint fresh strawberries, hulled and cut in half
1 tablespoon sugar
1 tablespoon fresh lemon juice
1 pound peaches, pitted and sliced
  Juice of 1 orange
2 tablespoons chopped fresh mint

Place the strawberries in a nonreactive bowl. Add the sugar and lemon juice and toss. Let sit for 30 minutes, in or out of the refrigerator. Add the peaches and orange juice, sprinkle on the mint, and toss. Serve immediately, or refrigerate and serve cold.

Makes 4 servings

ADVANCE PREPARATION
This will keep for a few hours in the refrigerator.

KEY NUTRIENTS
Folacin
Vitamin C
Manganese

ADVANCE
PREPARATION
The strawberries can
be tossed with the
sugar hours before
serving.

KEY NUTRIENTS
Folacin
Vitamin C
Manganese

Strawberries with Mint and Citrus Juice

Just before serving, add lemon, lime, or orange juice and mint, and you'll get the best out of even ordinary strawberries.

1 pint fresh strawberries, hulled and cut into quarters or halves
2 teaspoons sugar
Juice of $^1/_2$ lemon, lime, or orange
1 tablespoon slivered fresh mint leaves

Toss the strawberries with the sugar in a medium bowl. Let sit for 1 hour or longer, in or out of the refrigerator. Just before serving, toss with the citrus juice and mint. Serve immediately.

ADVANCE
PREPARATION
The strawberries can
be prepared a few
hours ahead, but the
juice should be
squeezed close to serv-
ing time and the mint
added at the last
minute.

KEY NUTRIENTS
Folacin
Vitamin C
Manganese

Strawberry Orange Soup

This dessert is very high in vitamin C.

2 pints fresh strawberries, hulled and quartered
2 tablespoons sugar, plus more to taste
2 tablespoons fresh lemon or lime juice
$1^1/_2$ cups fresh orange juice
2 tablespoons slivered fresh mint leaves plus a few whole leaves for garnish

1. Place the strawberries in a nonreactive bowl. Add the sugar and lemon or lime juice and toss. Let sit for 1 hour, in or out of the refrigerator, tossing gently from time to time.

2. Squeeze the orange juice and add to the strawberries. Taste and add a little more sugar, if desired. Chill until ready to serve.

3. Serve, garnishing each bowl with the slivered and whole mint leaves.

Eating Plans for Individual Needs

The prospect of gaining a certain number of pounds, getting a set number of calories, and sticking to a particular diet can be daunting. It's also the last thing you want to think about when you're pregnant. That's why we've come up with these meal plans. Eating for pleasure and good health, not eating by numbers, should be your focus. You'll get lots and lots of suggestions and menus from the following pages.

The first set of plans includes one week of meal ideas for breakfast, lunch, dinner, and snacks that are tailored to individual needs, such as lower-carb, higher-carb, and vegetarian and vegan plans, along with menus for the noncook. In the second set of eating plans, the menus are geared toward women with special needs, such as those who are lactose intolerant or have gestational diabetes. The third section includes plans for each trimester. Finally, there are suggestions for nursing mothers. In all of these sections, we use the same dishes but modify the menus to meet specific needs.

Some of the meals include ordinary dishes such as soft-boiled eggs, peanut butter sandwiches, or vanilla yogurt, which don't require recipes. Others include recipes in this book, which are easy to make, healthful, and tasty. And a number of meals are based on prepared or packaged foods that you can buy in the supermarket. We know that not everybody cooks, but if you're pregnant, you'll still want to know how to eat well.

What's in a Serving?

Most dietitians, as well as the American College of Obstetricians and Gynecologists, make recommendations for the number of servings pregnant women should have from each of the various

Recommended Daily Food Choices

BREAD, CEREAL, RICE, PASTA: 9
(1 serving = 1 slice of bread; 1 cup cold cereal; $^1/_2$ cup cooked cereal, rice or other grain, or pasta)

VEGETABLES: 4
(1 serving = 1 cup salad greens, $^1/_2$ cup cooked vegetables, 1 cup raw vegetables, $^3/_4$ cup vegetable juice)

FRUIT: 3
(1 serving = 1 piece or 1 cup cut up fruit, $^1/_2$ cup berries)

POULTRY, FISH, DRIED BEANS, MEAT, EGGS, NUTS: 3
(1 serving = 2–3 ounces cooked lean poultry, fish, or meat — so a normal serving of 6–8 ounces at a meal would constitute 2 servings or more; 1–1$^1/_2$ cups cooked beans; 1 egg; 1 ounce cheese; 2 tablespoons peanut butter)

MILK, YOGURT, CHEESE: 3
(1 serving = 1 cup milk or yogurt, 1$^1/_2$ ounces cheese)

Source: American College of
Obstetricians and Gynecologists,
www.acog.org.

food groups throughout the day or at each meal. So that you can see how our menus correspond to those suggestions, we follow each day's menu with a food group breakdown for the day.

Don't Forget Snacks

Snacking is important when you're pregnant. It may be difficult for you to get enough calories and protein at a meal, either because of nausea or, later in your pregnancy, because of heartburn or fullness. Between-meal eating can help you fulfill your nutritional requirements. Or you may feel ravenous all the time. Some women have an easier time with steady, desirable weight gain if they eat smaller meals throughout the day. Snacking also can relieve morning sickness. If you're pregnant with multiples, you need to snack to get in those extra small meals that provide the considerable number of additional calories you'll need.

A Note About Serving Sizes

Where serving sizes are not indicated, here is what we recommend.

Almonds: 1/4 cup

Applesauce: 1/2–3/4 cup

Cereal: 1/2 cup with 1/2 cup milk

Frozen yogurt: 1/2 cup

Milk and juice: 3/4–1 cup

Tofu: 3–4 ounces

Yogurt: 1 cup

If You Are Trying to Keep Calories Down . . .

↬ Use nonfat or low-fat dairy products (milk, yogurt, cottage cheese, cream cheese, frozen yogurt).

↬ Omit butter from bread.

If You Need More Ideas for Bulking Up . . .

↬ Reduced-fat (2%) or full-fat (4%) dairy products

↬ Full-fat fruit-flavored yogurt

↬ 2 ounces cheese

↬ Smoothies with optional brewer's yeast (page 44)

↬ Red meat

↬ Power Bars

↬ Ice cream

↬ Nuts and peanut butter

↬ Fortified high-calorie drinks such as Ensure*

* The National Academy of Sciences discourages the use of protein powders and drinks, citing evidence suggesting that they may be harmful. However, some practitioners recommend nutritional supplements for pregnant women carrying multiples, who must consume many more calories than women carrying singletons.

Just as with your menu plan, the type of foods you snack on should correspond to your weight-gain needs. If you're gaining a lot of weight and want to slow it down, focus on high-protein snacks and lower-calorie fruit and vegetable snacks. If you need to gain more weight, snack on higher-calorie foods. And if you're

Eating Plans

for Individual

Needs

doing just fine, choose a balance of carbohydrate-rich snacks and protein-rich snacks. If you're carrying twins or more, the snacks should be more like little meals.

Healthy Snacks

BREAD AND CEREALS

1 slice whole grain toast with peanut butter (omit for low fat)

1 slice whole grain toast with peanut butter and unsweetened fruit preserves (omit for low fat)

1 slice whole grain toast with nonfat or low-fat cream cheese or Yogurt Cheese (page 65)

Whole grain toast with banana

Whole wheat English muffin with unsweetened fruit preserves and/or nonfat or low-fat cream cheese

Whole grain toast with tahini

Rye or pumpernickel bread with cheese or low-fat cream cheese and cucumber

Whole grain bread or crackers with hummus

Molasses Bread (page 53), with or without applesauce

Banana Bread (page 52), with or without applesauce

Bran Muffin (page 48), with or without applesauce

High-Protein Muffin (page 50), with or without applesauce

Crackers with Yogurt Cheese (page 65) or Herbed Yogurt Cheese (page 65), cottage cheese, nonfat or low-fat cream cheese, or 1 ounce cheese. Low-fat crackers* include:

    Wasa Multi Grain, Hearty Rye, or Light Rye Crispbread

    Ry-Krisp

    Ryvita Crispbread

    Finn Crisp

    Slightly higher-fat crackers include:

    Melba toast

    Carr's Table Water Crackers

    Saltines

Cereal ($^1/_3$–$^1/_2$ cup) with nonfat or 1% milk

Granola ($^1/_4$–$^1/_2$ cup) with nonfat or 1% milk

Power Bars

Fig bars

Graham crackers

*If you are insulin-sensitive or overweight, note that all of these crackers, despite being low in fat, have very high glycemic indexes. Don't binge on them.

DAIRY PRODUCTS AND EGGS

Nonfat or low-fat fruit-flavored yogurt

$^1/_2$–1 cup nonfat or low-fat vanilla or plain yogurt, with or without fruit or applesauce

$^1/_2$–1 cup nonfat or low-fat plain or vanilla yogurt with 2 teaspoons ground flax seeds or wheat germ

Low-fat ice cream

Frozen yogurt

1 cup nonfat or 1% milk

1 cup low-fat buttermilk

1 cup soy milk or rice milk or rice drink

$^1/_2$–1 cup nonfat or low-fat cottage cheese

Deviled Eggs (page 54)

FRUITS AND FRUIT JUICES

Smoothies (page 44)

Fresh fruit, with or without 1 ounce cheese

Frozen grapes

Frozen berries

Canned fruit in juice

Fruit juice with optional brewer's yeast

Dried fruit (apricots, prunes, figs, raisins)

Dried Fruit Compote (page 42)

Dried Figs in Orange Juice (page 277)

Cheese-Stuffed Figs or Prunes (page 56)

Baked Apple (page 276)

Fruit ices or sherbet

Fruit Popsicles

VEGETABLES AND PICKLES

Carrot sticks, celery, raw peas with dip

Cucumbers with hummus

Dill pickles

Quick Cucumber Pickles (page 126)

Edamame. These are fresh green soybeans, boiled in the pod and eaten like peanuts as a snack. They are increasingly available at farmers' markets, natural food stores, and supermarkets and make a marvelous, nutritious snack.

NUTS AND CHIPS

2–4 tablespoons roasted almonds (omit for low fat)

2–4 tablespoons roasted pistachios (omit for low fat)

Oven-baked or microwaved tortilla chips with salsa

Eating Plans

for Individual

Needs

CAKES, COOKIES, AND COFFEE
  Angel food cake with berries
  Biscotti
  Nonfat or low-fat decaf latte (hot or iced)

LOWER-CARB, HIGH-PROTEIN PLAN

If you're gaining weight too quickly, are overweight to begin with, or don't want to gain as much weight as you did in your last pregnancy, these plans are for you. They're designed to give you the calories and nutrients you need, with an emphasis on protein. They're *not* modeled after the current popular low-carb diets: there are more carbohydrates here than those diets would allow. But dieting and pregnancy do not go together. Diets are designed for weight loss, and this shouldn't be your focus when you're pregnant. Rather, you should be getting the biggest nutritional bang for your buck from the foods you eat. And complex carbohydrates are good for you in many ways, providing fiber, some protein, vitamins, minerals, and little fat. Guidelines for reducing fat further are included. Bear in mind, however, that some fat is vital during pregnancy.

BREAKFASTS

NOTE: For a low-fat plan, yogurt and cottage cheese should be low fat or nonfat; milk can be 1%.

The following breakfast main dishes can be accompanied by a piece of fresh fruit, a glass of juice (see the list on page 9 for calories and sugar content), and a beverage. A glass of milk or soy milk or a cup of yogurt, preferably low fat, can be added. Milk can take the form of a nonfat or low-fat decaf latte or hot cocoa sweetened with a sugar substitute. Try to buy free-range eggs for their higher omega-3 content. For toast, seek out dense, mixed-grain breads. Regular whole wheat toast has a high glycemic index; the carbohydrates are quickly absorbed and encourage your body to store too much fat (see page 382). The denser the bread, the better. Butter is optional for a moderate-fat plan; omit for a low-fat plan. Other options are nonfat cream cheese or cottage cheese, Yogurt Cheese (page 65), or sesame tahini.

1 or 2 scrambled eggs with 1 slice whole grain toast

1 or 2 poached eggs with 1 slice whole grain toast

1 or 2 soft-boiled eggs with 1 slice whole grain toast

Quick Individual Omelet (page 34); plain, Swiss chard or spinach, broccoli or asparagus, tomato, mushroom, or cheese with 1 slice whole grain toast

1 or 2 Fried Eggs with Spicy Cooked Tomato Sauce (page 40) with 2 corn tortillas

Nonfat or low-fat yogurt (1 cup) or soy yogurt with fresh fruit, Dried Fruit Compote (page 42), dried fruit, or unsweetened fruit preserves

Banana or Strawberry Smoothie (page 44 or 45)

Nondairy Banana or Strawberry Smoothie (page 44 or 45)

2 slices whole grain toast with Apple-Cinnamon Tofu Spread (page 46)

Melon and cottage cheese with 1 slice whole grain toast

Vanilla yogurt with berries and high-protein cereal

Microwave Oatmeal with Raisins and Milk (page 31)

2 slices whole wheat toast with peanut butter or sesame tahini (omit for low fat)

High-Protein Muffin (page 50) and 1 cup nonfat or low-fat plain yogurt or soy yogurt

Kellogg's All-Bran Bran Buds or Kellogg's All-Bran with milk and blueberries

SANDWICHES AND PITA POCKETS

To keep carbohydrates under control with sandwiches, use a dense whole grain sliced bread or whole wheat pita. To reduce carbs further, if it's convenient, make open-faced sandwiches, using only one slice of bread. (This works only if you don't have to transport the sandwiches.) If you have a problem with extreme overweight or obesity, consider using lettuce and making roll-ups instead of sandwiches (see page 71).

Club Sandwich (page 72)

Tuna Sandwich (page 74)

Tofu and Spinach Pita Pocket (page 80)

Simple, Quick Tofu Sandwich (page 79) or Tofu Sandwich with Avocado and Tomato (page 79; omit for low fat)

Lower-Carb,

High-Protein

Plan

289

Roast Beef Sandwich (page 78; omit for low fat)

My Egg Salad Sandwich (page 77)

Tomato, Mozzarella, and Basil Sandwich (page 85)

Chicken Breast and Red Pepper Sandwich (page 73)

Creamy Cucumber Sandwich (page 125)

Grilled Portobello and Cheese (or Miso) Sandwich (page 83)

Sardine Spread and Cucumber Sandwich (page 76)

Hummus Pita Pocket (page 82)

White Bean or Black-Eyed Pea Pâté Sandwich (page 82)

LIGHT SOUPS

Mexican Chicken Soup with Zucchini, Chickpeas, and Tomatoes (page 90)

Gazpacho (page 106)

Chilled Cucumber Yogurt Soup (page 107)

Miso Soup with Tofu (page 96)

Italian Spinach and Egg Soup (page 97)

Garlic Soup with Broccoli (page 98)

Hot and Sour Soup (page 94)

Winter Vegetable Soup (page 102)

Chicken Soup with Egg and Lemon (page 93)

MAIN-DISH SALADS

These can also be served as starter salads in smaller portions.

Egg Salad (page 146)

Tuna and Green Bean Salad (page 153)

Beef and Arugula Salad (page 147)

Asian Chicken Salad (page 158) or Curried Chicken Salad (page 156)

Quinoa and Black Bean Salad with Lime Dressing (page 140)

Niçoise Salad (page 150)

Cobb Salad (page 154)

Broccoli and Chickpea Salad with Egg (page 141)

Frisée, Poached Egg, and Bacon Salad (page 148)

French Lentil Salad (page 136)

MAIN DISHES

Roast Chicken (page 171; remove skin for low fat)

Asian, Indian, or Mediterranean Chicken Breast (page 169)

Grilled or Pan-Seared Porterhouse Steak (page 179)

Pan-Seared or Grilled London Broil (page 180)

Roast Turkey with Wild Rice Stuffing (pages 186 and 187)

Steak or Chicken Fajitas (page 182; omit steak for low fat plan)

Mediterranean Chicken Stew (page 172)

Soft Tacos or Tostadas with Chicken, Corn, and Avocado (page 233)

All-Beef Burger (page 178)

Turkey Burger (page 178)

Soy burger, garden burger, or soy hot dog

Grilled or Broiled Fish Steak with Asian Flavors (page 195)

Snapper or Sole with Lemon, Capers, Oregano, and Olive Oil (page 194)

Grilled Tuna with Tomato-Balsamic Salsa (page 196)

Whole Trout Baked in Foil (page 192)

Salmon Fillet Cooked in the Microwave (page 190)

Halibut Cooked in the Microwave (page 189)

Red Snapper Fillet Baked in Foil (page 191)

Sole with Olive Oil, Lemon, and Scallions (page 193)

Hot or Cold Spinach Frittata (page 220)

Zucchini "Pasta" (page 205)

Spinach, Broccoli, or Asparagus Flan (page 228)

Stir-Fried Pork and Greens (page 185)

Stir-Fried Chicken and Broccoli (page 176)

Quesadilla (page 216; plain, black bean, or with greens)

Pan-Cooked Tofu (page 223) or Broiled or Grilled Tofu (page 224)

Stir-Fried Tofu with Red Chard (page 225)

Stir-Fried Tofu with Broccoli and Mushrooms (page 226)

Roast Pork Loin with Fennel-Pepper Rub (page 184)

VEGETABLE DISHES

Roasted Beets and Beet Greens (page 243)

Asian Greens (page 238)

Tomato Gratin (page 251)

Southern Italian–Style Broccoli Rabe (page 241)

Steamed Artichokes with Dips (page 244)

Zucchini and Rice Gratin (page 249)

Lower-Carb,

High-Protein

Plan

291

Baked Sweet Potato (page 256)
Broccoli with Garlic and Lemon (page 242)
Summer Vegetable Gratin (page 248)
Pan-Cooked Summer Squash (page 247)
Dry-Roasted Waxy Potatoes (page 253)
Baked Potato Skins (page 254)
Braised Red Cabbage (page 246)

SALADS

Green Salad with Vinaigrette (page 164)
Baby Greens Salad (page 110)
Creamy Cucumber Salad (page 125)
Tomato and Arugula Salad with Feta Cheese (page 116)
Greek Salad (page 115)
Beet and Orange Salad (page 117)
Coleslaw (page 127)
Asian Coleslaw (page 128)
Arugula or Baby Greens and Beet Salad (page 112)
Baby Spinach Salad with Mushrooms (page 111)
Grapefruit and Avocado Salad (page 118)
Quick Cucumber Pickles (page 126)
Classic Tabbouleh (page 138)
Grated Carrots in Vinaigrette (page 122)
Marinated Carrots (page 124)
Moroccan Cooked Carrot Salad with Cumin (page 123)
Guacamole (page 121; omit for low fat)
Three Omega-3 Salad (page 114)

DESSERTS

Fresh fruit
Strawberry or peach frozen yogurt
Melon with Mint and Lime (page 277)
Pineapple with Mint (page 277)
Orange and Mint Salad (page 281)
Biscotti
Baked Apple (page 276)
Strawberry Orange Soup (page 282)
Berry Cream (page 271)
Strawberries and Peaches with Mint (page 281)

Lower-Carb, High-Protein Menus

Bear in mind that some of the protein in these menus will come from dairy products, which are high in complete protein, and from grains. If you are overweight or insulin-sensitive, omit bread and make wrap versions of the sandwiches (see page 71). Water, mineral water, or iced herbal teas are recommended beverages with meals. Because these menus are useful if you have to watch your weight gain, we have specified amounts of some items, such as milk and yogurt.

DAY 1

Breakfast

1 or 2 scrambled eggs

1–2 ounces turkey or soy breakfast links (optional)

1 slice whole grain toast

³/₄–1 cup orange juice (fresh or commercial), ¹/₂ grapefruit, or 1 piece melon

Snack

Apple

1 ounce cheese

Lunch

Club Sandwich (page 72) or Tuna Sandwich (page 74)

Dill pickle

Coleslaw (store-bought or homemade, page 000)

1 cup nonfat or 1% milk or soy milk

1 piece fruit

Snack

1 cup nonfat or low-fat vanilla yogurt with blueberries

Dinner

Grilled or Broiled Fish Steak with Asian Flavors (page 195)

Steamed broccoli

Brown rice (page 266)

Green salad or Grated Carrots in Vinaigrette (page 122)

Snack

Pear

FOOD GROUP BREAKDOWN	
BREAD, CEREAL, RICE, PASTA	4
VEGETABLES	4
FRUIT	5
POULTRY, FISH, DRIED BEANS, MEAT, EGGS, NUTS	3–5
MILK, YOGURT, CHEESE	3

Lower-Carb,

High-Protein

Plan

DAY 2

**FOOD GROUP
BREAKDOWN**

Bread, Cereal,
  Rice, Pasta   3
Vegetables   4
Fruit   4
Poultry, Fish, Dried
  Beans, Meat,
  Eggs, Nuts   3
Milk, Yogurt,
  Cheese   3

Breakfast

Cereal, such as Kellogg's All-Bran or Kellogg's All-Bran Bran Buds, with nonfat or 1% milk and bananas or peaches

$3/4$–1 cup orange or grapefruit juice (fresh or commercial)

Snack

Strawberry Smoothie (page 45)

Lunch

Beef and Arugula Salad (page 147)

1 piece whole grain bread

$3/4$–1 cup nonfat or 1% milk or soy milk

Snack

$1/4$ cup roasted almonds

$3/4$–1 cup nonfat or 1% milk or soy milk

Dinner

Gazpacho (page 106; make enough for 2 meals)

Roast Chicken (page 171; remove skin for low fat)

Steamed green beans

Wild rice (page 267), brown rice (page 266), or basmati rice (page 265)

Green salad (optional)

Melon with Mint and Lime (page 277)

Snack

$1/2$ cup unsweetened applesauce

DAY 3

**FOOD GROUP
BREAKDOWN**

Bread, Cereal,
  Rice, Pasta   4
Vegetables   4
Fruit   4
Poultry, Fish, Dried
  Beans, Meat,
  Eggs, Nuts   2
Milk, Yogurt,
  Cheese   4

Breakfast

Banana Smoothie with optional flax seeds (page 44)

1 slice whole grain toast with low-fat cream cheese

Nonfat or low-fat decaf latte

Snack

Grapefruit

Lunch

Gazpacho (page 106)

Asian Chicken Salad (page 158)

1 cup nonfat or 1% milk or soy milk

1 piece fruit

Snack

Crudités with Curried Yogurt Dip (page 61)

2–4 Wasa or Ryvita crackers

Dinner

Grilled or Pan-Seared Porterhouse Steak (page 179) or Pan-Seared
or Grilled London Broil (page 180)

Mediterranean Greens (page 239)

Three Omega-3 Salad (page 114)

Strawberry frozen yogurt

Snack

1 slice whole grain toast with sesame tahini or peanut butter

DAY 4

Breakfast

1 or 2 poached eggs

1 slice whole grain toast

$^3/_4$–1 cup orange juice (fresh or commercial), $^1/_2$ grapefruit, or
1 piece melon

Snack

Frozen grapes

Lunch

Tomato, Mozzarella, and Basil Sandwich (page 85)

Quick Cucumber Pickles (page 126)

$^3/_4$–1 cup nonfat or 1% milk or soy milk

1 piece fruit

Snack

$^3/_4$–1 cup carrot juice

$^1/_4$ cup almonds

Dinner

Garlic Soup with Broccoli (page 98)

Spaghetti with commercial tomato sauce

Baby Greens Salad (page 110)

1 slice whole grain bread

1 ounce cheese

1 piece fruit

Snack

$^1/_2$ cup vanilla yogurt

FOOD GROUP
BREAKDOWN

BREAD, CEREAL, RICE, PASTA	4
VEGETABLES	5
FRUIT	4
POULTRY, FISH, DRIED BEANS, MEAT, EGGS, NUTS	2–5
MILK, YOGURT, CHEESE	3

Lower-Carb,

High-Protein

Plan

FOOD GROUP BREAKDOWN

Bread, Cereal, Rice, Pasta	4
Vegetables	4
Fruit	3½
Poultry, Fish, Dried Beans, Meat, Eggs, Nuts	2
Milk, Yogurt, Cheese	3

Breakfast

1 cup nonfat vanilla or plain yogurt with raisins or chopped dried apricots and 2 teaspoons ground flax seeds

1 slice whole grain toast

½ grapefruit

Nonfat or low-fat decaf latte

Snack

Strawberry Smoothie (page 45)

Lunch

Tuna Sandwich (page 74)

Coleslaw (store-bought or homemade, page 127)

Dill pickle

¾–1 cup nonfat or 1% milk or soy milk

Snack

Apple

Dinner

Mexican Chicken Soup with Zucchini, Chickpeas, and Tomatoes (page 90)

Quesadilla with Black Beans (page 217)

Baby Spinach Salad with Mushrooms (page 111)

Orange and Mint Salad (page 281)

Snack

½ cup nonfat or low-fat plain or vanilla yogurt with ¼–½ cup unsweetened applesauce

FOOD GROUP BREAKDOWN

Bread, Cereal, Rice, Pasta	4
Vegetables	5
Fruit	4
Poultry, Fish, Dried Beans, Meat, Eggs, Nuts	3
Milk, Yogurt, Cheese	3

DAY 6

Breakfast

Quick Individual Omelet with Cheese (page 36)

1 slice whole grain toast

¾–1 cup orange juice (fresh or commercial), ½ grapefruit, or 1 piece melon

Snack

High-Protein Muffin (page 50)

¾–1 cup low-fat buttermilk

Lunch

Crudités with Curried Yogurt Dip (page 61)

1 cup nonfat or low-fat cottage cheese with avocado

1 slice whole grain bread

1 cup nonfat vanilla or plain yogurt with berries, or 1 piece fruit

Snack

1/2 toasted whole grain English muffin with nonfat cream cheese
and unsweetened jam

3/4–1 cup nonfat or 1% milk or soy milk

Dinner

Salmon Fillet Cooked in the Microwave (page 190)

Tomato Gratin (page 251)

Corn on the cob

Creamy Cucumber Salad (page 125)

Peach frozen yogurt or fresh fruit

Snack

1 piece melon

DAY 7

Breakfast

High-Protein Muffin (page 50)

Banana Smoothie (page 44)

3/4–1 cup orange juice (fresh or commercial), 1/2 grapefruit, or 1
piece melon

Snack

Deviled Egg (page 54)

Lunch

Cucumber slices with Hummus (page 57)

Couscous Tabbouleh (page 139)

1 ounce cheese, 1/2–1 cup nonfat vanilla or plain yogurt, or 3/4–1 cup
nonfat or 1% milk or soy milk

1 piece fruit

Snack

1 cup low-fat plain yogurt with 1/4–1/2 cup unsweetened applesauce

Dinner

Hot and Sour Soup (page 94)

Stir-Fried Pork and Greens (page 185)

Asian Coleslaw (page 128)

Orange and Mint Salad (page 281)

Snack

Strawberries with milk

FOOD GROUP BREAKDOWN	
BREAD, CEREAL, RICE, PASTA	3
VEGETABLES	4
FRUIT	5
POULTRY, FISH, DRIED BEANS, MEAT, EGGS, NUTS	3
MILK, YOGURT, CHEESE	4

Lower-Carb,

High-Protein

Plan

HIGHER-CARB, HIGH-PROTEIN PLAN

This eating plan includes all of the dishes in the lower-carb plan, plus higher-carb dishes such as pasta, potatoes, and rice. I've listed a number of bean dishes here, because beans are relatively high in complex carbohydrates. (Because they have a low glycemic index, or GI, they are also appropriate for lower-carbohydrate menus.) This is still a moderately low-fat diet, with about 30% of calories from fat. Carbohydrates are a good choice for getting more calories into your diet, but make sure you don't overlook protein calories. The obvious high-carb foods, sweets, won't do you or your baby any good, but sometimes a dish of ice cream is just what the doctor ordered, hitting the spot, combating nausea, and helping to put on weight.

To the suggestions on pages 288–292 add the following:

BREAKFASTS

Whole grain toast can accompany all the breakfasts on pages 293–297.

Cereal with milk and bananas or peaches (Low-GI cereal choices include Kellogg's All-Bran Extra Fiber, Kellogg's All-Bran Bran Buds, and Kellogg's Special K. Intermediate-GI breakfast cereals include shredded wheat and puffed wheat.)

Buttermilk Pancakes (page 39) with maple syrup or canned peaches

Bran Muffin (page 48), yogurt, and fruit

Wheatena or Cream of Wheat with milk and raisins

Whole wheat bagel with low-fat cream cheese

Cornbread with butter and honey; plain or flavored yogurt

French Toast (page 38)

Muesli (page 33) with milk

Mango Smoothie (page 44)

SANDWICHES

Grilled Cheese Sandwich (page 84)

Bruschetta with Tomatoes and Parmesan (page 86), Mozzarella or Goat Cheese and Roasted Peppers (page 87), or Beans and Sage (page 87)

HEARTY SOUPS

Asian Noodle Soup with Spinach and Salmon (page 92)

Asian Noodle Soup with Tofu and Spinach (page 92)

Chicken Noodle or Tofu Noodle Soup (page 89)

Minestrone (page 100)

Lentil Soup (page 103)

Mushroom and Barley Soup (page 104)

MAIN-DISH SALADS

Bean Salad with Cumin Vinaigrette (page 134)

Tuna and Bean Salad (page 152)

Curried Mixed-Grain Salad (page 142)

Wild Rice Salad (page 144)

Potato and Green Bean Salad (page 130)

Warm Potato and Goat Cheese Salad (page 132)

Asian Noodle Salad (page 160)

Couscous Tabbouleh (page 139)

Chickpea Salad (page 133)

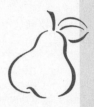

MAIN DISHES

Pasta with Pesto and Green Beans (page 199)

Creamy Pasta with Broccoli (page 197)

Creamy Pasta with Greens (page 198)

Quick Spinach and Tomato Lasagna (page 206)

Summer Pasta with Tomatoes and Green Beans or Peas (page 200)

Pasta with Tomato Sauce (page 201; with chickpeas, goat cheese,
     tuna, broccoli, greens, or turkey sausage or ground turkey)

Spinach or mushroom quiche

Fried Brown Rice and Vegetables (page 222)

Simple Homemade Pizza (page 210)

Polenta with Tomato Sauce and Beans (page 261)

Strata with Tomatoes and Greens (page 218)

Simmered Black Beans or Pinto Beans with Cilantro (page 229)

Black Bean Tostadas (page 234)

Quick Black Bean Tacos (page 232)

Winter Vegetable Couscous (page 214)

Couscous with Chickpeas and Greens (page 212)

Chicken, Lemon, and Olive Stew with Couscous (page 174)

Higher-Carb,

High-Protein

Plan

Baked Russet Potato (page 253) or Dry-Roasted Waxy Potatoes
   (page 253)

Potato Gratin (page 255)

Corn Gratin (page 250)

Corn on the cob

Steamed New Potatoes or Fingerlings with Herbs (page 252)

Basmati Rice Pilaf with Chickpeas (page 257)

Basmati Rice Pilaf with Peas (page 258)

Bulgur (page 263), quinoa (page 265), rice (page 265), or wheat
   berries (page 267)

DESSERTS

Desserts should be fruit-oriented, but you have more options than
with the lower-carb plan.

Scandinavian Fruit Soup (page 43)

Low-fat ice cream

Frozen yogurt

Frozen Banana Yogurt (page 279)

Cherry Clafoutis (page 274)

Chocolate Pudding (page 270)

Dried Fruit Compote (page 42)

Pears Poached in Ginger Honey Syrup (page 278)

Rice Pudding (page 280)

Bread Pudding with Apples or Peaches (page 269)

Flourless Orange Cake (page 273)

Brownies (page 272)

Higher-Carb, High-Protein Menus

You can use any of the lower-carb, high-protein meals in the previous section and add a slice of bread or a grain; a soup, salad, or side
dish from the higher-carb list; or a dessert as desired. If you need
to keep calories down, use nonfat or low-fat milk, yogurt, cottage
cheese, and cream cheese.

DAY 1

Breakfast

Cereal with milk and bananas or peaches

Whole grain toast with cream cheese or Yogurt Cheese (page 65)

Orange juice (fresh or commercial), grapefruit, or melon

Snack

Crudités with Thai Peanut Sauce (page 55)

Lunch

Grilled Cheese Sandwich (page 84)

Greek Salad (page 115)

Fresh fruit

Snack

2 fig bars

Milk or buttermilk

Dinner

Asian Noodle Soup with Spinach and Salmon (page 92)

Creamy Cucumber Salad (page 125)

Whole grain bread

Berry Cream (page 271)

Biscotti

Snack

Molasses Bread (page 53)

Milk or soy milk

FOOD GROUP BREAKDOWN	
BREAD, CEREAL, RICE, PASTA	8
VEGETABLES	4
FRUIT	4
POULTRY, FISH, DRIED BEANS, MEAT, EGGS, NUTS	3
MILK, YOGURT, CHEESE	3½

DAY 2

Breakfast

Scrambled eggs

Turkey or soy breakfast links (optional)

Whole grain toast

Orange juice (fresh or commercial), grapefruit, or melon

Snack

Whole grain toast with peanut butter or sesame tahini

Milk or soy milk

Lunch

Hummus Pita Pocket (page 82)

Classic Tabbouleh (page 138)

Milk or vanilla or plain yogurt

Fresh fruit

FOOD GROUP BREAKDOWN	
BREAD, CEREAL, RICE, PASTA	9
VEGETABLES	4
FRUIT	4
POULTRY, FISH, DRIED BEANS, MEAT, EGGS, NUTS	3–3½
MILK, YOGURT, CHEESE	2

Higher-Carb,

High-Protein

Plan

301

Snack

Orange

Toasted whole grain English muffin with cream cheese or jam

Dinner

Bruschetta with Mozzarella and Roasted Peppers (page 87)

Creamy Pasta with Broccoli (page 197)

Baby Greens Salad (page 110)

Pears Poached in Ginger Honey Syrup (page 278)

Snack

Vanilla yogurt

DAY 3

Breakfast

Microwave Oatmeal with Milk and Raisins (page 31)

Whole grain toast with jam

Orange juice (fresh or commercial; optional)

Snack

Banana Smoothie (page 44)

Lunch

Niçoise Salad (page 150)

Whole grain bread

Milk or soy milk (optional)

Snack

Edamame (fresh green soybeans)

Crudités with Thai Peanut Sauce (page 55)

Dinner

Roast Chicken (page 171)

Steamed New Potatoes or Fingerlings with Herbs (page 252)

Steamed broccoli or green beans

Arugula or Baby Greens and Beet Salad (page 112)

Orange and Mint Salad (page 281)

Snack

Graham crackers

Milk or buttermilk

FOOD GROUP BREAKDOWN	
BREAD, CEREAL, RICE, PASTA	6–7
VEGETABLES	5
FRUIT	3½
POULTRY, FISH, DRIED BEANS, MEAT, EGGS, NUTS	2–3
MILK, YOGURT, CHEESE	4

DAY 4

Breakfast

Orange juice (fresh or commercial)

Bran Muffin (page 48)

Vanilla or plain yogurt with berries and optional flax seeds

Decaf latte

Snack

Carrot and celery sticks with Curried Yogurt Dip (page 61)

Crackers with cheese

Lunch

Lentil Soup (page 103)

Chicken Breast and Red Pepper Sandwich (page 73)

Cheese or yogurt

Snack

Tomato juice or V8

Oven-baked or microwaved tortilla chips with salsa

Dinner

Tuna and Bean Salad (page 152)

Minestrone (page 100)

Whole grain bread

Frozen Banana Yogurt (page 279)

Snack

Applesauce

FOOD GROUP BREAKDOWN	
BREAD, CEREAL, RICE, PASTA	7
VEGETABLES	5
FRUIT	3½
POULTRY, FISH, DRIED BEANS, MEAT, EGGS, NUTS	5
MILK, YOGURT, CHEESE	3½

DAY 5

Breakfast

Poached eggs

Whole grain toast

Orange juice (fresh or commercial), grapefruit, or melon

Snack

Strawberry Smoothie (page 45)

Lunch

Tomato, Mozzarella, and Basil Sandwich (page 85)

Baby Greens Salad (page 110)

Milk or soy milk

Fresh fruit

FOOD GROUP BREAKDOWN	
BREAD, CEREAL, RICE, PASTA	6
VEGETABLES	4
FRUIT	5
POULTRY, FISH, DRIED BEANS, MEAT, EGGS, NUTS	3½
MILK, YOGURT, CHEESE	4½

Higher-Carb,

High-Protein

Plan

303

Snack

Bran Muffin (page 48)

Buttermilk

Dinner

Stir-fried Pork and Greens (page 185)

Grapefruit and Avocado Salad (page 118)

Chocolate Pudding (page 270)

Snack

Vanilla frozen yogurt

FOOD GROUP
BREAKDOWN

BREAD, CEREAL,
   RICE, PASTA   5–6
VEGETABLES   4
FRUIT   4
POULTRY, FISH, DRIED
   BEANS, MEAT,
   EGGS, NUTS   3
MILK, YOGURT,
   CHEESE   3½

DAY 6

Breakfast

Banana, Mango, or Strawberry Smoothie (page 44 or 45)

Bran Muffin (page 48)

Decaf latte

Snack

Wasa or Ryvita crackers with cheese

Crudités with Curried Yogurt Dip (page 61)

Lunch

Miso Soup with Tofu (page 96)

Asian Noodle Salad (page 160)

Fresh fruit

Snack

Plain or vanilla yogurt with berries

Dinner

Red Snapper Fillet Baked in Foil (page 191)

Rice or baked potato

Southern Italian–Style Broccoli Rabe (page 241)

Three Omega-3 Salad (page 114)

Frozen yogurt or fresh fruit

Snack

Toasted whole grain English muffin with jam

DAY 7

Breakfast

Buttermilk Pancakes (page 39) with maple syrup or canned peaches and yogurt

Turkey bacon or sliced turkey sausage or breakfast links (optional)

Orange juice (fresh or commercial), grapefruit, or melon

Snack

Power Bar

Lunch

My Egg Salad Sandwich (page 77)

Coleslaw (store-bought or homemade, page 127) or green salad

Fresh fruit

Snack

Whole grain toast with peanut butter

Milk or buttermilk

Dinner

Lentil Soup (page 103)

Quick Spinach and Tomato Lasagna (page 206)

Beet and Orange Salad (page 117)

Fresh fruit

Snack

Hot cocoa

FOOD GROUP BREAKDOWN	
BREAD, CEREAL, RICE, PASTA	6
VEGETABLES	3
FRUIT	4
POULTRY, FISH, DRIED BEANS, MEAT, EGGS, NUTS	3½
MILK, YOGURT, CHEESE	4

VEGETARIAN PLANS

Ovo-Lacto Vegetarian Plan

Use all the meatless recipes from the two preceding sections, plus the dishes in the vegan list below. If you are concerned with gaining too much weight, concentrate on the lower-carb plan. If you need to gain weight, concentrate on the higher-carb plan. The biggest challenge is getting enough protein without increasing your carbohydrate intake too much.

Vegan Plan

Many of the dishes listed here also appear in the preceding sections, but this gives you an idea of the range you have even if you don't eat dairy products. The main challenge is getting enough calcium. Here are the best vegetarian, nondairy sources of calcium.[1]

Vegetarian Foods Equal to About ¹/₂ Cup Milk in Calcium Content

4 ounces tofu, if processed with calcium sulfate
4 ounces collard greens
4 corn tortillas, if processed with calcium salts

Vegetarian Foods Equal to About ¹/₃ cup Milk in Calcium Content

1 cup cooked dried beans
4 ounces bok choy, turnip greens, or kale

BREAKFASTS

Nondairy Banana, Mango, or Strawberry Smoothie (page 44 or 45)
Whole grain toast with Apple-Cinnamon Tofu Spread (page 46)
Microwave Oatmeal with Milk and Raisins (page 31; made with soy
   milk and served with apples)
Wheatena with soy milk, apples, and raisins
Cereal with soy milk or rice milk
Couscous with Oranges and Dates (page 32)
Whole wheat toast with peanut butter and honey
Bean and rice burritos
Egg and Bean Tacos (page 235)
Scrambled Tofu (page 37)

SANDWICHES

Peanut Butter and Banana Sandwich (page 78)
Tofu and Spinach Pita Pocket (page 80)
Simple, Quick Tofu Sandwich (page 79)

[1] Institute of Medicine, *Nutrition During Pregnancy and Lactation: An Implementation Guide* (Washington, D.C.: National Academy Press, 1992), p. 102.

Tofu Sandwich with Avocado and Tomato (page 79)

Barbecued Tempeh Sandwich (page 81)

Grilled Portobello and Miso Sandwich (page 83)

White Bean Pâté Sandwich (page 82)

Hummus Pita Pocket (page 82)

HEARTY SALADS

Bean Salad with Cumin Vinaigrette (page 134)

French Lentil Salad (page 136)

Couscous Tabbouleh (page 139)

Classic Tabbouleh (page 138)

Chickpea Salad (page 133)

Curried Mixed-Grain Salad (page 142)

Wild Rice Salad (page 144)

White Bean and Basil Salad (page 137)

Tempeh and Sesame Salad (page 162)

Asian Noodle Salad (page 160)

LIGHT AND HEARTY SOUPS

Vegetarian Mexican Soup (page 91)

Gazpacho (page 106)

Miso Soup with Tofu (page 96)

Tofu Noodle Soup (page 89)

Lentil Soup (page 103)

Minestrone (page 100)

Mushroom and Barley Soup (page 104)

MAIN DISHES

Garden burgers or soy burgers

Pasta with Tomato Sauce and Chickpeas (page 202), Broccoli (page 202), or Greens (page 202)

Zucchini "Pasta" with tomato sauce (page 205)

Stir-Fried Tofu with Red Chard (page 225) with brown rice (page 266) or bulgur (page 263)

Soft Tacos with Tofu and Tomatoes (page 211)

Quesadilla with Black Beans (page 217)

Tofu with Dipping Sauces (page 60); tofu may be plain, pan-cooked (page 223), or broiled or grilled (page 224)

Stir-Fried Tofu with Broccoli and Mushrooms (page 226)

Fried Brown Rice and Vegetables (page 222)

Couscous with Chickpeas and Greens (page 212)

Winter Vegetable Couscous (page 214)

Basmati Rice Pilaf with Peas (page 257)

Simmered Black Beans with Cilantro (page 229)

Black Bean Tostadas (page 234)

SIDE DISHES, SALADS, AND DESSERTS

Choose appropriate dishes from the lists on pages 288–305.

Ovo-Lacto Vegetarian Menus

FOOD GROUP BREAKDOWN

BREAD, CEREAL, RICE, PASTA	6–7
VEGETABLES	4
FRUIT	5
POULTRY, FISH, DRIED BEANS, MEAT, EGGS, NUTS	2–4
MILK, YOGURT, CHEESE	4–5

DAY 1

Breakfast

Cereal with milk and bananas or peaches

Whole grain toast with cream cheese or Yogurt Cheese (page 65)

Orange juice (fresh or commercial), grapefruit, or melon

Snack

Banana Smoothie (page 44)

Lunch

Grilled Cheese Sandwich (page 84)

Three Omega-3 Salad (page 114)

Fresh fruit

Snack

Vanilla yogurt or edamame (fresh green soybeans)

Dinner

Asian Noodle Soup with Tofu and Spinach (page 92)

Creamy Cucumber Salad (page 125)

Marinated Carrots (page 124)

Whole grain bread

Berry Cream (page 271)

Snack

Whole grain toast with peanut butter or cream cheese

Milk or soy milk

DAY 2

Breakfast

Scrambled eggs

Soy breakfast links (optional)

Whole grain toast

Orange juice (fresh or commercial), grapefruit, or melon

Snack

Whole grain toast with peanut butter

Milk or soy milk

Lunch

Hummus Pita Pocket (page 82)

Classic Tabbouleh (page 138)

Milk or soy milk, or vanilla or plain yogurt

Fresh fruit

Snack

Bran Muffin (page 48)

Milk or buttermilk

Dinner

Creamy Pasta with Broccoli (page 197)

Tomato and Arugula Salad with Feta Cheese (page 116)

Pears Poached in Ginger Honey Syrup (page 278)

Snack

Banana

FOOD GROUP
BREAKDOWN

BREAD, CEREAL, RICE, PASTA	5
VEGETABLES	4
FRUIT	4
POULTRY, FISH, DRIED BEANS, MEAT, EGGS, NUTS	3
MILK, YOGURT, CHEESE	4

DAY 3

Breakfast

Microwave Oatmeal with Milk and Raisins (page 31; served with apples)

Orange juice (fresh or commercial)

Snack

Cheese-Stuffed Figs or Prunes (page 56)

Whole grain toast with jam

Lunch

My Egg Salad Sandwich (page 77)

Coleslaw (store-bought or homemade, page 127)

Dill pickle

Milk or soy milk (optional)

Snack

Plain or vanilla yogurt with applesauce

FOOD GROUP
BREAKDOWN

BREAD, CEREAL, RICE, PASTA	5-7
VEGETABLES	4
FRUIT	4
POULTRY, FISH, DRIED BEANS, MEAT, EGGS, NUTS	2½
MILK, YOGURT, CHEESE	4

Ovo-Lacto

Vegetarian

Plan

Dinner

Lentil Soup (page 103; with Greens; make enough for 2 meals)

Whole grain bread

Arugula or Baby Greens and Beet Salad (page 112)

Orange and Mint Salad (page 281)

Snack

Graham crackers

Milk, soy milk, or buttermilk

DAY 4

Breakfast

Orange juice (fresh or commercial)

Bran Muffin (page 50)

Vanilla or plain yogurt with berries and optional flax seeds

Snack

Carrot and celery sticks with Curried Yogurt Dip (page 61)

Wasa or Ryvita crackers with Hummus (page 57)

Lunch

Lentil Soup (page 103; with greens)

Tomato, Mozzarella, and Basil Sandwich (page 85)

Milk or soy milk

Snack

Tomato juice or V8

Cottage cheese

Dinner

Three Omega-3 Salad (page 114)

Spinach, Broccoli, or Asparagus Flan (page 228)

Steamed New Potatoes or Fingerlings with Herbs (page 252)

Whole grain bread

Frozen Banana Yogurt (page 279)

Snack

Orange

2 biscotti

DAY 5

Breakfast

Poached eggs

Whole grain toast

Orange juice (fresh or commercial), grapefruit, or melon

Snack

Apple

Cheese

Lunch

Cottage cheese

Baked Sweet Potato (page 256)

Whole grain bread

Baby Greens Salad (page 110)

Milk or soy milk

Fresh fruit

Snack

Miso Soup with Tofu (page 96)

Dinner

Stir-Fried Tofu with Red Chard (page 225)

Brown rice (page 266) or bulgur (page 263)

Grapefruit and Avocado Salad (page 118)

Frozen yogurt

Snack

Graham crackers

Milk or soy milk

FOOD GROUP BREAKDOWN

BREAD, CEREAL, RICE, PASTA	4–5
VEGETABLES	4
FRUIT	5
POULTRY, FISH, DRIED BEANS, MEAT, EGGS, NUTS	2½–3½
MILK, YOGURT, CHEESE	4

DAY 6

Breakfast

Orange juice (fresh or commercial), grapefruit, or melon

Buttermilk Pancakes (page 39) with strawberries or canned peaches and plain or vanilla yogurt

Decaf latte

Snack

Banana, Mango, or Strawberry Smoothie (page 44 or 45)

Lunch

Miso Soup with Tofu (page 96)

Asian Noodle Salad (page 160)

Fresh fruit

FOOD GROUP BREAKDOWN

BREAD, CEREAL, RICE, PASTA	6
VEGETABLES	4
FRUIT	6
POULTRY, FISH, DRIED BEANS, MEAT, EGGS, NUTS	3
MILK, YOGURT, CHEESE	3

Ovo-Lacto

Vegetarian

Plan

Snack

Vanilla yogurt with blueberries

Dinner

Quick Individual Omelet with Mushrooms (page 36) or mushroom quiche (store-bought)

Rice or baked potato

Southern Italian–Style Broccoli Rabe (page 241)

Three Omega-3 Salad (page 114)

Frozen yogurt or fresh fruit

Snack

Whole grain toast with cream cheese

Milk or soy milk

<table>
<tr><td colspan="2">FOOD GROUP BREAKDOWN</td></tr>
<tr><td>Bread, Cereal, Rice, Pasta</td><td>7</td></tr>
<tr><td>Vegetables</td><td>4</td></tr>
<tr><td>Fruit</td><td>4</td></tr>
<tr><td>Poultry, Fish, Dried Beans, Meat, Eggs, Nuts</td><td>2</td></tr>
<tr><td>Milk, Yogurt, Cheese</td><td>5</td></tr>
</table>

DAY 7

Breakfast

Cereal with milk and bananas or peaches

Whole grain toast

Orange juice (fresh or commercial), grapefruit, or melon

Snack

Apple or pear

Cheese

Lunch

Quinoa and Black Bean Salad with Lime Dressing (page 140)

Quesadilla (page 216)

Fresh fruit

Snack

Tomato juice or V8

Edamame (fresh green soybeans) or Tofu with Dipping Sauces (page 60)

Dinner

Quick Spinach and Tomato Lasagna (page 206)

Beet and Orange Salad (page 117)

Strawberries or raspberries with milk or vanilla yogurt

Snack

Hot cocoa

Vegan Menus

DAY 1

Breakfast
Microwave Oatmeal with Milk and Raisins (page 31; made with soy milk and served with apples)
Whole grain toast with Apple-Cinnamon Tofu Spread (page 46)
Fortified orange juice, grapefruit, or melon

Snack
Nondairy Banana Smoothie (page 44)

Lunch
French Lentil Salad (page 136)
Greek Salad (page 115; omit feta)
Whole grain bread
Fresh fruit

Snack
Whole grain toast with peanut butter or sesame tahini
Crudités

Dinner
Asian Noodle Soup with Tofu and Spinach (page 92)
Quick Cucumber Pickles (page 126)
Whole grain bread
Orange and Mint Salad (page 281)
Tofutti

Snack
Rice drink

FOOD GROUP BREAKDOWN

BREAD, CEREAL, RICE, PASTA	6
VEGETABLES	4
FRUIT	4
POULTRY, FISH, DRIED BEANS, MEAT, EGGS, NUTS	5

DAY 2

Breakfast
Scrambled Tofu (page 37)
Soy breakfast links (optional)
Whole grain toast
Fortified orange juice, grapefruit, or melon

Snack
Edamame (fresh green soybeans) or Tofu with Dipping Sauces (page 61)
Fruit juice with optional brewer's yeast

FOOD GROUP BREAKDOWN

BREAD, CEREAL, RICE, PASTA	9
VEGETABLES	4
FRUIT	5–6
POULTRY, FISH, DRIED BEANS, MEAT, EGGS, NUTS	6–7

Vegan

Plan

Lunch

Hummus Pita Pocket (page 82)

Classic Tabbouleh (page 138)

Soy milk

Fresh fruit

Snack

Grapefruit or orange

Rice cakes or whole grain toast with honey

Dinner

Bruschetta with Beans and Sage (page 87)

Pasta with Tomato Sauce and Broccoli (page 202)

Baby Greens Salad (page 110)

Pears Poached in Ginger Honey Syrup (page 278)

Snack

Frozen grapes

FOOD GROUP
BREAKDOWN

BREAD, CEREAL,
RICE, PASTA   7

VEGETABLES   4

FRUIT   4

POULTRY, FISH, DRIED
BEANS, MEAT,
EGGS, NUTS   6½

DAY 3

Breakfast

Microwave Oatmeal with Milk and Raisins (page 31; made with soy milk and served with apples)

Whole grain toast with jam

Snack

Whole grain toast with peanut butter

Soy milk

Lunch

Barbecued Tempeh Sandwich (page 81)

Coleslaw (store-bought or homemade, page 127)

Dill pickle

Soy milk (optional)

Snack

Orange

Wasa or Ry-Krisp crackers with sesame tahini

Dinner

Lentil Soup (page 103)

Garden burger on whole grain bun

Beet and Orange Salad (page 117)

Baked Apple (page 276; make extra)

Snack

Almonds

Cantaloupe

Breakfast

Whole grain toast with Apple-Cinnamon Tofu Spread (page 46) or peanut butter

Nondairy Banana, Mango, or Strawberry Smoothie with optional flax seeds (page 44 or 45)

Snack

Baked Apple (page 276) with granola and soy milk

Lunch

Quick Black Bean Tacos (page 232; omit cheese)

Baby Spinach Salad with Mushrooms (page 111)

Fresh fruit

Snack

Wasa or Ry-Krisp crackers

Tofu with Dipping Sauces (page 61)

Dinner

Three Omega-3 Salad (page 114)

Minestrone (page 100)

Whole grain bread

Fresh fruit

Tofutti

Snack

Whole grain toast with peanut butter or sesame tahini

FOOD GROUP BREAKDOWN	
BREAD, CEREAL, RICE, PASTA	4
VEGETABLES	5
FRUIT	4
POULTRY, FISH, DRIED BEANS, MEAT, EGGS, NUTS	6

Breakfast

Wheatena with raisins, apples, and soy milk (sweeten with honey or brown sugar)

Whole grain toast

Fortified orange juice, 1/2 grapefruit, or melon

Snack

Power Bar

Soy milk or rice milk

Lunch

Peanut Butter and Banana Sandwich (page 78)

Marinated Carrots (page 124)

Soy milk

Fresh fruit

FOOD GROUP BREAKDOWN	
BREAD, CEREAL, RICE, PASTA	6–7
VEGETABLES	4
FRUIT	6
POULTRY, FISH, DRIED BEANS, MEAT, EGGS, NUTS	7

Vegan

Plan

Snack

Crudités with Tofu Green Goddess (page 67)

Rice drink or soy milk

Dinner

Miso Soup with Tofu (page 96)

Stir-Fried Tofu with Red Chard (page 225)

Brown rice (page 266) or bulgur (page 263)

Grapefruit and Avocado Salad (page 118)

Dried Fruit Compote (page 42)

Snack

Fruit ice or Popsicle

FOOD GROUP
BREAKDOWN

BREAD, CEREAL,
  RICE, PASTA   7

VEGETABLES   4

FRUIT   4

POULTRY, FISH, DRIED
  BEANS, MEAT,
  EGGS, NUTS   5

DAY 6

Breakfast

Nondairy Banana, Mango, or Strawberry Smoothie (page 44 or 45)

Dried Fruit Compote (page 42)

Whole grain toast with Apple-Cinnamon Tofu Spread (page 46) or
  peanut butter

Snack

Wasa or Ry-Krisp crackers

Tofu with Dipping Sauces (page 61)

Lunch

Grilled Portobello and Miso Sandwich (page 83)

Asian Noodle Salad (page 160)

Fresh fruit

Snack

Toasted whole wheat English muffin with jam

Soy milk or rice milk

Dinner

Southern Italian–Style Broccoli Rabe (page 241)

Polenta with Tomato Sauce and Beans (page 261)

Baby Greens Salad (page 110)

Strawberry Orange Soup (page 282)

Snack

Banana

Breakfast

Cereal with soy milk or rice milk

Whole grain toast with unsweetened fruit preserves

Fortified orange juice, grapefruit, or melon

Snack

Crudités with Thai Peanut Sauce (page 61)

Wasa or Ry-Krisp crackers

Lunch

Tofu Sandwich with Avocado and Tomato (page 79)

Coleslaw (store-bought or homemade, page 127) or green salad

Fresh fruit

Soy milk or rice milk

Snack

Apple

Almonds

Dinner

Simmered Black Beans or Pinto Beans with Cilantro (page 229)

Corn tortillas

Guacamole (page 121)

Cantaloupe and berries

Snack

Tofutti

FOOD GROUP
BREAKDOWN

BREAD, CEREAL, RICE, PASTA	8
VEGETABLES	3
FRUIT	4
POULTRY, FISH, DRIED BEANS, MEAT, EGGS, NUTS	5

PLAN FOR THE NONCOOK OR THE RELUCTANT COOK

If you don't cook, you probably won't feel inclined to learn when you're feeling nauseous and/or exhausted. And even if you do cook, you may not want to.

Luckily, you can eat well on prepared foods during your pregnancy, provided you choose them carefully. It's crucial that you read labels for fats, protein, and overall calories. The percentage of calories from fats should be no more than 30%. Fortunately, there are now many brands of frozen and packaged dinners that follow

Plan for the

Noncook or the

Reluctant Cook

these guidelines. You also need to supplement prepared meals with fresh fruits and vegetables and dairy products. A salad; steamed broccoli, peas, or green beans; some cut-up raw vegetables such as carrots and red bell peppers; and a glass of milk or a bowl of yogurt will often do the trick.

Delis and deli sections of natural food stores and supermarkets are often stocked with an array of nutritious dishes, such as lentil salads, Chinese vegetables and rice, chicken salads, pasta dishes, and grain dishes. The fat content may be higher than it would be if you cooked these dishes yourself, but they are still good foods to eat. For example, our local natural food store carries a number of appropriate prepared dishes, including the following:

Asian cucumber salad
Greek orzo salad
Fresh sautéed spinach with garlic
Vegetable tamales
Vegetable quesadillas
Spinach quesadillas
Chicken quesadillas
Zucchini latkes
Autumn puree
Quinoa cakes
Lemon herb tofu
Asparagus with sesame dressing
Turkey burgers
Stuffed chicken breasts
Rosemary lemon chicken
Vegetable fried rice
Green beans with red pepper dressing
Sonoma chicken salad
Tuna salad
Teriyaki chicken skewers
Vegetarian chili
Vegetable gumbo with tofu
Beef stew with vegetables

The range at our local supermarket is not quite as good, but it includes choices such as bean salad, tabbouleh, Szechuan chicken salad, brown rice with vegetables, and roasted vegetables with balsamic vinaigrette.

What if take-out is your staple? This is doable, as long as you keep your kitchen stocked with fresh fruits and vegetables for between-meal snacks. Again, choice is the key word. Even fast food is viable, although we don't recommend it on a steady basis, because the caloric and fat content is generally very high and the fiber content low. You do get a lot of nutritious protein calories for your buck when you eat a hamburger. Relatively healthy fast-food choices include bean and rice burritos, chicken burritos, chicken fajitas, and steak fajitas. Some fast-food choices may be high in vitamin C, calcium, zinc, folate, vitamin B_6, and other nutrients.

Hazards

You take certain risks when you eat prepared foods, so you must choose carefully and be confident about the sanitary conditions of the places you shop. Deli meats, hot dogs and undercooked meats, poultry, and seafood can contain listeria bacteria, which can cause flu-like symptoms in pregnant women. Infection with these bacteria, listeriosis, can be treated with antibiotics, but it also can be passed to the fetus, resulting in miscarriage, premature birth, or stillbirth. Listeria also can be found in soft cheeses such as Brie, Camembert, and Mexican-style fresh cheese (queso fresco), as well as in unpasteurized milk products. Another parasite, *Toxoplasma gondii*, which causes a mild flu-like infection called toxoplasmosis, can contaminate undercooked meat and poultry and unwashed fruits and vegetables.

The Center for Science in the Public Interest and the U.S. Department of Agriculture (USDA) advise you to select only ready-to-eat foods that can be reheated, and then to reheat them to at least 165°F. Reheat hot dogs and deli meats until steaming. Avoid pâtés, unpasteurized juices, and products made with unpasteurized milk.

We would also caution you against self-serve salad bars, because the food practices there are often questionable. Produce is left out for too long and handled by too many people, which can cause contamination.

You may, however, use prewashed, precut salad greens and vegetables (if the convenience is worth the price) and low-fat prepared dressings. But do give prewashed greens a second rinse at home. This is important, as outbreaks of *E. coli* originating from unwashed greens have occurred in the past.

Your best all-around bet for safety and convenience is to choose foods that require cooking or thawing by exposure to high heat, or foods that you reheat. Frozen foods, such as pasta dishes and prepared meals, fit nicely into this category, as do packaged grain, bean, and pasta dishes. The downside is that many of these products are expensive, and many contain additives, preservatives, and flavor enhancers that may not be harmful to your baby but don't have any food value either. Following are some suggestions for prepared foods. Some of the brands and products in these lists and menus might be unavailable in your supermarket. However, you will probably be able to find a similar product made by a different company. Packaged rice pilafs, for example, are made by more than one food company, and with more than one style of seasoning. Choose what appeals to you. If a menu lists "Wolfgang Puck's Frozen Lasagna Dinner," and that product is not sold in your supermarket, choose another frozen lasagna dinner or another prepared pasta as your main dish.

FROZEN MEALS

BOBOLI PIZZA CRUSTS; top with commercial tomato sauce, vegetables, and grated cheese

EL CHARRITO LEAN OLÉ!

Bean & Cheese Burrito

Steak, Beans & Rice Burrito

HEALTHY CHOICE

Country Herb Chicken

Salisbury Steak

MICHAEL ANGELO'S

Vegetable Lasagna

Chicken Lasagna

Lasagna with Meat Sauce

Chicken Parmesan

STOUFFER'S LEAN CUISINE

Chicken in Peanut Sauce

Chicken Carbonara

Herb Roasted Chicken

Beef Peppercorn

STOUFFER'S LEAN CUISINE HEARTY PORTIONS MEAL

Chicken Fettucini with Broccoli

Jumbo Rigatoni with Meatballs

STOUFFER'S LEAN CUISINE SKILLET SENSATIONS

Herb Chicken and Roasted Potatoes

Chicken Oriental

Beef Teriyaki and Rice

Garlic Chicken

Chicken Primavera

VEGETARIAN BURGERS, HOT DOGS, AND SAUSAGES

Boca Burgers

Gardenburgers

Morningstar Farm Veggie Dogs

Morningstar Farms Breakfast Strips

WEIGHT WATCHERS SMART ONES

Santa Fe Style Rice and Beans

Lasagna Florentine

Lemon Herb Chicken Piccata

Fettuccini Alfredo with Broccoli

WOLFGANG PUCK'S MEALS (these meals contain no preservatives and many are low in fat)

PACKAGED MEALS

FARMHOUSE

Fettuccine Alfredo

Rice Pilaf

Spanish Style Rice

Brown and Wild Rice

Broccoli au Gratin Rice

Long Grain and Wild Rice

KNORR RICE MATES SEASONING PACKS

MAHATMA

Long Grain & Wild Rice with Seasonings

Plan for the
Noncook or the
Reluctant Cook

Saffron Yellow Seasonings & Long Grain Rice

Authentic Spanish Seasonings & Long Grain Rice

Red Beans and Rice with Seasonings

MARRAKESH EXPRESS

Couscous

Risotto

NEAR EAST COUSCOUS

Mediterranean Curry

Herbed Chicken

NEAR EAST PASTA

Spicy Tomato

Roasted Garlic & Olive Oil

NEAR EAST PILAFS

THE SPICE HUNTER QUICK POT PASTA

Roasted Pepper & Garlic

Sun Dried Tomato & Basil

THE SPICE HUNTER QUICK POT RISOTTO

Wild Mushroom

Classic Cheese

ZATARAIN'S NEW ORLEANS STYLE RICE MIXES

Zatarain's Spanish Rice

Zatarain's Red Beans & Rice

RICE A RONI RICE PILAF

ONE-PORTION MEALS AND SOUPS IN A CUP, VARIOUS BRANDS

THE SPICE HUNTER

Three Cheese Risotto

Spinach & Garlic Risotto

Minestrone

Split pea soup

Vegetarian chile

Rice and red beans

OTHER OPTIONS

Healthy Choice canned soups

Pasta and tomato sauces; serve with Boboli pizza crusts, pasta, chicken breasts, or fish

Menus for the Noncook or the Reluctant Cook

These menus combine prepared foods and some homemade dishes with fresh fruits, salads, and vegetables. For breakfasts and snacks, use any of the menus on pages 293–317.

Lentil Soup (canned, in a cup, or homemade, page 103)
Frozen lasagna
Baby Greens Salad (page 110)
Orange and Mint Salad (page 281)

Tortilla soup in a cup or Mexican Chicken Soup with Zucchini,
    Chickpeas, and Tomatoes (page 90)
Weight Watchers Smart Ones Santa Fe Style Rice and Beans
Green salad or Guacamole (page 121)
Fresh fruit

Weight Watchers Smart Ones Lasagna Florentine
Marinated Carrots (page 124)
Green salad
Pears Poached in Ginger Honey Syrup (page 278)

Weight Watchers Smart Ones Lemon Herb Chicken Piccata
Steamed broccoli
Baby Spinach Salad with Mushrooms (page 111)
Vanilla yogurt with berries

Crudités with Herbed Yogurt Cheese (page 65)
Weight Watchers Smart Ones Fettuccini Alfredo with Broccoli
Green salad
Strawberries with milk

Boca Burger, Gardenburger or Morningstar Farms Veggie Dog on
    whole wheat bun
Roasted Pepper and Mozzarella Antipasto (page 120)
Corn on the cob
Frozen yogurt

Tortilla soup in a cup or Gazpacho (page 106)
El Charrito Lean Olé! Bean & Cheese Burrito or Steak, Beans & Rice
    Burrito
Fresh Tomato Salsa (store-bought or homemade, page 63)
Guacamole (page 121) or Baby Greens Salad (page 110)
Fruit Popsicle

Frozen ravioli
Steamed green beans or broccoli
Arugula or Baby Greens and Beet Salad (page 112)
Plain or vanilla yogurt with fresh fruit

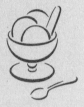

Stouffer's Lean Cuisine Chicken in Peanut Sauce
Creamy Cucumber Salad (page 125)
Bottled, canned, or homemade roasted red peppers (see page 119)
Frozen Banana Yogurt (page 279)

Minestrone (canned, in a cup, or homemade, page 100)
Stouffer's Lean Cuisine Chicken Carbonara
Southern Italian–Style Broccoli Rabe (page 241)
Baby Greens Salad (page 110)
Orange and Mint Salad (page 281)

Stouffer's Lean Cuisine Herb Roasted Chicken
Pan-Cooked Summer Squash (page 247)
Green salad
Piece of cheese
Fresh fruit

Stouffer's Lean Cuisine Beef Peppercorn
Steamed broccoli
Sliced tomatoes
Green salad
Strawberry frozen yogurt

Marinated Carrots (page 124)
The Spice Hunter Quick Pot Wild Mushroom Risotto
Three Omega-3 Salad (page 114)
Fresh fruit

Near East Spicy Tomato Pasta
Chicken Breasts with Mediterranean Flavors (page 170)
Steamed broccoli
Baby Spinach Salad with Mushrooms (page 111)
Melon with Mint and Lime (page 277)

Packaged Tomato and Lentil or Rice Pilaf
Spinach quiche
Greek Salad (page 115)
Vanilla frozen yogurt

Gazpacho with optional shrimp (page 106)
Packaged Red Beans and Rice
Quick Cucumber Pickles (page 126)
Watermelon with mint

Miso Soup with Tofu (page 96)
Frozen pork and vegetable pot stickers or Stouffer's Lean Cuisine
    Skillet Sensations Chicken Oriental
Farmhouse Long Grain and Wild Rice
Steamed broccoli or Chinese greens
Asian Coleslaw (page 128)
Fresh pineapple

Roast Chicken (store-bought or homemade, page 171)
Marrakesh Express Couscous
Green salad
Plain or vanilla yogurt with berries

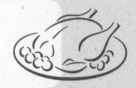

Middle Eastern Take-out
    Hummus
    Baba ghanoush
    Middle Eastern meatballs
    Tabbouleh
    Labne (Yogurt Cheese)
    Pita bread, preferably whole wheat
Fresh fruit

Eating Plans for Special Needs and High-Risk Pregnancies

CALCIUM-RICH PLAN
FOR THE LACTOSE-INTOLERANT

Many people, particularly those of African American, Asian, Native American, and Hispanic descent, have trouble digesting lactose, the sugar in milk. Lactose intolerance occurs in people who lack the enzyme lactase. Lactase can be purchased in pharmacies, either in drops that are added to milk or in pill form that is taken before eating or drinking dairy products. Lactase brand names include Lactaid, Lactrace, and Dairy Ease. You will also find Lactaid milk in your supermarket dairy case. This is milk to which the enzyme has been added.

Research indicates that lactose intolerance eases during the third trimester of pregnancy, so you might try milk at this time. The breaking down of lactose also appears to be enhanced by the cocoa in chocolate, which stimulates the body to make more lactase. Try drinking chocolate milk instead of plain, but keep in mind that 1 cup of chocolate milk contains 60 calories more than the equivalent amount of plain milk. You may also tolerate milk better when you drink it with other foods and when you choose 2% or whole milk. Milk with a higher fat content is digested more slowly, and this improves lactose digestion for some people.[1] Yogurt, buttermilk, sweet acidophilus milk, and cheese have a lower lactose content than milk.

If you cannot tolerate dairy products no matter what you try, you'll need a calcium-rich eating plan that is high in nondairy

[1] Bridget Swinney, *Eating Expectantly* (New York: Meadowbrook Press, 1996), p. 60.

sources of this important mineral. But even these foods will not yield nearly as much calcium as ³/₄ to 1 cup of milk, so your doctor also will probably advise you to take a calcium supplement. The best nondairy sources of calcium are, from highest to lowest:

Sardines with bones
Tofu processed with calcium sulfate
Canned salmon with bones
Fortified soy milk (varies with brand)
Fortified orange juice
Green leafy vegetables, especially collard greens but also broccoli, kale, bok choy, and mustard greens
Navy beans, pinto beans, and chickpeas
Corn tortillas processed with calcium salts
Sesame seeds and sesame tahini (made with roasted or toasted sesame seeds)

RECIPES THAT ARE HIGH IN CALCIUM

These recipes use the calcium-rich foods listed above. Some of them may contain a small amount of yogurt or cheese. You can omit these ingredients if you are sensitive to them. For example, a salad that contains a little bit of cheese will still be delicious without that ingredient. If yogurt is used as a liquid in a puree, the quantities will be so low that you probably won't have a reaction to it. If you do, try substituting mayonnaise or soy milk.

Three Omega-3 Salad (page 114)
Asian Greens (page 238)
Asian Noodle Soup with Tofu and Spinach (page 92)
Simmered Black Beans or Pinto Beans with Cilantro (page 229)
Roasted Beets and Beet Greens (page 243)
Broccoli and Chickpea Salad with Egg (page 141)
Broccoli with Garlic and Lemon (page 242)
Quesadilla with Greens (if you can tolerate the cheese; page 217)
Quesadilla with Black Beans (if you can tolerate the cheese; page 217)
Chickpea Salad (page 133)

Couscous with Chickpeas and Greens (page 212)

Creamy Pasta with Broccoli (if you can tolerate the cottage cheese; page 197)

Creamy Pasta with Greens (if you can tolerate the cottage cheese; page 198)

Garlic Soup with Broccoli (page 98)

Greek Spinach Pie (if you can tolerate the feta; page 208)

Nondairy Smoothie (page 44)

Hummus (page 57)

Lentil Soup (page 103; with greens)

Mediterranean Greens (page 239)

Miso Soup with Tofu (page 96)

Apple-Cinnamon Tofu Spread (page 46)

Refried Beans (page 230)

Sardine Spread (page 76)

Scrambled Tofu (page 37)

Southern Italian–Style Broccoli Rabe (page 241)

Baby Spinach Salad with Mushrooms (page 111)

Hot or Cold Spinach Frittata (page 220)

Stir-Fried Chicken and Broccoli (page 176)

Stir-Fried Tofu with Broccoli and Mushrooms (page 226)

Stir-Fried Tofu with Red Chard (page 225)

Soft Tacos with Tofu and Tomatoes (page 211)

Tofu with Dipping Sauces (page 61)

Tofu and Spinach Pita Pocket (page 80)

Tomato and Arugula Salad with Feta Cheese (page 116) (omit feta if you can't tolerate it)

White Bean and Basil Salad (page 137)

White Bean or Black-Eyed Pea Pâté (page 58)

White Bean Puree (page 62)

CALCIUM-RICH MENUS
FOR THE LACTOSE-INTOLERANT

DAY 1

Breakfast
Scrambled eggs

Turkey or soy breakfast links (optional)

Whole grain toast

Fortified orange juice, grapefruit, or melon

Snack
Whole grain toast with sesame tahini

Apple

Lunch
Club Sandwich (page 72) or Tuna Sandwich (page 73)

Baby Spinach Salad with Mushrooms (page 111)

Fresh fruit

Snack
Edamame (fresh green soybeans) or Tofu with Dipping Sauces (page 61)

1 slice whole grain toast with Hummus (page 195)

Dinner
Grilled or Broiled Fish Steak with Asian Flavors (page 195)

Steamed broccoli

Brown rice (page 266)

Green salad or Grated Carrots in Vinaigrette (page 122)

Snack
Pear

FOOD GROUP BREAKDOWN

BREAD, CEREAL, RICE, PASTA	8
VEGETABLES	5
FRUIT	4
POULTRY, FISH, DRIED BEANS, MEAT, EGGS, NUTS	7½

DAY 2

Breakfast
Cereal, such as Kellogg's All-Bran or Kellogg's All-Bran Buds, with soy milk and bananas or peaches

Fortified orange or grapefruit juice

Snack
Nondairy Strawberry Smoothie (page 45)

Lunch
Tofu and Spinach Pita Pocket (page 80)

Chickpea Salad (page 133)

Fresh fruit

FOOD GROUP BREAKDOWN

BREAD, CEREAL, RICE, PASTA	5
VEGETABLES	4
FRUIT	6
POULTRY, FISH, DRIED BEANS, MEAT, EGGS, NUTS	6

Calcium-Rich Plan

for the Lactose-

Intolerant

Snack

Toasted almonds

Soy milk or rice milk

Dinner

Gazpacho (page 106; make enough for 2 meals)

Roast Chicken (page 171; remove skin for low-fat)

Mediterranean Greens (page 239)

Wild rice (page 267), brown rice (page 266), or basmati rice (page 265)

Green salad (optional)

Melon with Mint and Lime (page 277)

Snack

Applesauce

Whole grain toast with roasted sesame tahini

FOOD GROUP
BREAKDOWN

BREAD, CEREAL, RICE, PASTA	4
VEGETABLES	5
FRUIT	4
POULTRY, FISH, DRIED BEANS, MEAT, EGGS, NUTS	6

DAY 3

Breakfast

Nondairy Banana Smoothie with optional flax seeds (page 44)

Whole grain toast with Apple-Cinnamon Tofu Spread (page 46)

Melon

Snack

Grapefruit

Lunch

Miso Soup with Tofu (page 96)

Asian Chicken Salad (page 158)

Fresh fruit

Snack

Crudités with Tofu Green Goddess (page 67)

Wasa or Ryvita crackers with Hummus (page 57)

Dinner

Gazpacho (page 106)

Grilled or Pan-Seared Porterhouse Steak (page 179) or Pan-Seared or Grilled London Broil (page 180)

Broccoli with Garlic and Lemon (page 242)

Three Omega-3 Salad (page 114)

Frozen soy yogurt

Snack

Whole grain toast with sesame tahini

DAY 4

Breakfast

Poached eggs

Whole grain toast

Fortified orange juice, grapefruit, or melon

Snack

Frozen grapes

Lunch

Beef and Arugula Salad (page 147)

Sardine Spread and Cucumber Sandwich (page 76) or Miso Soup
with Tofu (page 96)

Fresh fruit

Snack

Carrot juice

Almonds

Dinner

Bruschetta with Beans and Sage (page 87)

Spaghetti with commercial tomato sauce and broccoli

Baby Greens Salad (page 110)

Whole grain bread

Fresh fruit

Snack

Tofutti

FOOD GROUP BREAKDOWN	
BREAD, CEREAL, RICE, PASTA	10
VEGETABLES	5
FRUIT	4
POULTRY, FISH, DRIED BEANS, MEAT, EGGS, NUTS	6

DAY 5

Breakfast

Whole grain toast with Apple-Cinnamon Tofu Spread (page 46)

Microwave Oatmeal with Milk and Raisins (page 31; made with soy
milk or rice milk)

Grapefruit

Snack

Nondairy Strawberry Smoothie (page 45)

Lunch

Tuna Sandwich (page 74) or Sardine Spread and Cucumber Sandwich (page 76)

Coleslaw (store-bought or homemade, page 127)

Dill pickles

Fresh fruit

FOOD GROUP BREAKDOWN	
BREAD, CEREAL, RICE, PASTA	7
VEGETABLES	5
FRUIT	4
POULTRY, FISH, DRIED BEANS, MEAT, EGGS, NUTS	5

Calcium-Rich Plan

for the Lactose-

Intolerant

Snack

Power Bar

Dinner

Mexican Chicken Soup with Zucchini, Chickpeas, and Tomatoes
(page 90)

Quesadilla with Greens (page 217)

Refried Beans (page 230)

Baby Spinach Salad with Mushrooms (page 111)

Orange and Mint Salad (page 281)

Snack

Whole grain toast with sesame tahini

DAY 6

FOOD GROUP
BREAKDOWN

BREAD, CEREAL,
RICE, PASTA   7

VEGETABLES   4

FRUIT   5

POULTRY, FISH, DRIED
BEANS, MEAT,
EGGS, NUTS   7¹/₂

Breakfast

Quick Individual Omelet with Spinach or Broccoli (page 35)

Whole grain toast

Fortified orange juice, grapefruit, or melon

Snack

High-Protein Muffin (page 50)

Soy milk or rice milk

Lunch

Asian Noodle Soup with Tofu and Spinach (page 92)

Whole grain bread

Fruit Popsicle

Snack

Toasted whole grain English muffin with White Bean Pâté (page 58)
or sesame tahini

Soy milk or rice milk

Dinner

Salmon Fillet Cooked in the Microwave (page 190)

Tomato Gratin (page 251)

Corn on the cob

Baby Spinach Salad with Mushrooms (page 111)

Peach Tofutti or fresh fruit

Snack

Cantaloupe or watermelon

Breakfast

High-Protein Muffin (page 50)

Nondairy Banana Smoothie (page 44)

Fortified orange juice, grapefruit, or melon

Snack

Deviled Egg (page 54)

Lunch

Cucumber slices and whole wheat pita with Hummus (page 57)

Couscous Tabbouleh (page 139)

Fresh fruit

Snack

Tofu with Dipping Sauces (page 61)

Dinner

Hot and Sour Soup (page 94)

Stir-Fried Pork and Greens (page 185)

Rice

Asian Coleslaw (page 128)

Orange and Mint Salad (page 281)

Snack

Chocolate milk or soy milk

Graham crackers

FOOD GROUP BREAKDOWN	
BREAD, CEREAL, RICE, PASTA	3
VEGETABLES	4
FRUIT	4
POULTRY, FISH, DRIED BEANS, MEAT, EGGS, NUTS	6

PLAN FOR MULTIPLES

If you're expecting multiples, gaining weight is particularly important for the outcome of your pregnancy. Practitioners at the University of Michigan Multiples Clinic recommend that women gain 24 pounds by 24 weeks for twins, 36 pounds for triplets, and 50 pounds for quadruplets. You can do this by following a diet plan that includes three substantial meals and four or five substantial snacks.

Realistically, though, you may not be able to cope with this much food during the first trimester if you are suffering from extreme morning sickness — and morning sickness is much more likely to occur in women carrying multiples. In this case, you

Plan

for

Multiples

should eat those foods you can tolerate every couple of hours —
crackers, fruit, toast, juice, lemonade, ice cream, even potato chips.
But once you begin feeling better in the second trimester, you'll
have to catch up. Use the 10 weeks between week 14 and 24 to accomplish your weight-gain goals. If you aren't suffering from
morning sickness, you will probably feel much hungrier than
you've ever felt before, since increased hunger can accompany
multiples pregnancies. The ideal goal is to eat something every two
hours. If you are underweight to begin with, you need to eat even
more often — every hour and a half. Expectant mothers of multiples have reported successful pregnancy outcomes when they've
adhered to an eat-every-two-hours schedule.[2]

One of the common complaints in multiples pregnancies is
excess swelling, which can be greater than in singleton pregnancies. This is partly due to the fact that your large uterus inhibits
blood flow to the heart. Lying down can ease this problem. Carbohydrates can contribute to swelling, as each gram of carbohydrate
holds two grams of water. If you are suffering from swelling, you
might want to reconfigure the menus so that you are limiting your
carbohydrate intake at night.

Iron deficiency anemia is another common problem for
women carrying more than one baby. Since your iron stores are required for more than one fetus, you have to take in quite a lot of
iron and will probably need supplementation as well. An iron-rich
diet that includes red meat and liver can help. Your diet also will be
closely monitored by your health care team if you develop gestational diabetes (see page 341).

The menus that follow are based on the higher-carb, high-
protein menu plan beginning on page 298, with added between-
meal mini-meals or snacks. Since calorie requirements are so
much higher for multiples pregnancies, you may want to opt for
2% or full-fat dairy products.

[2] Barbara Luke and Tamara Eberlein, *When You're Expecting Twins, Triplets, or
Quads* (New York: Harper Perennial, 1999), pp. 62–63.

Ways to Increase Calorie Intake

- Drink and eat 2% or full-fat dairy products.
- Eat more high-fat, nutritious foods, such as salmon, red meat, cheese, avocados, nuts, sesame tahini, peanut butter and other nut butters, and pizza.
- Eat sweets that have food value, such as ice cream, milk shakes, and peanut butter or oatmeal cookies.
- Use butter on bread and toast.
- Toss vegetables with olive oil or butter.
- Drink supplements such as Ensure, or add protein powder to juices and smoothies.
- Drink lots of fruit juice and carbonated fruit drinks, as well as high-carb drinks such as Jamba Juice.
- Eat meal-size snacks, such as frozen entrees like macaroni and cheese.
- Keep your desk at work stocked with crackers and cheese, Power Bars, peanut butter, cookies, dried fruit, and nuts. If there is a refrigerator, bring in yogurt, cottage cheese, milk, and other cold snacks.

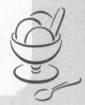

Menus for Multiples

DAY 1

Breakfast

Cereal with milk and bananas or peaches

Whole grain toast with cream cheese or Yogurt Cheese (page 65)

Orange juice (fresh or commercial), grapefruit, or melon

Snack

Crudités with Thai Peanut Sauce (page 55)

Milk

Toast or crackers with smoked trout or ham

Lunch

Grilled Cheese Sandwich (page 84) or All-Beef Burger (page 178)

Greek Salad (page 115)

Fresh fruit

Snack

1–1½ ounces cheese

2–4 fig bars

Milk or buttermilk

FOOD GROUP BREAKDOWN	
BREAD, CEREAL, RICE, PASTA	8
VEGETABLES	4
FRUIT	6½
POULTRY, FISH, DRIED BEANS, MEAT, EGGS, NUTS	4½
MILK, YOGURT, CHEESE	8½

Plan

for

Multiples

Snack

Apple

Vanilla, fruit-flavored, or plain yogurt

Dinner

Asian Noodle Soup with Spinach and Salmon (page 92)

Creamy Cucumber Salad (page 125)

Whole grain bread

Cheese

Raspberries with vanilla ice cream

Snack

Molasses Bread (page 53)

Milk

Snack

Peanut Butter and Banana Sandwich (page 78)

FOOD GROUP BREAKDOWN	
BREAD, CEREAL, RICE, PASTA	11
VEGETABLES	3½
FRUIT	5
POULTRY, FISH, DRIED BEANS, MEAT, EGGS, NUTS	7
MILK, YOGURT, CHEESE	4½

DAY 2

Breakfast

Scrambled eggs

Turkey or soy breakfast links

Whole grain toast with butter or jam

Orange juice (fresh or commercial), grapefruit, or melon

Snack

Whole grain toast with peanut butter or sesame tahini

Milk or soy milk

Snack

Apple

Bran Muffin (page 48)

Plain, vanilla, or fruit-flavored yogurt

Lunch

Hummus Pita Pocket (page 82) or Roast Beef Sandwich (page 78)

Classic Tabbouleh (page 138)

Milk or vanilla or plain yogurt

Fresh fruit

Snack

Orange

Toasted whole grain English muffin with cream cheese

Dinner
Bruschetta with Mozzarella and Roasted Peppers (page 87)

Creamy Pasta with Broccoli (page 197)

Grilled pork chops

Baby Greens Salad (page 110)

Pears Poached in Ginger Honey Syrup (page 278)

Snack
Vanilla yogurt or ice cream

DAY 3

Breakfast
Microwave Oatmeal with Milk and Raisins (page 31; served with apples)

Whole grain toast with jam and butter or cream cheese

Orange juice (fresh or commercial)

Snack
Banana Smoothie (page 44)

Lunch
Niçoise Salad (page 150)

Whole grain bread

Milk or soy milk (optional)

Cheese

Fresh fruit

Snack
Bean and cheese burrito

Snack
Fruit-flavored yogurt

Dinner
Roast Chicken (page 171)

Steamed New Potatoes or Fingerlings with Herbs (page 252) or
Potato Gratin (page 255)

Steamed broccoli or green beans

Arugula or Baby Greens and Beet Salad (page 112)

Orange and Mint Salad (page 28)

Snack
Graham crackers

Milk or buttermilk

Snack
Chocolate milk shake

FOOD GROUP BREAKDOWN	
Bread, Cereal, Rice, Pasta	5
Vegetables	4
Fruit	3
Poultry, Fish, Dried Beans, Meat, Eggs, Nuts	8
Milk, Yogurt, Cheese	5½

Plan

for

Multiples

FOOD GROUP
BREAKDOWN

BREAD, CEREAL,
  RICE, PASTA   8
VEGETABLES   7
FRUIT   4¹/₂
POULTRY, FISH, DRIED
  BEANS, MEAT,
  EGGS, NUTS   5¹/₂
MILK, YOGURT,
  CHEESE   6

Breakfast

Orange juice (fresh or commercial), grapefruit, or melon

Bran Muffin (page 48)

Vanilla or plain yogurt with berries and optional flax seeds

Decaf latte

Snack

Deviled Egg (page 54)

Whole grain bread with butter

Snack

Carrot and celery sticks with Guacamole (page 121)

Crackers with cheese

Lunch

Lentil Soup (page 103)

Chicken Breast and Red Pepper Sandwich (page 73)

Cheese or yogurt

Milk or soy milk

Fresh fruit

Snack

Tomato juice or V8

Oven-baked or microwaved tortilla chips with bean dip and salsa

Dinner

Steamed Artichokes with Dips (page 244)

Grilled or Pan-Seared Porterhouse Steak (page 179) or Pan-Seared
  or Grilled London Broil (page 180)

Baked potato with butter and sour cream

Mediterranean Greens (page 239)

Frozen Banana Yogurt (page 279)

Snack

Applesauce

Snack

Cereal with milk and bananas

DAY 5

Breakfast
Dried Fruit Compote (page 42)
Poached eggs
Whole grain toast with butter
Orange juice (fresh or commercial), grapefruit, or melon

Snack
Banana Strawberry Smoothie (page 44)

Snack
Apple
Cheese

Lunch
Tomato, Mozzarella, and Basil Sandwich (page 85)
Beef and Arugula Salad (page 147)
Milk or soy milk
Fresh fruit

Snack
Tuna Sandwich (page 74)
Milk or buttermilk

Dinner
Stir-Fried Pork and Greens (page 185)
Grapefruit and Avocado Salad (page 118)
Chocolate Pudding (page 270)

Snack
Vanilla frozen yogurt with canned peaches or apricots

Snack
Bran Muffin (page 48)
Milk or soy milk

FOOD GROUP BREAKDOWN	
Bread, Cereal, Rice, Pasta	7
Vegetables	4
Fruit	7
Poultry, Fish, Dried Beans, Meat, Eggs, Nuts	7
Milk, Yogurt, Cheese	8

DAY 6

Breakfast
Banana, Mango, or Strawberry Smoothie (page 44 or 45)
Bran Muffin (page 48)
Decaf latte

Snack
Peanut Butter and Banana Sandwich (page 78)
Milk or soy milk

FOOD GROUP BREAKDOWN	
Bread, Cereal, Rice, Pasta	10
Vegetables	3
Fruit	$4\frac{1}{2}$
Poultry, Fish, Dried Beans, Meat, Eggs, Nuts	6
Milk, Yogurt, Cheese	7

Plan

for

Multiples

Lunch

Miso Soup with Tofu (page 96)

Asian Noodle Salad (page 160)

Whole grain bread

Fresh fruit

Snack

Plain or vanilla yogurt with berries or canned peaches

Whole grain toast with butter or High-Protein Muffin (page 50)

Dinner

Salmon Fillet Cooked in the Microwave (page 190)

Rice or baked potato

Southern Italian–Style Broccoli Rabe (page 241)

Three Omega-3 Salad (page 114)

Frozen yogurt or fresh fruit

Snack

Cottage cheese

Sliced pineapple

Snack

Toasted whole grain bagel or English muffin with butter or cream cheese and jam

Milk or soy milk

FOOD GROUP
BREAKDOWN

Bread, Cereal, Rice, Pasta	8 1/2
Vegetables	3
Fruit	4
Poultry, Fish, Dried Beans, Meat, Eggs, Nuts	5
Milk, Yogurt, Cheese	5

DAY 7

Breakfast

Buttermilk Pancakes (page 39) with maple syrup and yogurt

Turkey bacon or sliced turkey sausage or breakfast links

Orange juice (fresh or commercial), grapefruit, or melon

Snack

Power Bar

Vanilla milk shake

Snack

Cottage cheese with avocado

Lunch

My Egg Salad Sandwich (page 77) or cheeseburger

Coleslaw (store-bought or homemade, page 127) or green salad

Fresh fruit

Snack

Whole grain toast with peanut butter or sesame tahini

Milk or buttermilk

Dinner

Lentil Soup (page 103)

Frozen Lasagna

Whole grain bread

Beet and Orange Salad (page 117)

Fresh fruit

Snack

Ice cream

Snack

Hot cocoa

2 oatmeal cookies

PLAN FOR GESTATIONAL DIABETES

Gestational diabetes, which is characterized by higher-than-normal levels of blood sugar, affects 3% to 5% of pregnant women in this country, according to the National Institutes of Health.[3] The statistics are higher for women of African American, Mexican American, South or East Asian, Pacific Islander, or Native American descent.

If you are diagnosed with gestational diabetes, you will probably be referred to a nutrition counselor, a registered dietitian, or a diabetes specialist, who will put you on a special diet to control weight gain and maintain normal blood-sugar levels and to help you monitor those levels. The condition needn't cause complications as long as your blood-sugar levels are controlled, and this can usually be accomplished through diet.

The body obtains most of its energy from a simple sugar called glucose, which comes either from simple carbohydrates, such as sugar, honey, molasses, and the sugars in fruit and milk, or from the breakdown of complex carbohydrates. Glucose enters the bloodstream after food is digested and is transported to the tissues and cells. The hormone insulin, which is created in the pancreas, carries the glucose to the cells and docks with tiny receptors called

[3] U.S. Department of Health and Human Services, *Understanding Gestational Diabetes*, NIH Publication No. 93-2788, February 1993, p. 3

insulin receptors on the cell membranes. This signals the cells to let the glucose in, so that it can be used as energy. If insulin does not do its job, glucose accumulates in the bloodstream and eventually spills into the kidneys.

Unlike type 1 diabetes (previously known as juvenile diabetes), gestational diabetes is not caused by an inability of the pancreas to produce enough insulin. In gestational diabetes, the pancreas produces plenty of insulin, but the various pregnancy hormones in the placenta inhibit the insulin receptors on the cell membranes from responding properly to the insulin, so glucose backs up in the blood.

The condition usually shows up about halfway or two thirds of the way through pregnancy. This is because, by 20 to 24 weeks, the placenta has grown quite large, and the larger the placenta, the more insulin-blocking hormones it creates. If the pancreas is not able to make extra insulin to deal with the blocking effect of the hormones, gestational diabetes results. The problem usually disappears after delivery.

Risk Factors

Any woman can develop gestational diabetes, but an increased risk appears to be associated with the following factors:

- Obesity
- History of diabetes in immediate family
- Gestational diabetes in a previous pregnancy
- Age 26 years and up
- Native American, Hispanic, South or East Asian, Pacific Islander, or African American ancestry

Most doctors and clinics routinely screen for gestational diabetes after the 24th week of pregnancy. However, if you have a history of gestational diabetes or you are at high risk, you may be screened earlier. The initial test to determine blood-sugar levels is a simple one in which you drink a glucose drink and have your blood-sugar level measured an hour later. If the results are abnormally high, a more elaborate three-hour test must be performed, since not everyone with a positive screening has diabetes.

Risks to the Baby

Unlike pregestational type 1 and type 2 diabetes, gestational diabetes does not cause birth defects. That's because birth defects occur during the first trimester, and gestational diabetes doesn't show up until the third.

High blood-sugar levels do pose several risks to the fetus, however. One is a condition called *macrosomia,* in which the fetus grows too large. Because the maternal blood carries too much glucose to the baby, his or her pancreas produces more insulin, which in response acts as a growth hormone, converting the extra glucose to fat. If the baby grows too large, a cesarean section may be necessary for delivery.

Another risk is that the newborn baby may develop low blood sugar, or hypoglycemia, which can affect the baby's brain function. If the mother's blood-sugar levels have been high throughout the last trimester, the fetus also will have a high level of insulin in its blood. Those high insulin levels can cause a significant drop in the baby's blood sugar once it is born. The newborn's blood-sugar levels will be checked, and if they are low, the baby will be given glucose, either intravenously or orally.

High blood-sugar levels in the mother can result in other complications in the newborn, such high bilirubin, low serum calcium, and low serum magnesium levels. The baby also can develop mild to severe breathing difficulties. In addition, studies have indicated that children of women who develop gestational diabetes may be at risk for developing type 2 diabetes in childhood.

Risks to the Mother

Although gestational diabetes usually disappears once the baby is born, it can indicate a predisposition for future adult-onset, or type 2, diabetes. If you are at risk for type 2 diabetes, you should have your blood-sugar levels monitored at your routine checkups. Most important, you should try to maintain a normal body weight through diet and exercise, because obesity is one of the greatest risk factors for diabetes. If you develop gestational diabetes, you will have a 50% greater risk of gestational diabetes in a subsequent pregnancy.

Plan for

Gestational

Diabetes

Foods to Avoid

SIMPLE SUGARS AND SYRUPS

Sugar

Honey

Molasses

Corn syrup

Maple syrup

OTHER SIMPLE SUGARS

(Look for these ingredients on product labels. If any of these is listed in the first through fifth positions, the food should be avoided.)

Corn sweetener

Dextrose

Disaccharide

Fructose

Glucose

High-fructose corn syrup

Juice concentrates

Lactose

Maltose

Natural sweeteners

Sucrose

SWEETS

Candy

Jelly

Cakes, cookies, and pastries

Soda

Fruit drinks

Fruit juice (6 ounces of most fruit juices contains 4–5 teaspoons of sugar)

Ice cream and other frozen desserts

Fruit-flavored yogurt

SOME COMMON STORE-BOUGHT FOODS

Commercial pizza (tomato sauces and crusts often contain sugar)

Some tomato sauces and pasta sauces (check labels for sugars)

Ketchup

Sugar-frosted cereals and cereals with raisins or other dried fruits

Peanut butter with sugar added

Muffins

Bagels (very high in carbohydrates and calories; 1 regular bagel is equivalent to 4 slices of bread)

Chinese food (sauces usually contain sugar)

Sushi (the vinegar in the rice is sweetened)

Managing Gestational Diabetes Through Diet

Your nutritional counselor will teach you how to monitor your blood-sugar levels at home. You test at specific times throughout the day — usually first thing in the morning before you eat and two hours after each meal, sometimes more often. You record the results in a diary, along with your meals and your exercise. Using those results, your health care provider can determine whether

Foods to Avoid in the Morning
and to Eat in Moderation

Fruit (very high in sugar)

Milk

Yogurt

Many dietitians are adamant about avoiding fruit, milk, and yogurt in the morning, when blood-sugar levels can be higher. They recommend a reduced-carbohydrate morning meal that may be higher in protein and fats. However, opinions among diabetes specialists differ. Some meal plans prepared by respected diabetes authorities allow small amounts of fruit and milk in the morning. You should consult with your specialist.

Certain fruits, such as bananas, are very sweet. Bananas can be included, but they should not be too ripe; the riper the banana, the more it can raise blood-sugar levels. No more than three inches of a banana should be eaten at one time.

Complex carbohydrates and foods that are high in fiber decrease the body's need for insulin and help keep blood-sugar levels within the normal range. The American Diabetes Association recommends that you get at least half of your daily calories from complex carbohydrates. Some complex carbohydrates, however, have higher glycemic indexes (see pages 382–83) than others and can raise blood-sugar levels in certain individuals. You should minimize your intake of floury potatoes (the kind used for baked potatoes) and white bread. You may eat pasta, white rice, and waxy potatoes, but in moderation.

Soluble fiber, the type found in oat bran, appears to help lower glucose and insulin in the blood.[*] Insoluble fiber, the type found in wheat bran, vegetables, and beans, has also been found to reduce the risk of developing type 2 diabetes.[†] Protein and fats have less effect on blood sugar than carbohydrates, but saturated fats can decrease insulin's efficiency, which can lead to excessive weight gain and thus contribute to diabetes. However, some types of fats can be beneficial. These are the monounsaturates in olive oil and canola oil and the omega-3 rich fats found in cold-water fish, flax seeds, canola oil, and walnuts. New research has indicated that a diet low in omega-3s may contribute to insulin resistance. Cell membranes are largely made up of fatty acids, and when they are rich in omega-3s, they have more insulin receptors,[††] which facilitates the efficient use of glucose.

[*] Elizabeth Hiser. *The Other Diabetes: Living and Eating Well with Type 2 Diabetes* (New York: William Morrow, 1999), p. 50.

[†] Ibid., p. 51.

[††] Ibid., p. 65.

Plan for

Gestational

Diabetes

Foods to Emphasize

Complex carbohydrates (vegetables, grains, beans, peas, and pasta)
High-fiber foods
Protein
Low-fat foods and monounsaturates (such as olive oil and canola oil)
Foods high in omega-3s (such as fatty fish, flax seeds, and greens)

your diet and weight gain need further adjusting. Weight control is essential: excess calories will lead to weight gain, which can lead to elevated insulin requirements.

Another test you may be required to do regularly is a urine test for ketones. *Ketones* are a byproduct of the breakdown of fat, and inadequate insulin or inadequate calories in the diet may result in their presence in the blood. Large amounts of ketones can be harmful to the fetus.

To keep your blood-sugar levels within the normal range — which is less than 90 mg/dl before breakfast and no higher than 120 mg/dl after meals — avoid foods that are high in simple sugars. It's very important to eat regular meals that include foods from the different food groups (complex carbohydrates, protein, fats, vegetables). You'll need to eat substantial between-meal snacks, especially at bedtime. Because blood-sugar levels tend to be higher in the morning, you should keep carbohydrates to a minimum at breakfast. In most cases, fruits, which are very high in sugar, and milk and yogurt, which contain lactose, a simple sugar, are not allowed until later in the day. (Unlike milk and yogurt, cheese is not high in lactose and is considered a protein and also a fat, unless it is a low-fat cheese.)

Eating a bedtime snack is extremely important if you have gestational diabetes. You need protein and complex carbohydrates to stabilize your blood sugar throughout the night, when levels tend to be low. If your blood-sugar levels fall below normal during the night, your body will use fats as a fuel source, resulting in the production of ketones. This condition is called *starvation ketosis* and can be harmful to the fetus. If you are taking insulin, a bedtime snack eaten two to three hours after dinner is particularly critical. Starch will stabilize your blood sugar early in the evening, and protein will have a longer stabilizing effect.

Some women are so fatigued during their pregnancy that they come home from work, eat, and go straight to bed. This makes it very difficult to have a nighttime snack. If this is the case with you, eat a snack during the night when you get up to go to the bathroom. Prepare the snack before you go to bed. If heartburn is a problem, propping yourself up on pillows might help.

Managing Gestational Diabetes Through Exercise

Exercise not only helps you to maintain a healthy weight, but it also can help regulate your blood-sugar level, particularly shortly after a meal. Gentle exercise, such as walking and swimming, are better than more rigorous activities, such as jogging or aerobics, especially if you have not exercised previously. You should check and record your blood-sugar level before and after exercising.

Other Types of Diabetes

If you suffer from type 1 or type 2 diabetes, discuss this matter with your doctor, preferably before you become pregnant. Because of the hormones your body produces during pregnancy, diabetes usually becomes more acute during pregnancy, so it is very important to monitor your blood sugar and ketones regularly and to stick to the diet plan prescribed by your health care provider. It is essential not to skip meals, especially if you are taking insulin.

Gestational Diabetes Menus

Most diets for diabetes of all kinds are based on the Exchange Lists for Meal Planning from the American Diabetes Association and the American Dietetic Association. An *exchange* is a given quantity of a particular food in a food group that has approximately the same number of calories and nutrients as a given quantity of another food in the same group; thus these foods can be exchanged for each other. This system of menu planning can be confusing, but you will probably be given a menu plan and a complete list of exchanges when you meet with your dietitian. The important thing is to be aware of the serving size for each food (see the exchange list on page 350).

Physicians and nutritionists emphasize the importance of having a variety of food groups at each meal. They should include complex carbohydrates, protein, and some fats, preferably monounsaturated. Fats help stabilize sugar in the blood. The distribution of calories should be roughly 45% to 50% carbohydrate, 20% protein, and 30% fats.

Following is a typical basic meal plan that a California hospital might offer patients with gestational diabetes. It may be tailored to more specific needs and tastes. California practitioners are influenced by a state diabetes and pregnancy program called Sweet Success, which does not advocate the consumption of any juice, or of fruit or milk (including yogurt) in the morning, because blood-sugar levels are at their highest in many women at that time of day and the glycemic indexes for these foods is high. However, not all dietitians and nutritionists adhere to these rules. The insulin response to foods appears to be highly individualized, and by monitoring your blood sugar, you can work with your health care provider to create a meal plan that suits your needs.[4]

Along with the individualized nature of insulin response, caloric needs vary according to size, ideal weight, and activity level. It is important to work closely with a dietitian to create a meal plan that works for you. You can use the plan and menu suggestions that follow to devise a program with your diabetes counselor.

[4]Anna Maria Siega-Riz, Assistant Professor of Maternal and Child Health and Nutrition, University of North Carolina School of Public Health, Chapel Hill, correspondence with author.

Basic Meal Plan

Breakfast (7:30 a.m.)

1 serving starch (complex carbohydrate) group

1 serving protein/meat substitute group

0 servings fruit group

0 servings milk (milk, yogurt) group

2 servings fat group

Midmorning Snack (10 a.m.)

1 serving starch (complex carbohydrate) group

1 serving protein/meat substitute

Lunch (12–1 p.m.)

2 servings starch (complex carbohydrate) group

3 servings protein/meat substitute group

1 serving vegetable group

1 serving fruit group

$^{1}/_{2}$ serving milk group

1 serving fat group

Midafternoon Snack (3–4 p.m.)

1 serving starch (complex carbohydrate) group

1 serving protein/meat substitute group

1 serving fruit group

1 serving fat group

Dinner (6–8 p.m.)

2 servings starch (complex carbohydrate) group

3 servings protein/meat substitute group

1 serving vegetable group

1 serving fruit group

$^{1}/_{2}$ serving milk group

1 serving fat group

Bedtime Snack (10 p.m.)

2 servings starch (complex carbohydrate) group

1 serving protein/meat substitute group

$^{1}/_{2}$ serving milk group

1 serving fat group

Plan for

Gestational

Diabetes

Exchange List*

1 STARCH =

1 slice bread; 1 tortilla; 6 crackers; $\frac{1}{2}$ cup cooked pasta, bulgur, corn, potatoes, or hot cereal; $\frac{1}{3}$ cup cooked rice; $\frac{3}{4}$ cup cooked beans, peas, or lentils (also counts as 1 protein); $\frac{3}{4}$ cup flaked but not instant cereal

1 FAT =

1 teaspoon butter, oil, mayonnaise, or low-fat mayonnaise; 1 tablespoon salad dressing or 2 tablespoons low-fat dressing; $\frac{1}{8}$ avocado; 20 small peanuts; 8 large olives; 2 tablespoons sour cream; 1 slice bacon

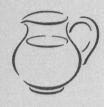

1 MILK =

SKIM/VERY LOW-FAT: 1 cup skim, $\frac{1}{2}$%, or 1% milk or buttermilk; 1 cup nonfat or low-fat sugar-free yogurt; $\frac{3}{4}$ cup nonfat plain yogurt
LOW-FAT: 1 cup 2% milk or $\frac{3}{4}$ cup low-fat plain yogurt
WHOLE: 1 cup whole milk or 1 cup kefir (a fermented milk product)

1 MEAT/MEAT SUBSTITUTE =

VERY LEAN: 1 ounce fish, shellfish, chicken or turkey breast, nonfat cheese, or sandwich meat with 1 gram or less fat per ounce; $\frac{1}{4}$ cup nonfat or low-fat cottage cheese; $\frac{1}{2}$ cup cooked beans, peas, or lentils (also counts as 1 starch)
LEAN: 1 ounce round, sirloin, or flank steak; pork tenderloin; ham; veal; leg of lamb; dark-meat chicken without skin; cheese or lunch meat with 3 grams of fat or less per ounce; or water-packed tuna
MEDIUM FAT: 1 ounce most other beef, mozzarella cheese, cheese with less than 5 grams of fat per ounce, dark-meat chicken with skin, salmon, tuna in oil (drained), or ground turkey; 1 egg; $\frac{1}{2}$ cup tofu
HIGH FAT: 1 ounce sparerib, sausage, regular cheese, hot dog, or sandwich meat with 8 grams of fat or less per ounce

1 FRUIT =

1 medium fresh fruit; 3 inches banana; 12 cherries; 15 small grapes

1 VEGETABLE =

$\frac{1}{2}$ cup cooked vegetable; $\frac{1}{2}$ cup vegetable juice; 1 cup raw vegetable

*Exchange Lists for Meal Planning, American Diabetes Association and American Dietetic Association, 1995.

Sample Breakfast
No Fruit, Milk, or Yogurt Allowed (7:30 a.m.)

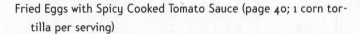

1 scrambled egg cooked in 1 teaspoon butter or olive oil
1 slice whole grain toast with 1 teaspoon butter

1 slice whole grain toast
1/2 cup low-fat cottage cheese

Fried Eggs with Spicy Cooked Tomato Sauce (page 40; 1 corn tortilla per serving)

1 or 2 poached eggs
1 slice whole grain toast

1/2 toasted whole wheat English muffin
1/3 cup nonfat or low-fat cottage cheese

Quick Individual Omelet with Cheese (page 36)
1 slice whole grain toast

Oatmeal with slivered almonds, moistened with 1/2 cup rice milk or
soy milk and sweetened with aspartame

Sample Breakfast
Some Fruit, Milk, or Yogurt Allowed (7:30 a.m.)

1 cup cooked oatmeal with 1/2 apple and up to 1/2 cup nonfat
or 1% milk

Nondairy Banana Strawberry Smoothie with flax seeds (page 44;
use only 3 inches not-too-ripe banana)

1/2 cup Muesli (page 33; omit raisins or currants with up to 1/2 cup
nonfat or 1% milk)

1/2 cup yogurt with ground flax seeds and 1 sliced peach

Sample Midmorning Snacks
No Fruit, Milk, or Yogurt Allowed (10 a.m.)

1 slice whole grain toast or 2–4 Ry-Krisp crackers
1 ounce cheese

1 slice whole grain toast
Hard-cooked egg (see page 155)

$^1/_4$ cup roasted almonds
Carrot sticks

1 slice whole grain bread or toast
$^1/_4$–$^1/_2$ cup low-fat cottage cheese

$^1/_2$ Grilled Cheese Sandwich (page 84)

2–4 Ry-Krisp crackers
2 ounces Tofu with Dipping Sauces (pages 60; don't use dips that
     call for sugar, or substitute aspartame)

$^1/_2$ Tuna Sandwich (page 74)

1 slice whole grain bread or toast with 1 ounce tofu or 1 tablespoon
     peanut butter
$^1/_2$ cup crudités

Sample Midmorning Snacks
Fruit, Milk, and Yogurt Allowed (10 a.m.)

1 small apple or pear
1 ounce cheese

$^1/_2$ cup roasted almonds
1 orange
Carrot sticks

$^1/_2$ cup nonfat or low-fat cottage cheese
1 slice whole grain bread
1 orange or tangerine

Sample Lunches (12–1 p.m.)

Tuna Sandwich (page 74)
Baby Greens Salad (page 110)
1 small apple
1/2 cup nonfat or 1% milk

Roast Beef Sandwich (page 78) with sliced tomatoes
1/2 cup nonfat or 1% milk or soy milk
1 small pear

Gazpacho (page 106)
Asian Chicken Salad (page 158)
2 slices whole grain bread
1/2 cup nonfat or 1% milk or soy milk
1 orange

Tomato, Mozzarella, and Basil Sandwich (page 85)
Baby Greens Salad (page 110)
1/2 cup nonfat or 1% milk or soy milk
1 peach

Crudités with Curried Yogurt Dip (page 61)
1 cup nonfat or low-fat cottage cheese with avocado
1 slice whole grain bread
1/2 cup blueberries with 1/2 cup nonfat or 1% milk

Cucumber slices with Hummus (page 57) or Hummus Pita Pocket
    (page 82)
Couscous Tabbouleh (page 139)
1 slice whole grain bread (omit if choice is pita pocket)
1 piece of fruit or 1/2 cup nonfat or low-fat plain yogurt with 1/2 cup
    blueberries

Niçoise Salad (page 150)
1 slice whole grain bread
1/2 cup nonfat or 1% milk or soy milk
1 piece fruit

Plan for

Gestational

Diabetes

Sample Midafternoon Snacks (3–4 p.m.)

2–4 Ry-Krisp crackers
1 ounce cheese
1 small apple

Quesadilla (page 216)
1 small orange

Crudités
2–4 Wasa or Ryvita crackers with 1 tablespoon peanut butter
Tofu with Dipping Sauces (page 61)
1/2 banana (not too ripe; no more than 3 inches)

Edamame (fresh green soybeans)
1 slice whole grain bread
1 ounce cheese
1 small apple

1/3 cup unsweetened cereal with 1/2 cup nonfat or 1% milk and 1
    sliced peach

1/2 toasted whole wheat English muffin with nonfat cream cheese
    and unsweetened jam
3/4–1 cup nonfat or 1% milk or soy milk

Banana Strawberry Smoothie (page 45; use only 3 inches of not-
    too-ripe banana)

1/2 Grilled Cheese Sandwich (page 84)
1 small apple or pear

Sample Dinners (6–8 p.m.)

Grilled or Broiled Fish Steak with Asian Flavors (page 195; omit
    sugar, or substitute aspartame)
Steamed broccoli (1/2 cup)
Brown rice (page 266)
Green salad
1/2 cup low-fat yogurt with 3/4 cup blueberries

Grilled or Pan-Seared Porterhouse Steak (page 179) or Pan-Seared
or Grilled London Broil (page 180)
Mediterranean Greens (page 239)
Three Omega-3 Salad (page 114)
1/2 cup low-fat vanilla yogurt with strawberries

Gazpacho (page 106; make enough for 2 meals)
Roast Chicken (page 171; remove skin for low-fat)
Steamed green beans
Wild rice (page 267), brown rice (page 266), or basmati rice (page
265)
Green salad (optional)
Melon with Mint and Lime (page 277)

Garlic Soup with Broccoli (page 98)
Salmon Fillet Cooked in the Microwave (page 190)
Baby Greens Salad (page 110)
Bulgur (page 263) or quinoa (page 265)

Mexican Chicken Soup with Zucchini, Chickpeas, and Tomatoes
(page 90)
Quesadilla with Black Beans (page 217)
Baby Spinach Salad with Mushrooms (page 111)
Orange and Mint Salad (page 281)

Chicken Breast with Mediterranean Flavors (page 170)
Tomato Gratin (page 251)
Corn on the cob or Mediterranean Greens (page 239)
Creamy Cucumber Salad (page 125)
1 small pear

Hot and Sour Soup (page 94)
Stir-Fried Pork and Greens (page 185)
1 ounce cheese
Orange and Mint Salad (page 281)

Sample Bedtime Snacks (10 p.m.)

2 slices whole wheat toast with 1 tablespoon sesame tahini or
peanut butter
1/2 cup nonfat or 1% milk or soy milk

Plan for

Gestational

Diabetes

$^1\!/_2$ chicken sandwich

$^1\!/_2$ to 1 cup nonfat or 1% milk or soy milk

$^1\!/_2$ cup Muesli (page 33; omit raisins or currants) with $^1\!/_2$ cup nonfat or 1% cup milk

$^1\!/_2$ cup nonfat or low-fat plain yogurt with 1 tablespoon toasted almonds

2 slices whole wheat toast

2 slices whole grain toast with $^1\!/_4$ cup Yogurt Cheese (page 65)

2 tablespoons toasted almonds

$^1\!/_2$ cup unsweetened cereal with $^1\!/_2$ cup nonfat or 1% milk

1 slice whole wheat toast with 1 ounce melted cheese

$^1\!/_2$ cup buttermilk

2 slices whole wheat bread

1 ounce chicken

EATING WHILE ON BED REST

A number of pregnancy complications can result in a prescription for bed rest. These include complications from diabetes, hypertension, preeclampsia (pregnancy-induced hypertension), vaginal bleeding, premature labor (a frequent complication of multiples), and poor growth of the baby (intrauterine growth retardation, or IUGR).

Types of Bed Rest

There are three degrees of bed rest. All of them should be taken seriously, as they are intended to save your pregnancy. You will be instructed to lie on your side, preferably the left side, and to avoid lying on your back. Lying on your back puts an undue amount of weight on your back, your intestines, and, most important, the vein that returns blood from the lower body to the heart. Being horizontal on your back can inhibit circulation and digestion. Lying on your side, however, can improve blood flow, both to your own organs and to the fetus, reduce strain on your heart, reduce the levels of stress hormones that may be responsible for contractions, and take pressure off your cervix. Contractions may stop simply as a result of eliminating activity. Depending on your symptoms, you may be ordered to stay in bed only until they go away or until near the end of your pregnancy (which can mean several weeks or months), when the risks associated with preterm labor are at a minimum.

Modified bed rest means that you will be able to sit up and get out of bed from time to time. A small amount of activity is allowed, but you will be instructed to lie down on your side for several hours a day, which means you will not be able to go to work.

Strict bed rest is just that: you will be required to lie down (again, in a lateral position) almost all the time. A daily shower and trips to the bathroom may or may not be permitted. Some women on strict bed rest set up a rented hospital bed or a couch in a central area of the house, such as a family room or dining room off the kitchen. It helps to be in a place that is accessible to other members of the family. A radio, cordless phone, laptop computer, and television and VCR with a remote can all help pass the time. An intercom system — buy the baby monitor now — is also useful. No matter where in the house you choose to be, set up a cooler or mini-refrigerator within reach, and have somebody fill it with drinks and snacks.

Hospital bed rest is the strictest kind. It can last from a day or two to several months, depending on your symptoms. You may have to take medication to stop contractions. Many women who are required to be on hospital bed rest are not even allowed bathroom privileges.

Eating While on Bed Rest

Keeping your spirits up and feeding yourself properly are among the biggest challenges of bed rest. You will need help, not only from your partner but also from friends and family. Because you are not allowed to get out of bed, you will need food delivered to your bedside and snacks at your fingertips. One of the tricks is obtaining adequate nutrition for your growing baby or babies (particularly if you are carrying twins or more), while not obtaining too many calories and gaining too much weight due to reduced activity. Since being on bed rest can be incredibly tedious and eating is an age-old antidote for boredom, you may have to double your efforts when it comes to maximizing your nutrition. Dietitians do not recommend special eating plans for women on bed rest, but they do emphasize the importance of avoiding empty calories.

Whether on hospital bed rest or strict home bed rest, you should have a large bowl of fresh fruit within reach and cut-up vegetables in your bedside refrigerator or in a bowl of ice water. You also should have bottles or a pitcher of water next to your bed. Some of the most useful menus for bed rest are in the plan for the noncook or the reluctant cook (pages 323–25). You may find grocery shopping services on the Internet, which can be a godsend. From your position in bed, you can order food for the week, as well as ready-made meals from the deli. There are also a number of meal delivery services — type in "meal delivery services" on your computer to see what is available in your area — and many restaurants now have online take-out services as well. Browsing the Net for these online food services is not just a useful way to nourish yourself; it also helps pass the time. Just make sure that there is someone at home to answer the doorbell or that the delivery service knows where to leave your order.

If you are on hospital bed rest, do not despair. You don't *have* to stick to the hospital menus. Find out what the hospital cafeteria offers and request options from there. Also, you can have those meal delivery services bring food to you in the hospital as well as at home. Call on family and friends to bring you things you especially like to eat. Get to know the nurses; they will have access to drinks and snacks and will have a refrigerator that you should be able to use.

Eating Plans
for the Trimesters

THE FIRST TRIMESTER:
MENUS FOR THE NAUSEOUS AND TIRED

These menus assume that you might not be up to a large meal but that you will need to eat often. If you find that you're hungry, add food from any of the lists on pages 288–356.

DAY 1

Snack before breakfast
Whatever works for you — crackers, matzo, almonds, hard candy such as lemon drops, pretzels, apple juice, or carbonated fruit drinks

Breakfast
Fruit-flavored yogurt or plain or vanilla yogurt with dried fruit, Dried Fruit Compote (page 42), fresh fruit, or applesauce

Snack
Bran Muffin (page 48)
Milk

Snack
Watermelon

Lunch
Club Sandwich (page 72)
Milk

Snack
Apple

Dinner
Chicken Noodle or Tofu Noodle Soup (page 89)
Baby Greens Salad (page 110)
Whole grain bread
Pears Poached in Ginger Honey Syrup (page 278)

FOOD GROUP BREAKDOWN	
BREAD, CEREAL, RICE, PASTA	5
VEGETABLES	2
FRUIT	4
POULTRY, FISH, DRIED BEANS, MEAT, EGGS, NUTS	2
MILK, YOGURT, CHEESE	4

Eating Plan

for the

First Trimester

359

Snack

Vanilla frozen yogurt

DAY 2

FOOD GROUP BREAKDOWN

Bread, Cereal, Rice, Pasta	8
Vegetables	3
Fruit	4
Poultry, Fish, Dried Beans, Meat, Eggs, Nuts	3
Milk, Yogurt, Cheese	3

Snack before breakfast (whatever works)

Breakfast

Poached egg

Whole grain toast

Melon

Snack

Crackers with cheese

Apple juice

Snack

Lemonade (page 69) or carbonated fruit drink

Lunch

Tuna Sandwich (page 74) with lettuce and tomato on whole grain or rye bread

Pickle

Fresh fruit

Snack

Apple

Dinner

Chicken, pork, or vegetarian pot stickers or Chicken Breast with Asian Flavors (page 170)

Farmhouse Brown and Wild Rice

Steamed green beans

Fruit sherbet

Snack

Cereal with milk

FOOD GROUP BREAKDOWN

Bread, Cereal, Rice, Pasta	6
Vegetables	3
Fruit	4
Poultry, Fish, Dried Beans, Meat, Eggs, Nuts	1
Milk, Yogurt, Cheese	5

DAY 3

Snack before breakfast (whatever works)

Breakfast

Toasted whole grain English muffin with low-fat cream cheese and jam

Cottage cheese

Cantaloupe

Snack

Banana Smoothie (page 44)

Snack

Pretzels, bagel chips, or crackers

Milk

Lunch

Grilled Cheese and Tomato Sandwich (page 84)

Coleslaw (store-bought or homemade, page 127) or Baby Greens
Salad (page 110)

Snack

Melon

Snack

Milk or chocolate milk

Dinner

Spinach tortellini

Steamed broccoli

Strawberry frozen yogurt

Snack

Jell-O

Biscotti or graham crackers

DAY 4

Snack before breakfast (whatever works)

Breakfast

Cereal with milk and peaches or bananas

Snack

Power Bar

Snack

Grapefruit

Lunch

Couscous Tabbouleh (page 139) or store-bought tabbouleh

Hummus Pita Pocket (page 82)

Snack

Lemonade (page 69), carbonated fruit drink, or ginger ale

Graham crackers or Bran Muffin (page 48)

FOOD GROUP BREAKDOWN	
BREAD, CEREAL, RICE, PASTA	5
VEGETABLES	3
FRUIT	2
POULTRY, FISH, DRIED BEANS, MEAT, EGGS, NUTS	3
MILK, YOGURT, CHEESE	1 OR 2

Eating Plan

for the

First Trimester

Dinner

Scrambled eggs or Quick Individual Omelet with Spinach (page 36)

Greek Salad (page 115)

Fresh fruit

Snack

Fruit Popsicle or vanilla frozen yogurt

Snack before breakfast (whatever works)

Breakfast

Toasted whole grain bagel

Fresh or frozen fruit, such as melon

Plain or vanilla yogurt with Dried Fruit Compote (page 42; optional)

Snack

Crackers

Jicama with Lime Juice and Salt (page 56)

Snack

Fruit juice or carbonated fruit drink

Cheese

Lunch

Cottage cheese with fruit or avocado

Whole grain bread, toast, or crackers

Snack

Mango Smoothie (page 44)

Dinner

Roast Chicken (store-bought or homemade, page 171)

Farmhouse Brown and Wild Rice

Steamed frozen or fresh peas

Sliced tomatoes

Pear

Snack

Molasses Bread (page 53) or Bran Muffin (page 48)

Milk

FOOD GROUP
BREAKDOWN

Bread, Cereal, Rice, Pasta	6
Vegetables	3
Fruit	5
Poultry, Fish, Dried Beans, Meat, Eggs, Nuts	2
Milk, Yogurt, Cheese	5

DAY 6

Snack before breakfast (whatever works)

Breakfast
Fruit-flavored yogurt

Whole grain toast

Snack
Banana

Milk

Snack
Rice cakes or crackers with cottage cheese (optional)

Lunch
Chicken Breast and Red Pepper Sandwich (page 73)

Quick Cucumber Pickles (page 126)

Milk

Fresh fruit

Snack
Pretzels or fat-free tortilla chips with Fresh Tomato Salsa (page 63)
or store-bought salsa

Lemonade (page 69)

Dinner
Packaged Red Beans and Rice

Grated Carrots in Vinaigrette (page 122)

Apple

Cheese

Snack
Jell-O with fruit, or frozen grapes

Biscotti or graham crackers

DAY 7

Snack before breakfast (whatever works)

Breakfast
Poached eggs

Whole grain toast

Snack
Bran Muffin (page 48)

Grapefruit

FOOD GROUP
BREAKDOWN

BREAD, CEREAL, RICE, PASTA	7
VEGETABLES	3½
FRUIT	4
POULTRY, FISH, DRIED BEANS, MEAT, EGGS, NUTS	3
MILK, YOGURT, CHEESE	5

FOOD GROUP
BREAKDOWN

BREAD, CEREAL, RICE, PASTA	7
VEGETABLES	2
FRUIT	3½
POULTRY, FISH, DRIED BEANS, MEAT, EGGS, NUTS	3
MILK, YOGURT, CHEESE	4

Eating Plan

for the

First Trimester

Snack

Fruit-flavored yogurt

Lunch

Lentil Soup (canned, in a cup, or homemade, page 103)

Whole grain bread

Orange and Mint Salad (page 281)

Snack

Applesauce

Biscotti

Dinner

Creamy Pasta with Broccoli (page 197)

Baby Greens Salad (page 110)

Frozen Banana Yogurt (page 279) or fruit Popsicle

Snack

Cereal with milk

THE SECOND TRIMESTER: MENUS FOR THE HUNGRY

These menus are much the same as the lower-carb, high-protein and higher-carb, high-protein menus on pages 282–304, except there is a bit more food. If you are already suffering from heartburn and indigestion, see the third-trimester little-meal menus beginning on page 370.

FOOD GROUP
BREAKDOWN

BREAD, CEREAL,
  RICE, PASTA   4
VEGETABLES   5
FRUIT   5
POULTRY, FISH, DRIED
  BEANS, MEAT,
  EGGS, NUTS   4 TO 6
MILK, YOGURT,
  CHEESE   6½

DAY 1

Breakfast

Scrambled eggs

Turkey or soy breakfast links (optional)

Whole grain toast

Orange juice (fresh or commercial), grapefruit, or melon

Snack

Apple

Cheese

Snack

Ryvita crackers with peanut butter or cottage cheese

Edamame (fresh green soybeans) or crudités

Lunch
- Club Sandwich (page 72)
- Dill pickle
- Coleslaw (store-bought or homemade, page 127)
- Milk or soy milk
- Fresh fruit

Snack
- Vanilla or fruit-flavored yogurt

Dinner
- Grilled or Broiled Fish Steak with Asian Flavors (page 195)
- Steamed broccoli
- Brown rice (page 266) or basmati rice (page 265)
- Green salad or Grated Carrots in Vinaigrette (page 122)
- Berries with milk, or pear

Snack
- Milk or soy milk
- Banana

DAY 2

Breakfast
- Vanilla or plain yogurt with granola
- Whole grain toast with butter or honey
- Grapefruit
- Decaf latte

Snack
- Blueberry Peach Frappe (page 68)

Snack
- Graham crackers
- Mint tea

Lunch
- Tuna Sandwich (page 74)
- Coleslaw (store-bought or homemade, page 127)
- Sliced tomatoes
- Pear
- Milk or soy milk

Snack
- Whole grain toast with peanut butter
- Milk or soy milk

FOOD GROUP BREAKDOWN	
BREAD, CEREAL, RICE, PASTA	7
VEGETABLES	4
FRUIT	5
POULTRY, FISH, DRIED BEANS, MEAT, EGGS, NUTS	4
MILK, YOGURT, CHEESE	5

Eating Plan

for the

Second Trimester

Dinner
Gazpacho (page 106; make enough for 2 meals)
Roast Chicken (store-bought or homemade, page 171)
Basmati rice (page 265) or couscous (page 263)
Baby Spinach Salad with Mushrooms (page 111)
Orange and Mint Salad (page 281)

Snack
Applesauce
Molasses Bread (page 53) or Banana Bread (page 52)

FOOD GROUP
BREAKDOWN

BREAD, CEREAL, RICE, PASTA	5
VEGETABLES	7
FRUIT	2
POULTRY, FISH, DRIED BEANS, MEAT, EGGS, NUTS	5
MILK, YOGURT, CHEESE	5

DAY 3

Breakfast
Banana Strawberry Smoothie with optional flax seeds (page 44)
Whole grain toast with peanut butter or cream cheese
Decaf latte

Snack
Grapefruit
Biscotti

Lunch
Gazpacho (page 106)
Asian Chicken Salad (page 158)
Whole grain bread
Milk
Fresh fruit

Snack
Crudités with Curried Yogurt Dip (page 61)
Wasa or Ry-Krisp crackers or rice cakes

Dinner
Grilled or Pan-Seared Porterhouse Steak (page 179) or Pan-Seared
    or Grilled London Broil (page 180)
Roasted Beets and Beet Greens (page 243)
Baked potato or corn on the cob (optional)
Tomato Gratin (page 251)
Baby Greens Salad (page 110)
Frozen yogurt

Snack
Milk
Banana Bread (page 52) or Molasses Bread (page 53)

DAY 4

Breakfast
- Buttermilk Pancakes (page 39) with maple syrup or strawberries and yogurt
- Orange juice (fresh or commercial)
- Decaf latte

Snack
- Carrot and celery sticks with Curried Yogurt Dip (page 61)
- Crackers with cheese

Snack
- Apple

Lunch
- Cottage cheese with avocado
- Whole grain bread
- Baby Spinach Salad with Mushrooms (page 111)
- Milk
- Orange

Snack
- Tomato juice or V8
- Oven-baked or microwaved tortilla chips with Fresh Tomato Salsa (page 63) or store-bought salsa

Dinner
- Tuna and Bean Salad on optional bed of greens (page 152)
- Minestrone (page 100)
- Whole grain bread
- Frozen Banana Yogurt (page 279)

Snack
- Milk or soy milk
- Biscotti

FOOD GROUP BREAKDOWN

BREAD, CEREAL, RICE, PASTA	7
VEGETABLES	5½
FRUIT	4
POULTRY, FISH, DRIED BEANS, MEAT, EGGS, NUTS	4
MILK, YOGURT, CHEESE	4½

DAY 5

Breakfast
- Poached eggs
- Whole grain toast
- Orange juice (fresh or commercial)
- Melon

Snack
- Strawberry Smoothie (page 45)

FOOD GROUP BREAKDOWN

BREAD, CEREAL, RICE, PASTA	6
VEGETABLES	4
FRUIT	6
POULTRY, FISH, DRIED BEANS, MEAT, EGGS, NUTS	3
MILK, YOGURT, CHEESE	5

Eating Plan

for the

Second Trimester

Lunch

Tomato, Mozzarella, and Basil Sandwich (page 85)

Baby Greens Salad (page 110)

Milk or soy milk

Fresh fruit

Snack

Bran Muffin (page 48)

Buttermilk

Dinner

Stir-Fried Pork and Greens (page 185)

Rice

Grapefruit and Avocado Salad (page 118)

Chocolate Pudding (page 270)

Snack

Applesauce

FOOD GROUP
BREAKDOWN

BREAD, CEREAL, RICE, PASTA	6
VEGETABLES	3
FRUIT	6
POULTRY, FISH, DRIED BEANS, MEAT, EGGS, NUTS	3½
MILK, YOGURT, CHEESE	3½

DAY 6

Breakfast

Microwave Oatmeal with Milk and Raisins (page 31)

Melon

Whole grain toast

Orange or grapefruit juice (fresh or commercial)

Snack

Cheese-Stuffed Figs or Prunes (page 56)

Lunch

Beef and Arugula Salad (page 147)

Whole grain bread

Milk

Fresh fruit

Snack

Toasted almonds

Milk

Snack

Toasted whole grain bagel with cream cheese

Dinner

Salmon Fillet Cooked in the Microwave (page 190)

Steamed green beans

Wild rice (page 267) or brown rice (page 266)

Baby Greens Salad (page 110)

Melon with Mint and Lime (page 277)

Snack

Banana

DAY 7

Breakfast

High-Protein Muffin (page 50)

Vanilla or plain yogurt

Orange juice (fresh or commercial) or grapefruit

Melon

Snack

Crackers

Hard-cooked egg (see page 155) or cheese

Lunch

Creamy Cucumber Sandwich (page 125)

Couscous Tabbouleh (page 139)

Milk

Fresh fruit

Snack

Mango Smoothie (page 44)

Dinner

Hot and Sour Soup (page 94)

Stir-Fried Tofu with Red Chard (page 225)

Brown rice (page 266) or bulgur (page 263)

Grated Carrots in Vinaigrette (page 122)

Frozen yogurt

Snack

Fruit Popsicle

FOOD GROUP
BREAKDOWN

BREAD, CEREAL, RICE, PASTA	6
VEGETABLES	4
FRUIT	4
POULTRY, FISH, DRIED BEANS, MEAT, EGGS, NUTS	5
MILK, YOGURT, CHEESE	5

Eating Plan

for the

Second Trimester

THE THIRD TRIMESTER: LITTLE MEALS

You should continue to gain about a pound a week (less if you are overweight, more if you are underweight) during the third trimester, or up until the final weeks, when weight gain can slow down or even reverse itself. This can be difficult, as eating large meals is not possible for most women at this time — there is just no room. The eating suggestions in this section focus on little meals that provide maximum nutrition for you and your baby. For more complete menus with snacks, those listed for the first trimester (pages 359–64) might be most suitable, as the meals are relatively small. If you have room for larger meals, use menus from the meal plans that work best for you.

LITTLE MEALS

Supplement meals with milk or soy milk whenever possible. Eat fruit, yogurt, and other snacks (see pages 286–88) between meals.

Scrambled, poached, or soft-boiled eggs
Whole grain bread
Baby Greens Salad (page 110)

Cheese
Apple or pear
Whole grain bread

Cereal with milk and fruit

Whole grain crackers or bread with Sardine Spread (page 76) or peanut butter
Quick Cucumber Pickles (page 126)

Salmon Fillet Cooked in the Microwave (page 190)
Steamed New Potatoes or Fingerlings with Herbs (page 252)
Steamed broccoli

Niçoise Salad (page 150)
Whole grain bread

Marinated Carrots (page 124)
Cheese
Whole grain bread

Banana Smoothie (page 44)

Tuna Sandwich (page 74)
Grated Carrots in Vinaigrette (page 122)

Lentil Soup (page 103)
Baby Greens Salad (page 110)
Whole grain bread

Pan-cooked chicken breast (see page 169) or a few slices roast
    chicken
Steamed broccoli, green beans, or greens
Basmati rice (page 265)

Greek Salad (page 115)
Whole grain bread

Quiche
Baby Greens Salad (page 110)

Plain or vanilla yogurt with applesauce
Whole grain bread

Cottage cheese with avocado or fruit

Quesadilla (page 216)
Baby Spinach Salad with Mushrooms (page 111)

Grilled Cheese Sandwich (page 84)
Sliced tomatoes

Caesar salad
Whole grain bread

Spinach tortellini
Steamed broccoli
Baby Greens Salad (page 110)

Edamame (fresh green soybeans) or Crudités with Thai Peanut
    Sauce (page 55)
Miso Soup with Tofu (page 96)

Tofu with Dipping Sauces (page 60)

Steamed spinach or broccoli

Basmati rice (page 265), brown rice (page 266), or buckwheat noodles (page 262)

Stir-Fried Tofu with Red Chard (page 225)

Brown rice (page 266) or bulgur (page 263)

Stir-Fried Pork and Greens (page 185)

Brown rice (page 266) or bulgur (page 263)

Egg Salad (page 146) on a bed of greens or My Egg Salad Sandwich (page 77)

Apple

Asian Chicken Salad (page 158)

Fresh fruit

Tomato, Mozzarella, and Basil Salad (page 85)

Pan-cooked, grilled, or poached chicken breast (see page 169 or 156)

Classic Tabbouleh (page 138)

Bread, pita bread, or crackers with Hummus (page 57)

Quick Individual Omelet with Spinach (page 35)

Green salad

Eating Plan
for Nursing
Mothers

Congratulations! You did it! Now that you've had your baby, your energy needs while you are nursing are even greater than during pregnancy — about 500 to 640 calories a day over prepregnancy intake, as opposed to 200 to 300 calories a day during the last two trimesters of pregnancy. No wonder so much of the folk wisdom concerning what to eat to ensure an adequate milk supply during this period focuses on high-calorie, nutrient-dense foods.

In fact, the extra calories are for your benefit, not your infant's. They do not increase milk supply, according to studies of well-nourished lactating women in industrialized countries.[1] Even when nutrient intake is low, mothers who breastfeed without giving any supplemental formula to their infants during the first four to six months can supply adequate nutrition. It's your nutrient stores that are at risk of being depleted through your milk. The extent to which they are depleted is directly related to how much and how long you breastfeed. That's why Recommended Dietary Allowances (RDAs) for all of the nutrients are higher during lactation. They are not difficult to meet if your caloric intake is sufficient. But if your daily caloric intake is less than 2,700 calories and you are consuming less than the RDAs, the nutrients that you risk becoming deficient in are calcium, zinc, magnesium, vitamin B_6, and folate.[2] The best food sources for these nutrients are listed in A Nutritional Primer (page 381).

---

[1] Subcommittee on Nutrition During Lactation, Committee on Nutritional Status During Pregnancy and lactation, Food and Nutrition Board, Institute of Medicine, and National Academy of Sciences, *Nutrition During Lactation* (Washington, D.C.: National Academy Press, 1991), p. 5.

[2] Ibid., p. 4.

Nutrition and Mother's Milk

Although the *quantity* of milk you produce does not appear to be affected by your caloric intake, its nutritional *quality* can be altered if your nutritional status is low. If you don't get enough vitamins in particular, the vitamin content of your milk can be depleted. (Most vitamins are stored in very small amounts and must be replenished daily.)[3] With the exception of selenium and iodine, minerals and trace minerals in milk do not appear to be affected by your daily consumption. Some studies suggest that poor maternal nutrition can deprive milk of its ability to provide an infant with resistance to disease, which is among the greatest benefits of breastfeeding.

Weight Loss (or Gain) During Lactation

Even with the extra calories, most women lose weight at a rate of about 1 to 2 pounds per month during the first 4 to 6 months of lactation. If you drop below your prepregnancy weight or you breastfeed for more than six months, you will need to consume 650 or more calories a day above your prepregnancy consumption. To ensure that you are obtaining enough nutrients, your daily caloric intake should not drop below 1,800 calories a day, no matter how determined you are to lose your pregnancy weight. Although weight loss does not appear to affect milk production, it can have a negative effect on your nutrient stores. For example, studies have indicated that calcium depletion during lactation can lead to short-term bone loss.

It probably won't be difficult for you to find nutritious ways to add 300 calories to your postpregnancy diet. A couple of nutritious snacks or glasses of milk should do it. The real challenge of those early weeks and months after childbirth may be finding the time to cook, and you may need to rely on more take-out and prepared foods for dinner.

If you find that you are not losing weight, are gaining it, or are losing too much, you should seek individualized counseling with a registered dietitian.

[3] Ibid., p. 6.

Multiples

Your caloric needs will be even greater if you have given birth to twins or more. However, the caloric demands for multiples are lower during lactation than they were during pregnancy.

Should You Avoid Certain Foods?

Much has been written and passed down from mother to daughter, from clinic to patient, about foods that are thought to give a breastfed baby colic. The medical literature supports none of these hypotheses. The truth is, nobody understands what causes colic — why some babies get it and some don't. If your baby has gas or colic, you can try playing around with your diet. You may find that eliminating one type of food or another helps. Or you may find yourself walking the halls with a screaming baby at night no matter what you cut out of your diet.

Menus for Nursing Mothers

Any of the menu plans for pregnancy in this book also will work for lactation, as long as you add a few extra snacks. You will find suggestions for more between-meal snacks on page 000. The emphasis should be on foods that are nutrient-dense rather than foods that get their calorie boost from fats. The following menus include a mix of ready-to-eat meals and home-cooked ones.

DAY 1

Breakfast
High-fiber cereal with milk and bananas
Whole grain toast with cream cheese
Orange juice (fresh or commercial), grapefruit, or melon

Snack
Apple
Cheese

Lunch
Club Sandwich (page 72) or Tuna Sandwich (page 74)
Dill pickle
Milk or soy milk
Fresh fruit

FOOD GROUP
BREAKDOWN

BREAD, CEREAL, RICE, PASTA	5
VEGETABLES	3
FRUIT	6
POULTRY, FISH, DRIED BEANS, MEAT, EGGS, NUTS	5 TO 6
MILK, YOGURT, CHEESE	6

Eating Plan

for Nursing

Mothers

Snack

Vanilla yogurt with blueberries

Almonds

Dinner

Grilled or Broiled Fish Steak with Asian Flavors (page 195) or
 scrambled eggs and toast

Blanched spinach or Swiss chard

Brown rice (page 266)

Baby Greens Salad (page 110) or Grated Carrots in Vinaigrette
 (page 122)

Vanilla frozen yogurt

Snack

Pear

Milk or plain or vanilla yogurt

Almonds (optional)

FOOD GROUP
BREAKDOWN

BREAD, CEREAL, RICE, PASTA	8
VEGETABLES	3
FRUIT	4
POULTRY, FISH, DRIED BEANS, MEAT, EGGS, NUTS	4
MILK, YOGURT, CHEESE	5

DAY 2

Breakfast

Toasted whole grain English muffin with cream cheese and jam

Cottage cheese

Melon

Orange juice (fresh or commercial)

Snack

Banana Smoothie (page 44)

Bran Muffin (page 48)

Lunch

Grilled Cheese and Tomato Sandwich (page 84)

Coleslaw (store-bought or homemade, page 127) or Baby Greens
 Salad (page 110)

Orange or melon

Snack

Whole grain toast with peanut butter

Milk or chocolate milk

Dinner

Chicken, pork, or vegetarian pot stickers or Chicken Breast with
 Asian Flavors (page 195)

Farmhouse Brown and Wild Rice

Steamed green beans

Fruit sherbet

Snack

High-fiber cereal with milk

DAY 3

Breakfast

Cereal, such as Kellogg's All-Bran or Kellogg's All-Bran Bran Buds, with milk and bananas or peaches

Orange or grapefruit juice (fresh or commercial)

Whole wheat bagel with cream cheese

Snack

Strawberry Smoothie (page 45)

Power Bar

Lunch

Couscous Tabbouleh (page 139) or store-bought tabbouleh

Hummus Pita Pocket (page 82)

Milk or soy milk

Fresh fruit

Snack

Toasted almonds

Milk or soy milk

Edamame (fresh green soybeans) or crudités with Curried Yogurt Dip (page 61)

Dinner

Gazpacho (page 106; make enough for 2 meals)

Roast Chicken (page 171; remove skin for low fat)

Steamed green beans or Mediterranean Greens (page 239)

Wild rice (page 267), brown rice (page 266), or basmati rice (page 265)

Green salad (optional)

Melon with Mint and Lime (page 277)

Snack

Applesauce

Vanilla yogurt

FOOD GROUP
BREAKDOWN

BREAD, CEREAL, RICE, PASTA	7
VEGETABLES	5
FRUIT	6
POULTRY, FISH, DRIED BEANS, MEAT, EGGS, NUTS	4 1/2
MILK, YOGURT, CHEESE	5

FOOD GROUP
BREAKDOWN

BREAD, CEREAL,
  RICE, PASTA   7
VEGETABLES   2
FRUIT   4
POULTRY, FISH, DRIED
  BEANS, MEAT,
  EGGS, NUTS   4½
MILK, YOGURT,
  CHEESE   6

DAY 4

Breakfast

Banana Smoothie with optional flax seeds (page 44)

Whole wheat toast with cream cheese or peanut butter

Snack

Plain or vanilla yogurt with blueberries

Bran Muffin (page 48)

Lunch

Chicken sandwich

Quick Cucumber Pickles (page 126)

Milk

Fresh fruit

Snack

Toasted almonds

Milk or soy milk

Dinner

Packaged Red Beans and Rice

Grated Carrots in Vinaigrette (page 122)

Cheese

Baked Apple (page 276)

Snack

Milk

Whole grain toast with peanut butter or sesame tahini

FOOD GROUP
BREAKDOWN

BREAD, CEREAL,
  RICE, PASTA   8
VEGETABLES   4
FRUIT   4
POULTRY, FISH, DRIED
  BEANS, MEAT,
  EGGS, NUTS   3½
MILK, YOGURT,
  CHEESE   5

DAY 5

Breakfast

Poached eggs

Whole grain toast

Orange juice (fresh or commercial), grapefruit, or melon

Snack

Blueberry Peach Frappe (page 68)

Lunch

Tomato, Mozzarella, and Basil Sandwich (page 85)

Quick Cucumber Pickles (page 126)

Milk or soy milk

Fresh fruit

Snack

Carrot juice

Almonds

Dinner

Spaghetti with commercial tomato sauce and Parmesan cheese

Baby Greens Salad (page 110)

Whole grain bread

Cheese or milk

Fresh fruit

Snack

Milk

Bran Muffin (page 48)

Breakfast

Vanilla or plain yogurt with raisins or chopped dried apricots and
2 teaspoons optional ground flax seeds

Whole grain toast

Grapefruit

Decaf latte

Snack

Edamame (fresh green soybeans) or crudités with Curried Yogurt
Dip (page 61)

Whole grain toast with sesame tahini

Lunch

Tuna Sandwich (page 74)

Coleslaw (store-bought or homemade, page 127)

Dill pickle

Milk or soy milk

Apple

Snack

Milk

Bran Muffin (page 48)

Dinner

Mexican Chicken Soup with Zucchini, Chickpeas, and Tomatoes
(page 90)

Grilled or Pan-Seared Porterhouse Steak (page 179) or Pan-Seared
or Grilled London Broil (page 180)

Baked Russet Potato (page 253), Dry-Roasted Waxy Potatoes (page
253), or Baked Potato Skins (page 254)

Baby Spinach Salad with Mushrooms (page 111)

Orange and Mint Salad (page 281)

FOOD GROUP
BREAKDOWN

BREAD, CEREAL, RICE, PASTA	6
VEGETABLES	6
FRUIT	5
POULTRY, FISH, DRIED BEANS, MEAT, EGGS, NUTS	4½
MILK, YOGURT, CHEESE	5

Eating Plan

for Nursing

Mothers

Snack

Plain or vanilla yogurt with applesauce

Almonds

DAY 7

Breakfast

Muesli (page 33) with milk

Whole grain toast with Yogurt Cheese (page 65) and jam

Orange juice (fresh or commercial), grapefruit, or melon

Snack

Hard-cooked egg (see page 155)

Milk or soy milk

Lunch

Warm Potato and Goat Cheese Salad (page 132)

Pan-cooked chicken breast (see page 169)

Whole grain bread

Milk or soy milk

Fresh fruit

Snack

Crackers with cheese

Crudités

Pear

Dinner

Lentil Soup (canned, in a cup, or homemade, page 103)

Frozen Lasagna

Baby Greens Salad (page 110)

Fruit Popsicle

Snack

High-fiber cereal with milk

FOOD GROUP
BREAKDOWN

Food Group	
Bread, Cereal, Rice, Pasta	8
Vegetables	3
Fruit	3
Poultry, Fish, Dried Beans, Meat, Eggs, Nuts	6
Milk, Yogurt, Cheese	5

A Nutrition Primer

This may be the first time in your life that you've taken an interest in what nutrients are. If you've struggled with weight and used or read about popular diets, you might have a notion that fats and carbs are "bad." In fact, fats and carbs have their place in a healthful diet. But if you are trying to maximize your nutrition while watching your caloric or sugar intake, you may need to restrict your consumption of some *types* of these nutritional elements to some degree.

Here we talk about what the nutritional elements are and what they do in your body and for your developing baby. A basic understanding of nutrition should help you with your choice of eating plans.

Macronutrients are the nutrients we get in the largest amounts — proteins, fats, carbohydrates, fiber. They provide energy and help maintain and repair body tissue.

Micronutrients include vitamins, minerals, and phytochemicals, which we get in smaller amounts but which are equally important in regulating chemical processes that take place in the body. Minerals play a role in regulating these processes and also in the formation and maintenance of new tissue — bones, teeth, blood, and muscle.

Water is the other essential nutrient. All chemical reactions within the body require the fluid medium that it provides. It's critical for circulation and for the removal of waste, for regulating body temperature, and for lubricating the body.

The Macronutrients

CARBOHYDRATES

Carbohydrates provide 40% to 50% of your body's energy. Most carbohydrates are supplied by plant-based foods. All sugars and starches, as well as dietary fiber, are carbohydrates.

Here is how carbohydrates work and why the overconsumption of certain carbohydrates can lead to weight gain. Starches and sugars are consumed and transformed by your body into a substance called glucose, a simple form of sugar that is transported in the blood to cells and used for energy. A substance called insulin, produced by the pancreas, is needed to transport glucose. The more glucose the body produces, the more insulin is required. The cells of the body take in as much glucose as they need for energy, and any that is left over is converted into another substance called glycogen. Some of the glycogen can be stored in the muscles and liver, but only about ¾ pound; the rest is converted to fat.

Nutritionists have long focused on two types of carbohydrates. *Simple carbohydrates* are sugars. They include white sugar, maple sugar and syrup, honey, corn syrup, and molasses. Sugars are often added to processed foods. Naturally occurring sugars are present in fruits. Dairy products, particularly milk, also contain sugars, as do many vegetables. But these foods also have other important nutrients. *Complex carbohydrates* are starches. These foods are a better nutritional package than simple carbohydrates because they contain vitamins, minerals, and often protein, as well as fiber and water. They are called complex because they consist of large chains of glucose molecules. Foods that are high in complex carbohydrates include bread, potatoes, sweet potatoes, grains, pasta, beans, and vegetables such as winter squash. The more refined the food is, the less nutrition it provides.

When it comes to your body's ability to metabolize carbohydrates, a more significant aspect of them is their *glycemic index (GI)*, which defines the rate at which they are digested and metabolized. Some starches, due to their structural characteristics, have a low GI and are digested more quickly than others. They affect blood-sugar levels, which can be toxic if too high, and tax the pancreas, which is required to produce more insulin in response. Insulin in turn promotes fat storage and can also be a factor in arterial damage. In some people who are considered insulin resistant, cells can respond to frequent bursts of insulin by becoming insensitive to the hormone. Insulin resistance has been associated with obesity. Other conditions associated with insulin resistance are abnormalities in blood fats, adult-onset (type 2) diabetes, and heart disease.

Insulin resistance, or a tendency to convert carbohydrates to fat instead of using them for energy, may be genetic, but a food's GI has a great deal to do with the way the body responds to carbohydrates. Interestingly, some complex carbohydrates, such as floury (russet) potatoes, white and whole wheat flour, and sticky short-grain rice, have a higher GI and are digested more quickly than simpler sugars and other starches. Even within food groups there is variation. Waxy potatoes, such as fingerlings and white rose, have a lower GI than russets. Basmati rice is much lower than Arborio or medium-grain rice. Pasta cooked al dente does not have a particularly high GI. And many vegetables that may have a high GI on a chart (such as carrots) would have to be eaten in much larger than normal quantities to have a significant effect on blood sugar.[1] The carbohydrate component of your diet should favor carbohydrates with a low GI.

No matter what the GI, both simple and complex carbohydrates, as well as protein, contain 4 calories per gram. Since protein requirements are greater during pregnancy, it makes sense to get the extra calories you need from protein rather than carbohydrates, or from a combination of protein and complex, low-GI carbohydrates, especially if you are one of those people who puts on weight merely by looking at a slice of bread. If you crave carbohydrates, you need to focus on low-GI carbohydrates, and you still need to get nutritionally dense calories from other foods.

FIBER

Fiber is the part of a plant that can't be digested by the enzymes in the human intestinal tract. Fiber lowers cholesterol and blood-sugar levels and helps remove waste through the intestines. For pregnant women, fiber's biggest benefit is preventing or treating constipation. Fiber is present in all fruits and vegetables, as well as in whole grains and particularly beans (one of the reasons beans cause flatulence). You'll need to drink plenty of fluids for fiber to work.

[1] Andrew Weil, *Eating Well for Optimum Health* (New York: Alfred A. Knopf, 2000), pp. 51–72.

PROTEIN

Seventy-five percent of our body tissue is protein. It is the basic material of life. Protein is the stuff of muscles, organs, antibodies, some hormones, and enzymes. This is why protein is so important when it comes to pregnancy, for both your own increasing tissues and your developing baby. You don't necessarily need more protein than the normal American diet supplies, but you do need adequate protein, about 50 to 100 grams a day. Nursing mothers need additional protein to keep up their milk stores.

Proteins are complex molecules that are made up of chains of amino acids in thousands of different configurations. They are constantly being broken down and reconstituted within the body. Some amino acids are reused, and some are lost — a process called *protein turnover*. For bodies to grow and function, protein turnover must occur, and thus we must obtain some of the replacement protein from foods.

We can obtain that replacement protein, or more specifically the amino acids that make up the protein, from animal- and plant-based foods. The *essential amino acids* must be supplied by foods, and both animal products and plant products are good sources. Protein from animal sources — meat, fish, poultry, eggs, and dairy products — is often referred to as *complete protein* because it contains all of the essential amino acids in comparable amounts, and the protein is thus readily available to the body. Protein in plants may be lower in some of the amino acids and higher in others, but that does not make the protein any less valuable to the body. The underrepresented amino acids will be obtained throughout the day at other meals or from some of the bacteria in the digestive tract.[2] Also, we instinctively combine foods that have complementary amino acids, such as beans and rice or corn tortillas, or pasta and cheese.

Animal products are made up of protein and fat, with relatively few carbohydrates, if any, and no dietary fiber. Red meats and dairy products have higher amounts of fat, with a higher proportion of saturated fat, than poultry and fish. But red meats and organ meats also provide a good dose of iron that is readily avail-

[2] Ibid., p. 104.

able to the body, and they are good sources of some of the B vitamins. Plant protein sources are relatively high in complex carbohydrates but low in fats.

FATS

The technical term for fats is *lipids*. Like amino acids, essential fatty acids, which are components in fats, must be obtained from foods and are vital to every cell in the body. They are the substance of some of our hormonelike compounds that help control blood pressure, blood clotting, and inflammation, among other functions. Fats help maintain healthy skin and hair and transport the fat-soluble vitamins — A, D, E, and K — through the bloodstream. They regulate blood-cholesterol levels and to some extent help make you feel satiated when you eat them, because they slow the emptying of food from the stomach. They also help make food taste good, partly because fat molecules convey the flavor molecules of many foods to our taste buds. We need fats for proper fetal growth and development. Cell membranes are composed primarily of lipids, and the fetal brain is 60% fat. Other essential fatty acids are important in the building of fetal eye tissue.

Extra calories from carbohydrates, protein, and fats are stored as fat in the adipose cells that insulate the body. When the body needs more energy than has been supplied by carbohydrates, it draws on this fat. So these stores are important for energy, especially for those who exercise. When you're pregnant, you produce hormones that tell the body to store more fat, which you need particularly in breast tissue.

A certain group of fatty acids called omega-3s appear to be very beneficial to health. Recent research has shown that omega-3s can protect people against heart disease and diabetes and are important for brain development and function in a developing fetus. The best source of omega-3 fatty acids is fatty cold-water fish, such as salmon, mackerel, sardines, and herring. Eggs from free-range chickens are also good sources. Capsules containing fish oil are now widely marketed, but it's best to go right to the source for omega-3s. The best plant sources are flax seeds (available in natural food stores), olive oil, canola oil, greens, legumes, nuts, and seeds. Canola oil and walnuts are particularly good plant sources, although you should make sure the canola oil is cold-processed, as heat can destroy the omega-3s in plant foods. Of equal importance is balancing the ratio of omega-3s with other essential fatty acids, the omega-6s, which are found in polyunsaturated oils (such as safflower oil, corn oil, and sunflower oil) and in meat from animals raised on grains. If the ratio of omega-6s is too high, the body is not able to obtain the omega-3 benefits.

One of the downsides of fats is that they contain twice as many calories per gram (9) as protein and carbohydrates. For that reason, controlling fat consumption is one of the easiest ways to control weight. Of greater significance to overall health is the *type* of fats you consume. All fats and oils contain varying amounts of three kinds of fatty acids: saturated, monounsaturated, and polyunsaturated. Saturated fatty acids predominate in animal fats, butter fat, coconut oil, palm oil, and palm kernel oil. Monounsaturated fatty acids are concentrated in olive oil, as well as in avocados, canola oil, and peanut oil. Large amounts of polyunsaturated fats are found in virtually all other oils made from seeds, nuts, and grains, as well as in cottonseed oil and fish oil.

Too much saturated fat and polyunsaturated fat in the diet can result in high blood cholesterol and triglycerides, a risk factor in heart disease. Too many polyunsaturates in the diet also can affect the delicate balance of omega-3s and omega-6s. Polyunsaturated fats are susceptible to oxidation and rancidity, which can be caused by exposure to light, heat, and air. Oxidation is harmful to cells and tissues; oxidized oils have been shown to severely restrict blood flow and are implicated in cancer, degenerative diseases, inflammation, and aging

Commercially produced polyunsaturated oils also can be hazardous because the structure of their fatty acids changes to an unnatural form when they are subjected to the heat, light, and chemical solvents used in processing. Called *trans-fatty acids*, these substances cannot produce membranes and hormones the way fatty acids in their natural form do, and they may even be damaging. Trans-fatty acids also result when oils are subjected to a type of processing called *hydrogenation*, which solidifies them and makes them more stable, so that foods made with them will have a longer shelf life. Most processed foods contain *partially hydrogenated vegetable oil*, and these foods, as well as margarine, contain

Sources of Fats

SATURATED FATS
(solid at room temperature)
- Animal fat
- Butter fat
- Coconut oil
- Palm kernel oil
- Palm oil

MONOUNSATURATED FATS
(liquid at room temperature)
- Avocado oil
- Canola oil
- Olive oil
- Peanut oil

POLYUNSATURATED FATS
(liquid at room temperature)
- Corn oil
- Cottonseed oil
- Fish oil
- Flax seed oil
- Grapeseed oil
- Safflower oil
- Sesame oil
- Soybean oil
- Sunflower oil
- Walnut oil

saturated fatty acids and trans-fatty acids, both of which can be harmful to your health.

Cholesterol is a fatty substance with hard, waxy characteristics found in the blood *(serum cholesterol)* and in animal fats. Although too much serum cholesterol can be a risk factor for or an indication of heart disease, some cholesterol is essential. It's a vital constituent of cell membranes and nerves and a building block for important hormones, including sex hormones and adrenal hormones such as cortisone. It's necessary for the metabolism of vitamin D and the manufacture of bile acids that aid in the digestion of dietary fats. It's also important for healthy skin. Our bodies manufacture most of the cholesterol we need. Recent research indicates that high levels of cholesterol are not so much a result of dietary cholesterol as of a diet high in saturated fat and high-GI carbohydrates.

After a meal, fatty acids and cholesterol are transported to the liver on droplets called *high-density lipoproteins (HDLs)*. The liver metabolizes the fatty acids and cholesterol, eliminating some of the cholesterol as bile, and sends them out to cells on another type of lipoprotein, a *low-density lipoprotein (LDL)*. The LDLs dock on the cells, the cells take what they need, and the LDLs reenter the bloodstream, carrying excess fat and cholesterol to fat cells for

A Nutrition Primer

storage or transferring them to HDLs, which return to the liver. Because LDLs indicate an excess of triglycerides and cholesterol in the blood stream, they are popularly known as "bad cholesterol," whereas HDLs are known as "good cholesterol." These are, in fact, misnomers, as HDLs and LDLs are transport vehicles for both cholesterol and triglycerides. Even so, high blood levels of LDLs and low levels of HDLs, as well as a low HDL-to-LDL ratio, are risk factors for heart disease, and saturated fats and high-GI carbohydrates raise LDL levels.

If you eat a lot of fast foods or commercially prepared foods, your diet is probably too high in fats. You should consume about 30% of your calories in the form of fats, primarily monounsaturates such as olive oil, avocados, nuts, and cold-pressed canola oil.

The Micronutrients

Vitamins, minerals, and a newly discovered group of compounds called phytochemicals are substances that, in minuscule amounts, perform important functions in the body. Vitamins and minerals are vital for maintaining health, and during pregnancy they play a role in the development of your baby and in keeping your own metabolism on track. Phytochemicals' role is more of a protective one, but this becomes increasingly important as we are bombarded with environmental and dietary hazards. Fruits and vegetables are the best sources of most vitamins and minerals, and the only sources of phytochemicals. Their importance in your diet cannot be overemphasized.

VITAMINS

Vitamins affect all of the body's functions. They are organic substances that help regulate cellular activity, and we cannot live or produce healthy babies without them. Except for vitamins D and K, they must be obtained from foods. Here are some of the functions that vitamins perform:

- Promote good vision
- Form normal blood cells
- Create strong bones and teeth
- Aid in the functioning of the circulatory and nervous systems
- Aid in the conversion of food to energy

The vitamins needed are A, C, D, E, and K, as well as the B vitamins thiamin, riboflavin, niacin, pantothenic acid, B_6, B_{12}, folacin, and biotin.

Fat-Soluble Vitamins

Some vitamins are fat-soluble and are stored in the liver and fat tissue, usually for relatively long periods. Fat-soluble vitamins can reach toxic levels if too many are consumed — something that can happen if you take them in the form of supplements.

Vitamin A

Vitamin A is important for:

- ❧ Development and function of eyes
- ❧ Growth and development of cells
- ❧ Development of bones
- ❧ Healthy skin, teeth, mucous membranes, bones, and soft-tissue linings
- ❧ Reproduction and lactation; the formation of sperm
- ❧ Strong immune system
- ❧ Metabolism of fat

Vitamin A found in animal foods is called *retinol*. It is readily usable by the body. Vitamin A found in plant foods is a precursor of vitamin A that comes in the form of compounds called *carotenoids* (the best known is *beta carotene*), which are converted to vitamin A by the body. Beta carotene provides about two thirds of the vitamin A in our diets. In addition to the benefits of vitamin A listed above, beta carotene provides antioxidant protection against free radicals, which are dangerous compounds that can break down cells. Orange and dark green fruits and vegetables are the best sources of beta carotene.

Because vitamin A is a fat-soluble vitamin, excessive amounts can accumulate in your system and be toxic. Your daily dose of vitamin A should come from food sources rather than vitamin supplements and should never exceed 5,000 IU a day. Vitamin A toxicity has been known to cause birth defects, such as head, heart, brain, facial, and spinal cord deformities. Medicines high in vitamin A, such as Accutane, which is used to treat skin disorders, must be avoided during pregnancy. The best source of vitamin A is

BEST SOURCES OF VITAMIN A

Carrots
Sweet potatoes
Spinach and other leafy greens, particularly kale
Winter squash
Romaine lettuce
Mangoes
Peaches and apricots
Whole and fortified milk
Eggs
Beef liver and organ meats
Fish oils

beta carotene from plant-based sources, which is converted by the body to safe levels of vitamin A.[3]

Vitamin D

The requirements for vitamin D increase during pregnancy and lactation by about 100 IU. Vitamin D is vital for the absorption of calcium and phosphorous and for their retention in the bones, blood, and other tissues. Deficiencies during pregnancy have been associated with neonatal hypocalcemia, convulsions, and decreased tooth enamel, as well as softening of the mother's bones.

Vitamin D does not occur naturally in foods. It is synthesized from a precursor in the skin after exposure to the sun's ultraviolet light. For this reason, people who live in northern climates have lower levels of this vitamin, particularly in winter. In the United States, milk is fortified with vitamin D, and this is the best dietary source. Vegans and people who don't consume milk or milk products because of lactose intolerance must be sure to get enough sunlight and should take a multivitamin containing vitamin D.

Vitamin E

Vitamin E is an important antioxidant, trapping potentially dangerous free radicals and preventing oxidation of polyunsaturated fatty acids. It is present in the polyunsaturated fatty acids of cell membranes, and in blocking their oxidation, it prevents the destruction of cell membranes and cells, intracellular structures, and enzymes. Its deficiency can lead to sterility, anemia, and neuromuscular abnormalities. Premature infants have decreased levels of vitamin E, which can result in anemia, and are routinely given supplements. There is no evidence that this condition could be altered if the pregnant mother were to take vitamin E supplements.

Vitamin K

Vitamin K is a fat-soluble vitamin that is required for proper clotting of the blood. There are also vitamin K–dependent proteins found in bone, plasma, kidney, and other tissues. Newborns, who

---

[3] drkoop.com/wellness/nutrition/vitamins_minerals/; Arlene Eisenberg et al., *What to Eat When You're Expecting* (New York: Workman Publishing, 1986), p. 326.

BEST SOURCES OF VITAMIN E

Wheat germ
Wheat germ oil
Polyunsaturated oils, such as soybean, corn, and cotton- seed oil
Mayonnaise
Nuts and seeds
Peanuts
Peanut butter
Whole grains
Seafood
Apples
Carrots
Celery
Green leafy vegeta- bles

are deficient in this vitamin, are routinely given vitamin K injections after birth. This condition has nothing to do with the mother's intake of vitamin K during pregnancy. The vitamin is produced largely in the flora of our own intestines.

Water-Soluble Vitamins

Unlike fat-soluble vitamins, most of the water-soluble vitamins are not stored in the body and should be obtained from foods every day. They should be exposed to a minimum of heat and light and will be lost in boiling water. Steaming and dry heat such as roasting are the best ways to prepare foods high in these vitamins.

Vitamin C

Vitamin C is a water-soluble vitamin that is essential for many metabolic processes. The need for this vitamin rises during pregnancy. Wounds, fevers, infections, smoking, rapid growth, and stress also increase the need for vitamin C, which is important for:

- ↣ Healthy gums and teeth; muscles, cartilage, and other tissue; and vascular system
- ↣ Iron absorption
- ↣ Healing of wounds
- ↣ Immune responses
- ↣ Allergic reactions
- ↣ Function of white blood cells[4]

Thiamin, Riboflavin, and Niacin
(Vitamins B_1, B_2, and B_3)

These water-soluble vitamins are instrumental in the release of energy in the cells.

Thiamin is essential for the metabolism of carbohydrates into energy. The higher your carbohydrate intake, the more thiamin you need. It is also used in brain and nerve cell function and in heart function, growth, and muscle tone.

Riboflavin is necessary for tissue function, oxygenation and

[4] Institute of Medicine *Nutrition During Pregnancy: Part I, Weight Gain; Part II, Nutrient Supplements* (Washington, D.C.: National Academy Press, 1990), p. 368.

BEST SOURCES OF VITAMIN K

Green leafy vegetables
Green beans
Dairy products
Eggs
Cereals
Meat
Beef liver
Olive oil
Soybean oil
Green tea

BEST SOURCES OF VITAMIN C

Green and red bell
  peppers
Tomatoes
Green leafy vegetables
Broccoli
Potatoes
Parsley
Citrus fruits
Strawberries
Cantaloupe
Kiwi fruit
Guavas

Best Sources of Thiamin

Whole and enriched
    grains
Enriched breads and
    cereals
Wheat germ
Dried beans
Peas
Pork
Liver
Seeds and nuts
Brewer's yeast

Best Sources of Riboflavin

Broccoli
Turnip greens
Asparagus
Spinach
Fortified cereals and
    grains
Milk
Cottage cheese
Eggs
Meat
Poultry
Liver

Best Sources of Niacin

Mushrooms
Peas
Dried beans
Whole and enriched
    grains
Meat
Poultry
Fish
Nuts

Best Sources of Pantothenic Acid (B$_5$)

Meat
Poultry
Fish
Cheese
Whole grains
Nuts
Legumes

Best Sources of Vitamin B$_6$

Tomatoes
Brown rice
Wheat bran and germ
Soybeans
Salmon
Poultry
Lamb
Veal
Organ meats
Blackstrap molasses
Brewer's yeast

respiration, protein and energy metabolism, and hormone synthesis. High doses of riboflavin may prevent migraines.

Niacin is present in all cells and aids in the release of energy from carbohydrates and protein, in the metabolism of fatty acids, and in tissue respiration. It is used in the synthesis of protein and fats and is needed for a healthy gastrointestinal tract. Niacin also benefits the skin and nervous system, circulation, appetite, and cell health. The requirement for niacin increases with caloric intake.

Pantothenic Acid (Vitamin B$_5$)

This vitamin is present in all living cells and is available in many foods, including meat, eggs, cheese, fish, whole grain cereals, nuts, vegetables, and legumes. It is needed for numerous functions, including the following:

- Antibody production
- Adrenal activity and hormone synthesis
- Energy metabolism
- Metabolism for growth in cells
- Metabolism of vitamin D and red blood cells

Vitamin B$_6$ (Pyridoxine, Pyridoxal, Pyridoxamine)

Vitamin B$_6$ plays a major role in protein metabolism, and because protein requirements are greater during pregnancy, a modest increase in vitamin B_6 is required. Recent studies indicate that 25 mg of vitamin B_6 every 8 hours can help alleviate severe morning sickness. This vitamin also is required for countless other cellular processes, including the following:

- Metabolism of carbohydrates and fats
- Immune and hormonal functions
- Formation of histamine, serotonin, and dopamine compounds that are vital to our bodies
- Synthesis of a component of red blood cells called heme compounds

High doses of vitamin B_6 can be harmful to the nervous system and can cause difficulties with balance.

Vitamin B_{12}

Vitamin B_{12} boosts the immune system and helps prevent heart disease. It is necessary for:

- Normal cell division and protein synthesis
- Healthy nervous system
- Red blood cell formation
- Synthesis of RNA and DNA
- Metabolism of energy

The vitamin is supplied by animal proteins such as meat, fish, eggs, milk, and cheese. Plant foods do not supply vitamin B_{12}.

Biotin

Biotin helps in the metabolism of proteins, carbohydrates, and fats. It is present in many foods and is also produced by intestinal flora.

Folic Acid

Folic acid is a water-soluble B vitamin. Also known as pteroylglutamic acid (PGA), folic acid from food sources is called folate or folacin. Because the vitamin is unstable, it breaks down easily when exposed to heat and air, so much is lost in cooking. For this reason, although folic acid is found in many foods, doctors often prescribe folate supplements to pregnant women.

BEST SOURCES OF VITAMIN B12

Beef
Fish
Pork
Poultry
Cheese
Eggs
Milk

BEST SOURCES OF BIOTIN

Spinach
Peas
Cauliflower
Mushrooms
Cheese
Egg yolks
Salmon
Chicken breasts
Organ meats
Peanuts
Nuts
Chocolate

BEST SOURCES OF FOLIC ACID

Green leafy vegetables
Broccoli
Asparagus
Oranges and orange juice
Oatmeal
Dried beans
Fortified cereals
Liver
Nuts
Brewer's yeast

Folic acid plays an important role in the metabolism of amino acids and the synthesis of nucleic acids. This is vital for normal cell division and replication. It is needed for fetal growth and for the formation of red blood cells. Scientific studies suggest that a deficiency in folate, particularly during the early weeks of pregnancy, can result in spontaneous abortion, small birth weight, or fetal malformation, particularly a defect in the neural tube called spina bifida. For this reason, health professionals recommend that women of reproductive age take a daily supplement of 0.4 mg of folate *prior to conception*.

MINERALS

Like vitamins, minerals are essential to your body for a number of metabolic processes, such as bone formation and maintenance, circulatory and heart function, and digestion. Some minerals are present in larger quantities than others; these are called macrominerals. Those that are present in minute quantities are called trace minerals or trace nutrients. They are just as essential to good health as the macrominerals.

Calcium

Calcium is essential for building and maintaining healthy bones and teeth. It also plays a role in these functions:

- Regulating heartbeat rhythm
- Lowering blood pressure
- Regulating muscle contraction
- Clotting blood
- Transmitting nerve impulses
- Maintaining cell membranes
- Absorbing vitamin B_{12}
- Stimulating enzyme activity

To meet the calcium requirements of your developing baby and the production of breast milk, your body will draw on the calcium from your bones if you don't get enough from your diet or from supplements. Vitamin D is also required for the absorption of calcium. Although diet is the best source of calcium, many doctors recommend supplementation.

BEST SOURCES OF CALCIUM

Green leafy vegetables
Fortified orange juice
Navy and pinto beans
Milk
Cheese
Part-skim ricotta cheese
Yogurt, especially low-fat and nonfat
Fortified soy milk
Tofu processed with calcium sulfate
Sardines with bones
Canned salmon with bones

Phosphorus

Phosphorus is a major component of bones and teeth. Its metabolism is closely linked with that of calcium. It is a component of DNA and RNA and is present in every cell in the body. It is also needed for:

- Energy metabolism in cells
- Absorption of glucose
- Transport of fatty acids
- Maintenance of acid balance in the body

Most people obtain enough phosphorus from their diets,[5] and there is some indication that excessive amounts in relation to calcium and vitamin D may result in the loss of calcium through the urine. Phosphorus is found in many foods.

Magnesium

Magnesium is necessary for:

- Release of parathyroid hormone, which regulates your calcium-phosphorus balance, and other metabolic and enzymatic processes
- Temperature control
- Nerve and muscle contraction
- Protein synthesis
- Bone growth

It is available from many foods, particularly grains, seafood, and green vegetables. Magnesium deficiency, which is rare, can be a factor in preeclampsia, a form of hypertension that occurs during pregnancy.

Iron

Iron is necessary for the production of hemoglobin, which transfers and transports oxygen in the blood, and the production of iron enzymes, which use oxygen to produce energy in the cells. It is needed during pregnancy to supply the growing fetus and placenta

[5] Ibid., p. 318.

BEST SOURCES OF
PHOSPHORUS

Whole grains
Dairy products
Eggs
Fish
Poultry
Meat
Nuts and seeds

BEST SOURCES OF
MAGNESIUM

Some green leafy
   vegetables, such as
   kale and spinach
Whole grains
Wheat germ and bran
Beans and legumes
Nuts
Meat

BEST SOURCES OF
IRON

Spinach and other
   leafy greens
Whole and enriched
   grains
Legumes
Eggs
Fish and shellfish
Meat
Poultry
Liver and other organ
   meats
Oysters
Blackstrap molasses

and to increase the mother's red blood cell mass, which will be a buffer when blood is lost during delivery.

Iron is present in food in two forms: *heme iron,* found in animal sources, and *nonheme iron,* found in plant sources. Most of the iron in our diets comes from vegetable sources, but this type of iron is not easily absorbed. Elements in whole grains and legumes, milk, tea, and many vegetables inhibit the absorption of nonheme iron. The inclusion of small amounts of meat and foods that contain ascorbic acid (such as orange juice) increases the absorption of nonheme iron greatly. Heme iron is easily absorbed by the body, and its absorption is unaffected by other foods eaten at the same time.

Pregnant women can easily become deficient in iron. Even if you're eating lots of iron-rich foods, you may be absorbing the iron inadequately. When iron stores are depleted, hemoglobin production can become impaired, resulting in iron deficiency anemia. Although prenatal vitamins usually provide enough iron, women are routinely assessed for iron deficiency at their monthly checkups, and many doctors recommend iron supplements. Because iron supplements can be toxic to young children, they should be kept out of their reach, as should all medications.

BEST SOURCES OF
POTASSIUM

Potatoes
Tomato juice
Winter squash
Most raw vegetables
Bananas
Melon
Orange juice
Dried fruit
Citrus fruit
Nectarines
Dried beans
Sunflower seeds
Nuts
Blackstrap molasses

Potassium
Potassium aids in:

- Regulating muscle activity and contractions
- Maintaining normal blood pressure
- Maintaining a normal fluid balance in the body
- Transmitting nerve impulses
- Sustaining heart rhythm
- Synthesizing protein

Zinc
Zinc is a key element in cell reproduction and differentiation, as it plays an important role in DNA and protein metabolism. It is needed for:

- Normal growth
- Brain development

- Healing of wounds
- Hair growth
- Development of taste perception
- Appetite regulation
- Night vision
- Hormonal activity, reproduction, and lactation
- Metabolism of carbohydrates

BEST SOURCES OF ZINC

Whole grains
Wheat germ
Eggs
Fish and shellfish
Oysters
Meat
Liver
Poultry
Popcorn

Most zinc in the American diet comes from animal products, although it is present in other foods. High doses of calcium can inhibit zinc absorption, as can large amounts of iron. Zinc from animal sources is probably more readily absorbed than zinc from vegetable sources.

Iodine

Iodine is necessary for healthy thyroid function and the production of the thyroid hormones that control metabolism. Iodine deficiency during pregnancy can result in a number of disorders in the fetus. Most people in this country obtain enough iodine from iodized salt. Seafood and sea vegetables, milk, and bread are also good sources.

Chromium

BEST SOURCES OF CHROMIUM

Asparagus
Peas
Mushrooms
Whole grains
Cheese
Meat
Blackstrap molasses
Brewer's yeast

Chromium is believed to play a role in the metabolism of sugars. A low chromium intake has been found to result in glucose intolerance.[6] There are studies currently under way to determine whether chromium deficiency is involved in gestational diabetes.

Manganese

Manganese is an important antioxidant. Manganese is important in:

- Development and function of the bones, cartilage, and pancreas
- Metabolism of glucose and fats
- Synthesis of fats and carbohydrates
- Reproduction

BEST SOURCES OF MANGANESE

Fruits
Peas
Whole grains and cereals
Beans
Nuts
Tea
Cloves

[6] Ibid., p. 310.

Seafood
Meat
Whole grains
Brazil nuts

+> Brain function

+> Growth

Selenium

Selenium acts as an important antioxidant against free-radical damage in the body. The body also needs it for proper immune response and functioning of the heart muscle.

Whole grains
Raisins
Nuts
Legumes
Shellfish
Liver and kidneys
Blackstrap molasses
Cocoa

Copper

Copper is found in nerve coverings and connective tissue. Copper-containing enzymes act as antioxidants against free radicals and help in other metabolic processes. Copper plays a key role in:

+> Production of energy required for metabolism

+> Transport and use of iron

+> Bone health

Fluoride

Fluoride is needed for strong teeth. The best source is fluoridated water and supplements.

Sulfur

Sulfur is present in all body tissues. It is derived from protein foods.

Sodium and Chloride

These components of salt are necessary for regulating electrolyte and fluid balance in the body. Sodium aids in muscle contraction and nerve function. Chloride is crucial for the formation of gastric juices and digestion and in maintaining the body's acid-base balance. Salt-restricted diets can lead to deficiencies in these trace minerals. Table salt and animal products are good sources of sodium and chloride.

Spinach
Lima beans
Cereals
Breads
Milk

Molybdenum

Molybdenum is a component of three enzymes and aids in:

+> Metabolism of DNA and RNA

+> Metabolism of food

+> Prevention of cavities

+> Breakdown of a toxic buildup of sulfites in the body

PHYTOCHEMICALS

Phytochemicals, a new area in nutritional research, are compounds found in plants that play a protective role in our bodies' defense against disease-causing agents such as carcinogens. Only a few types are now known, but many more probably have yet to be discovered. Their attributes underline how important fruits and vegetables are for a healthy diet. The fact that these elements are only beginning to be identified illustrates how much more there is to learn about the foods we eat.

Green tea, apples, olive oil, berries, cherries, red grapes, plums, pomegranates, red cabbage, some beans and grains, and yellow and orange fruits and vegetables are all sources of different types of phytochemicals that act as antioxidants. *Phytoestrogens*, found in soybeans and flax, interact with estrogen receptors on cells and may have a protective effect on hormones, perhaps fighting hormone-driven cancers, such as breast cancer and prostate cancer. Soy foods also may help prevent heart disease. Phytochemicals in wild mushrooms boost the immune system. Others in the cabbage family, broccoli, raspberries, blueberries, and citrus peel protect against cancer. Garlic contains a substance that lowers blood pressure and acts as a natural antibiotic, and ginger contains an anti-inflammatory phytochemical.

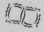

Selected Bibliography

BOOKS

Bowes & Church's Food Values of Portions Commonly Used, 17th ed. Revised by Jean A. T. Pennington. Philadelphia: Lippincott Williams & Wilkins, 1998.

Carper, Jean. *Jean Carper's Total Nutrition Guide*. New York: Bantam Books, 1987.

Erick, Miriam. *No More Morning Sickness: A Survival Guide for Pregnant Women*. New York: Plume, 1993.

Hiser, Elizabeth. *The Other Diabetes: Living and Eating Well with Type 2 Diabetes*. New York: William Morrow, 1999.

Luke, Barbara, and Tamara Eberlein. *When You're Expecting Twins, Triplets, or Quads: A Complete Resource*. New York: Harper Perennial, 1999.

Margen, Sheldon, M.D., and the Editors of the University of California at Berkeley *Wellness Letter*. *The Wellness Encyclopedia of Food and Nutrition: How to Buy, Store, and Prepare Every Fresh Food*. New York: Rebus, 1992.

Samuels, Mike, M.D., and Nancy Samuels. *The New Well Pregnancy Book*. New York: Simon & Schuster, 1996.

Subcommittee for a Clinical Application Guide, Committee on Nutritional Status During Pregnancy and Lactation, Food and Nutrition Board, Institute of Medicine, and National Academy of Sciences. *Nutrition During Pregnancy and Lactation: An Implementation Guide*. Washington, D.C.: National Academy Press, 1992.

Subcommittee on Nutritional Status and Weight Gain During Pregnancy, Subcommittee on Dietary Intake and Nutrient Supplements During Pregnancy, Committee on Nutritional

Status During Pregnancy and Lactation, Food and Nutrition Board, Institute of Medicine, and National Academy of Sciences. *Nutrition During Pregnancy: Part I, Weight Gain; Part II, Nutrient Supplements.* Washington, D.C.: National Academy Press, 1990.

Subcommittee on Nutrition During Lactation, Committee on Nutritional Status During Pregnancy and Lactation, Food and Nutrition Board, Institute of Medicine, and National Academy of Sciences. *Nutrition During Lactation.* Washington, D.C.: National Academy Press, 1991.

U.S. Department of Health and Human Services. *Understanding Gestational Diabetes: A Practical Guide to a Healthy Pregnancy.* NIH Publication No. 93-2788. February 1993.

Weil, Andrew, M.D. *Eating Well for Optimum Health: The Essential Guide to Food, Diet, and Nutrition.* New York: Alfred A. Knopf, 2000.

ARTICLES AND WEB SITES

Center for Science in the Public Interest. *Protect Your Unborn Baby: Important Food Safety Information to Help Avoid Miscarriage.*
www.cspinet.org/foodsafety/brochure_pregnancy.html.

Erick, Miriam. "Nausea & Vomiting in Pregnancy," *ACOG Clinical Review* (May/June 1997).

Kjos, S., M.D.; and T. Buchanan, M.D., "Gestational Diabetes Mellitus." *New England Journal of Medicine* 341 no. 23 (December 2, 1999).

Luke, B.; B. Gillespie; F.R. Witter, M.D.; R. D. Newman, M.D.; J. Mauldin, M.D.; F. Salmam, M.D.; and M.J. Sullivan, M.D.; "The Importance of Early Weight Gain in the Intrauterine Growth and Birth Weight of Twins." *American Journal of Obstetrics and Gynecology* 179, no. 5 (November 1998): 1155–61.

March of Dimes Birth Defects Foundation. *Healthy Eating During Pregnancy.* White Plains, New York: March of Dimes, Foundation, 1995.

Nutrition Center. drkoop.com.

Sahakian, V., M.D.; D. Rouse, M.D.; S. Sipes, M.D.; N. Rose; and J. Niebyl, M.D., "Vitamin B$_6$ Is Effective Therapy for Nausea and Vomiting of Pregnancy: A Randomized, Double-Blind Placebo-Controlled Study." *Obstetrics & Gynecology* 78, no. 1 (July 1991): 33–36.

U.S. Department of Agriculture. Food Safety and Inspection Service. *Listeriosis and Pregnancy.* www.fsis.usda.gov.

www.modimes.org.

Vutyavanich, T., M.D.; Wongtra-ngan, S. M.D.; R. Ruangsri. "Pyridoxine for Nausea and Vomiting of Pregnancy: A Randomized, Double-Blind, Placebo-Controlled Trial." *American Journal of Obstetrics and Gynecology* (September 1995): 881–84.

Index

age, weight gain and, 10–11
alcohol consumption, 17
amino acids, essential, 384
amniotic fluid, 11
anemia, iron deficiency, 14, 334, 396
antacids, 23
Apples
    Apple-Cinnamon Tofu Spread, 46
    Baked Apples, 276
    Bread Pudding with Apples or Peaches, 269
    Muesli, 33
    Scandinavian Fruit Soup, 43
Apricots
    Bran Muffins, 48–49
    Couscous with Oranges and Dates, 32–33
    Dried Fruit Compote, 42
    Scandinavian Fruit Soup, 43
Artichokes
    Simple Homemade Pizza, 210
    Steamed Artichokes with Dips, 244–45
Arugula
    Arugula or Baby Greens and Beet Salad, 112–13
    Beef and Arugula Salad, 147
    Beet and Orange Salad, 117
    Grapefruit and Avocado Salad, 118

Tomato and Arugula Salad with Feta Cheese, 116
Asian Chicken Salad, 158
Asian Coleslaw, 128
Asian Noodles, 262
Asian Noodle Salad, 160–61
Asian Noodle Soup with Spinach and Salmon, 92
Asian Noodle Soup with Tofu and Spinach, 92
Asparagus
    Asparagus Flan, 228
    Quick Individual Omelets, Flat or Folded, 35
aversions, 17–18
Avocados
    Avocado Sandwich, 75
    Chicken, Red Pepper, and Avocado Sandwich, 73
    Club Sandwich with Avocado, 72
    Cobb Salad, 154–55
    Grapefruit and Avocado Salad, 118
    Guacamole, 121
    Mexican Chicken Salad, 159
    Mexican Chicken Soup with Zucchini, Chickpeas, and Tomatoes, 90–91
    Salsa with Avocado, 63
    Soft Tacos or Tostadas with Chicken, Corn, and Avocado, 233

Tofu Sandwich with Avocado and Tomato, 79
Vegetarian Mexican Soup, 91

Baby salad greens
    Arugula or Baby Greens and Beet Salad, 112–13
    Baby Greens Salad, 110
Bacon
    Club Sandwich, 72
    Cobb Salad, 154–55
    Frisée, Poached Egg, and Bacon Salad, 148–49
Baked Apples, 276
Baked Potato Skins, 254
Baked Russet Potatoes, 253
Baked Sweet Potatoes, 256
balanced diet, 3
Balsamic vinegar
    Grilled Tuna with Tomato-Balsamic Salsa, 196
Bananas
    Banana Bread, 52
    Banana Smoothie, 44
    Banana Strawberry Smoothie, 44
    Frozen Banana Yogurt, 279
    Frozen Strawberry Banana Yogurt, 279
    Peanut Butter and Banana Sandwich, 78

Barbecued Tempeh Sandwich, 81

Barley
    Mushroom and Barley Soup, 104–5

Basil
    Pasta with Pesto and Green Beans, 199
    Tomato, Mozzarella, and Basil Sandwich, 85
    White Bean and Basil Salad, 137

beans, 24. *See also specific types of beans*

Bean Salad with Cumin Vinaigrette, 134–35

Beans and Sage, 87

bed rest, 356–58

bedtime snacks, 28, 346–47

Beef
    Beef and Arugula Salad, 147
    Beef Burgers, 178
    Grilled or Pan-Seared Porterhouse Steak, 179
    Pan-Seared or Grilled London Broil, 180–81
    Roast Beef Sandwich, 78
    Steak Fajitas, 182–83

Beet greens. *See* Greens

Beets
    Arugula or Baby Greens and Beet Salad, 112–13
    Beet and Orange Salad, 117
    Roasted Beets and Beet Greens, 243

Bell peppers. *See also* Roasted peppers
    Asian Coleslaw, 128
    Asian Noodle Salad, 160–61
    Chickpea Salad, 133
    Coleslaw, 127
    Couscous Tabbouleh, 139

Gazpacho, 106

Greek Salad, 115

Mediterranean Chicken Stew, 172–73

Quinoa and Black Bean Salad with Lime Dressing, 140

Simple Homemade Pizza, 210

Summer Vegetable Gratin, 248

Tempeh and Sesame Salad, 162–63

Tuna and Bean Salad, 152–53

Wild Rice Salad, 144–45

Berry Cream, 271

Beverages. *See also* Smoothies
    Blueberry Frappe, 68
    Blueberry Peach Frappe, 68
    caloric content of, 9
    Ginger Tea, 69
    Lemonade, Sparkling or Flat, 69
    Limeade, Sparkling or Flat, 69
    for nausea, 15

biotin, 393

Black beans
    Bean Salad with Cumin Vinaigrette, 134–35
    Black Bean Tacos, Quick, 232
    Black Bean Tostadas, 234–35
    Chalupas, 234–35
    Egg and Bean Tacos, 235
    Quesadillas with Black Beans, 217
    Quick Refried Beans, 231
    Quinoa and Black Bean Salad with Lime Dressing, 140

Refried Beans, 230–31

Simmered Black Beans with Cilantro, 229

Black-eyed peas
    Black-Eyed Pea Pâté Sandwich, 82
    White Bean or Black-Eyed Pea Pâté, 58–59

Black pepper
    Roast Pork Loin with Fennel-Pepper Rub, 184

bland foods, craving for, 19, 21

blood cholesterol, 386, 387

blood sugar. *See* gestational diabetes; glucose

blood volume, maternal, 21

Blueberries
    Blueberry Frappe, 68
    Blueberry Peach Frappe, 68

body fat stores, 3–4, 10–11

body mass index (BMI), 8

body weight. *See* weight gain; weight reduction

Borlotti beans
    Minestrone, 100–101
    Tuna and Bean Salad, 152–53

Braised Red Cabbage, 246

Bran Muffins, 48–49

Bread(s). *See also* Sandwiches
    Banana Bread, 52
    French Toast, 38
    Molasses Bread, 53

Bread Pudding with Apples or Peaches, 269

brewer's yeast in smoothies, 45

Broccoli
    Broccoli and Chickpea Salad with Egg, 141
    Broccoli Flan, 228
    Broccoli with Garlic and Lemon, 242

Creamy Pasta with Broc-
coli, 197
Curried Mixed-Grain
Salad, 142–43
Fried Brown Rice and Veg-
etables, 222
Garlic Soup with Broccoli,
98–99
Niçoise Salad, 150–51
Pasta with Tomato Sauce,
202
Quick Individual Omelets,
Flat or Folded, 35
Stir-Fried Chicken and
Broccoli, 176–77
Stir-Fried Tofu with Broc-
coli and Mushrooms,
226–27
Tortellini with Broccoli and
Sage, 203
Wild Rice Salad, 144–45
Broccoli rabe
Southern Italian–Style
Broccoli Rabe, 241
Broiled or Grilled Tofu, 224
Brownies, 272
Bruschetta, 86–87
Bulgur
Chicken Soup with Egg and
Lemon, 93
cooking directions for, 263
Tabbouleh, Classic, 138
Buttermilk
Banana Smoothie, 44
Banana Strawberry
Smoothie, 44
Bran Muffins, 48–49
Buttermilk Pancakes, 39
Buttermilk Vinaigrette, 165
Mango Smoothie, 44
Molasses Bread, 53
Peach Smoothie, 44

Strawberry Smoothie, 45

Cabbage
Asian Coleslaw, 128
Braised Red Cabbage, 246
Coleslaw, 127
Minestrone, 100–101
caffeine consumption, 17
Cakes
Flourless Orange Cake, 273
calcium, 394
eating plan rich in, for lac-
tose-intolerant women,
326–33
food content of, 306
need for, 22, 27
calories, 9, 386
increasing intake of, 335
needs for, 13, 374
cancer prevention, 399
Cannellini beans
Minestrone, 100–101
Polenta with Tomato Sauce
and Beans, 261
Capers
Simple Homemade Pizza,
210
Snapper with Lemon, Ca-
pers, Oregano, and Olive
Oil, 194
Sole with Lemon, Capers,
Oregano, and Olive Oil,
194
carbohydrates, 4, 381–83
complex, 345, 382
diabetes and, 345
simple, 382
swelling and, 334
weight gain and, 7, 8
Carrots
Coleslaw, 127
Gazpacho, 106

Grated Carrots in Vinai-
grette, 122
Marinated Carrots, 124
with garlic, 124
Mexican Chicken Soup
with Zucchini, Chick-
peas, and Tomatoes,
90–91
Minestrone, 100–101
Moroccan Cooked Carrot
Salad with Cumin, 123
Vegetarian Mexican Soup,
91
Winter Vegetable Couscous,
214–15
Winter Vegetable Soup, 102
Chalupas, 234–35
Chard. See Greens
Cheddar cheese
Classic Quesadilla, 216
Grilled Cheese and Sage
Sandwich, 85
Grilled Cheese and Tomato
Sandwich, 85
Grilled Cheese Sandwich,
84–85
Quesadillas with Black
Beans, 217
Quesadillas with Greens,
217
Quick Individual Omelets,
Flat or Folded, filling, 36
cheese. See also specific cheeses
soft, warning about, 17
Cheese-Stuffed Figs or
Prunes, 56
chemical pollutants in fish, 17
Cherries
Cherry Clafoutis, 274
Dried Fruit Compote, 42
High-Protein Muffins,
50–51

Cherries (*cont.*)
  Scandinavian Fruit Soup, 43
Chicken
  Asian Chicken Salad, 158
  Asian Noodle Salad, 160–61
  Chicken, Lemon, and Olive
    Stew with Couscous,
    174–75
  Chicken, Red Pepper, and
    Avocado Sandwich, 73
  Chicken Breast and Red
    Pepper Sandwich, 73
  Chicken Breasts with Asian
    Flavors, 169
  Chicken Breasts with In-
    dian Flavors, 170
  Chicken Breasts with
    Mediterranean Flavors,
    169
  Chicken Fajitas, 182–83
  Chicken Noodle Soup, 89
  Chicken Sandwich with
    Lettuce and Tomato, 73
  Chicken Soup with Egg and
    Lemon, 93
  Club Sandwich, 72
  Cobb Salad, 154–55
  Curried Chicken Salad,
    156–57
  Hot and Sour Soup, 94–95
  Mediterranean Chicken
    Stew, 172–73
  Mexican Chicken Salad, 159
  Mexican Chicken Soup
    with Zucchini, Chick-
    peas, and Tomatoes,
    90–91
  Poached Chicken Breasts,
    156
  Roast Chicken, 171
  Soft Tacos or Tostadas with
    Chicken, Corn, and Avo-
    cado, 233

Stir-Fried Chicken and
    Broccoli, 176–77
Chickpeas
  Basmati Rice Pilaf with
    Chickpeas, 257
  Broccoli and Chickpea
    Salad with Egg, 141
  Chickpea Salad, 133
  Couscous Tabbouleh, 139
  Couscous with Chickpeas
    and Greens, 212–13
  Curried Mixed-Grain
    Salad, 142–43
  Hummus, 57
  Mexican Chicken Soup
    with Zucchini, Chick-
    peas, and Tomatoes,
    90–91
  Pasta with Tomato Sauce,
    202
  Spinach Salad with Chick-
    peas, Walnuts, and Feta,
    114
  Three Omega-3 Salad, 114
  Tuna and Bean Salad,
    152–53
  Vegetarian Mexican Soup,
    91
  Winter Vegetable Couscous,
    214–15
Chilled Cucumber Yogurt
    Soup, 107
chloride, 398
Chocolate
  Brownies, 272
  Chocolate Pudding, 270–71
cholesterol, 387
chromium, 22, 397
cider, unpasteurized, 17
Cilantro
  Simmered Black Beans or
    Pinto Beans with
    Cilantro, 229

Cinnamon
  Apple-Cinnamon Tofu
    Spread, 46
Clafoutis
  Cherry Clafoutis, 274
Club Sandwich, 72
  with avocado, 72
Cobb Salad, 154–55
Coleslaw, 127
  Asian Coleslaw, 128
colic, 375
comforting foods, craving for,
    19
complete protein, 384
constipation, 23–24, 28
Cookies
  Brownies, 272
cooking
  eating plan not requiring,
    317–25
  to prevent foodborne ill-
    nesses, 29
copper, 398
Corn
  Corn Gratin, 250
  Soft Tacos or Tostadas with
    Chicken, Corn, and Avo-
    cado, 233
  Summer Vegetable Gratin,
    248
Cornmeal. *See* Polenta
Cottage cheese
  Berry Cream, 271
  Black Bean Tostadas,
    234–35
  Chalupas, 234–35
  Cheese-Stuffed Figs or
    Prunes, 56
  Creamy Cucumber Salad,
    125
  Creamy Cucumber Sand-
    wich, 125
  Creamy Garlic Dip, 245

Creamy Pasta with Broc-
coli, 197
Creamy Pasta with Greens,
198–99
Low-Fat, High-Protein
Quesadillas, 216–17
Low-Fat Green Mayon-
naise, 64
Low-Fat Mayonnaise, 64
Quesadillas with Black
Beans, 217
Quesadillas with Greens,
217
Quick Spinach and Tomato
Lasagna, 206–7
Couscous
Chicken, Lemon, and Olive
Stew with Couscous,
174–75
cooking directions for,
263–64
Couscous Tabbouleh,
139
Couscous with Chickpeas
and Greens, 212–13
Couscous with Oranges
and Dates, 32–33
Winter Vegetable Couscous,
214–15
cramps, muscular, 28
Cranberries
High-Protein Muffins,
50–51
cravings, 4, 14, 16, 17–18, 19,
20–21
Creamy Cucumber Salad, 125
Creamy Cucumber Sandwich,
125
Creamy Garlic Dip, 245
Creamy Pasta with Broccoli,
197
Creamy Pasta with Greens,
198–99

Crudités with Thai Peanut
Sauce, 55
crunchy foods, craving for, 19
Cucumbers
Asian Chicken Salad, 158
Chilled Cucumber Yogurt
Soup, 107
Creamy Cucumber Salad,
125
Creamy Cucumber Sand-
wich, 125
Gazpacho, 106
Greek Salad, 115
Quick Cucumber Pickles,
126
Sardine Spread and Cu-
cumber Sandwich, 76–77
Tuna and Bean Salad,
152–53
Cumin
Bean Salad with Cumin
Vinaigrette, 134–35
Chicken Breasts with In-
dian Flavors, 170
Moroccan Cooked Carrot
Salad with Cumin, 123
Curry
Broccoli and Chickpea
Salad with Egg, 141
Curried Chicken Salad,
156–57
Curried Mixed-Grain
Salad, 142–43
Curried Yogurt Dip, 61

Dates
Couscous with Oranges
and Dates, 32–33
deli meats, cold, warning
about, 17
Deviled Eggs, 54
diabetes. See gestational diabetes

diarrhea, 24
dietary fats, 4, 385–88
dietary fiber, 23, 28, 345, 383
digestive tract, 23–24
Dill
Yogurt Dip with Mint or
Dill, 245
Dipping sauces. See Sauces
Dressings
Buttermilk Vinaigrette, 165
Classic Vinaigrette, 164
Cumin Vinaigrette, 134–35
Lemon Buttermilk Vinai-
grette, 165
Lemon Vinaigrette,
164–65
Lemon Yogurt Vinaigrette,
165
Low-Fat Green Mayon-
naise, 64
Low-Fat Mayonnaise, 64
Tofu Green Goddess, 67
Tofu Mayonnaise, 66
Yogurt Vinaigrette, 165
Dried Figs in Orange Juice,
277
Dried Fruit Compote, 42
Drinks. See Beverages;
Smoothies
drugs, prescription and over-
the-counter, 6
Dry jack cheese
Grilled Cheese Sandwich,
84–85
Dry-Roasted Waxy Potatoes,
253
eating disorders, 5
eating habits, healthy, 3, 6
eating plans, 283–380
for bed rest, 356–58
for first trimester, 359–64
for gestational diabetes,
341–56

eating plans (*cont.*)
higher-carb, high-protein,
298–305
for lactose intolerance,
326–33
lower-carb, high-protein,
288–97
for multiple pregnancies,
333–41
for noncooks and reluctant
cooks, 317–25
for nursing mothers, 373–80
recommended daily food
choices for, 284
for second trimester,
364–69
snacks in, 284–88
for third trimester, 370–72
vegetarian, 305–17
Eggs
Broccoli and Chickpea
Salad with Egg, 141
Cherry Clafoutis, 274
Chicken Soup with Egg and
Lemon, 93
Chocolate Pudding, 270–71
Cobb Salad, 154–55
Corn Gratin, 250
Deviled Eggs, 54
Egg and Bean Tacos, 235
Egg Salad, 146
Egg Salad Sandwich, My,
77
Flourless Orange Cake, 273
French Toast, 38
Fried Brown Rice and Veg-
etables, 222
Fried Eggs with Spicy
Cooked Tomato Sauce,
40–41
Frisée, Poached Egg, and
Bacon Salad, 148–49

Garlic Soup with Broccoli,
98–99
Greek Spinach Pie, 208–9
Hot and Sour Soup, 94–95
Hot or Cold Spinach Frit-
tata, 220–21
Huevos Rancheros, 40–41
Italian Spinach and Egg
Soup, 97
Niçoise Salad, 150–51
Potato and Green Bean
Salad, 130–31
Potato Gratin, 255
Quick Individual Omelets,
Flat or Folded, 34–36
safety of, 29
Spanakopita, 208–9
Spinach, Broccoli, or As-
paragus Flan, 228
Strata with Tomatoes and
Greens, 218–19
Summer Vegetable Gratin,
248
Zucchini and Rice Gratin,
249
embryo, 12
emotional swings, 13
essential amino acids, 384
estrogen, 13, 23
exchange(s), 347
Exchange Lists, 347, 350
exercising, 6, 347
expiration dates on foods, 29

fast foods, 319
fat(s). *See* body fat stores; dietary fats
fatigue, 14, 26
fatty acids, 27, 385–86
Fennel
Roast Pork Loin with Fen-
nel-Pepper Rub, 184

ferritin test, 14
Feta cheese
Black Bean Tacos, Quick,
232
Black Bean Tostadas, 234–35
Chalupas, 234–35
Greek Salad, 115
Greek Spinach Pie, 208–9
Spanakopita, 208–9
Spinach Salad with Chick-
peas, Walnuts, and Feta,
114
Three Omega-3 Salad, 114
Tomato and Arugula Salad
with Feta Cheese, 116
fetal development, 12, 18–19,
21, 25–26
fetus, weight gain due to, 11
Figs
Bran Muffins, 48–49
Cheese-Stuffed Figs or
Prunes, 56
Dried Figs in Orange Juice,
277
Dried Fruit Compote, 42
first trimester, 12–18
caloric needs during, 13
cravings during, 14, 17–18
embryonic and fetal development during, 12
hormones during, 12–13
key nutrients for, 15
menus for, 359–64
problems during, 13–18
weight gain during, 13–14
Fish
Asian Noodle Soup with
Spinach and Salmon, 92
cautions regarding, 17
Grilled or Broiled Fish
Steaks with Asian Fla-
vors, 195

Grilled Tuna with Tomato-Balsamic Salsa, 196
Halibut Cooked in the Microwave, 189
Niçoise Salad, 150–51
Pasta with Tomato Sauce, 202
Red Snapper Fillets Baked in Foil, 191
Salmon Fillets Cooked in the Microwave, 190
Sardine Spread and Cucumber Sandwich, 76–77
Snapper with Lemon, Capers, Oregano, and Olive Oil, 194
Sole with Lemon, Capers, Oregano, and Olive Oil, 194
Sole with Olive Oil, Lemon, and Scallions, 193
Tuna and Bean Salad, 152–53
Tuna and Green Bean Salad, 153
Tuna for the Week, 74
Tuna Sandwiches, 74–75
Whole Trout Baked in Foil, 192
fish oil, 385
Flan
Spinach, Broccoli, or Asparagus Flan, 228
flatulence, 24
Flax seeds
Asian Chicken Salad, 158
Muesli, 33
in smoothies, 45
Flourless Orange Cake, 273
fluids, for constipation, 24
fluoride, 398
folate/folic acid, 5, 15, 393–94

Fontina cheese
Grilled Cheese Sandwich, 84–85
foodborne illnesses, 29
food safety and storage, 29, 319–20
French Lentil Salad, Warm or Cold, 136–37
French Toast, 38
Fresh Tomato Salsa, 63
Fried Eggs with Spicy Cooked Tomato Sauce, 40
Frisée, Poached Egg, and Bacon Salad, 148–49
Frittatas
Hot or Cold Spinach Frittata, 220–21
frozen foods, eating plan using, 317–25
Frozen yogurt
Blueberry Frappe, 68
Blueberry Peach Frappe, 68
Frozen Banana Yogurt, 279
Frozen Strawberry Banana Yogurt, 279
fruit. See also specific fruits
caution regarding, 17
craving for, 19
fruit juices, 9, 17. See also specific juices

Garbanzo beans. See Chickpeas
Garlic
Broccoli with Garlic and Lemon, 242
Creamy Garlic Dip, 245
Garlic Soup with Broccoli, 98–99
Gazpacho, 106
gestational diabetes, 341–56
management of, 344–47

menus for, 347–56
risk factors for, 342
risks associated with, 343, 347
Ginger
craving for, 19
Ginger Tea, 69
Pears Poached in Ginger Honey Syrup, 278
Soy Ginger Dipping Sauce, Simple, 60
glucose, 345, 382
gestational diabetes and, 341–42
glycemic index (GI), 382, 383
Goat cheese
Mozzarella or Goat Cheese and Roasted Peppers, 87
Pasta with Tomato Sauce, 202
Warm Lentil Salad with Goat Cheese, 137
Warm Potato and Goat Cheese Salad, 132
Grapefruit and Avocado Salad, 118
grape leaves as wraps, 71
Grated Carrots in Vinaigrette, 122
Gratins
Corn Gratin, 250
Potato Gratin, 255
Summer Vegetable Gratin, 248
Tomato Gratin, 251
Zucchini and Rice Gratin, 249
Greek Salad, 115
Greek Spinach Pie, 208–9
Green beans
Minestrone, 100–101
Niçoise Salad, 150–51

Green beans (*cont.*)
Pasta with Pesto and Green
Beans, 199
Potato and Green Bean
Salad, 130–31
Summer Pasta with Toma-
toes and Green Beans or
Peas, 200
Tuna and Green Bean
Salad, 153
White Bean and Basil Salad,
137
Wild Rice Salad, 144–45
Greens. *See also* Baby salad
greens; Spinach
Couscous with Chickpeas
and Greens, 212–13
Creamy Pasta with Greens,
198–99
Pasta with Tomato Sauce,
202
Quesadillas with Greens,
217
Quick Individual Omelets,
Flat or Folded, 35
Roasted Beets and Beet
Greens, 243
Stir-Fried Pork and Greens,
185
Stir-Fried Tofu with Red
Chard, 225
Strata with Tomatoes and
Greens, 218–19
Winter Vegetable Couscous,
214–15
Grilled Cheese Sandwich,
84–85
Grilled or Broiled Fish Steaks
with Asian Flavors, 195
Grilled or Pan-Seared Porter-
house Steak, 179
Grilled Portobello and Cheese

(or Miso) Sandwich, 83
Grilled Tuna with Tomato-
Balsamic Salsa, 196
Gruyère cheese, 36
Corn Gratin, 250
Grilled Cheese Sandwich,
84–85
Grilled Portobello and
Cheese (or Miso) Sand-
wich, 83
Potato Gratin, 255
Spinach, Broccoli, or As-
paragus Flan, 228
Strata with Tomatoes and
Greens, 218–19
Summer Vegetable Gratin,
248
Guacamole, 121

Halibut Cooked in the Mi-
crowave, 189
handwashing, 29
healthy diet, 3
heart, maternal, 21
heartburn, 23, 24, 26
heme iron, 396
hemorrhoids, 24, 28
Herbs. *See also specific herbs*
Herbed Yogurt Cheese, 65
Steamed New Potatoes or
Fingerlings with Herbs,
252
high-density lipoproteins
(HDLs), 387, 388
High-Protein Muffins, 50–51
Homemade Pizza, Simple, 210
Honey
Pears Poached in Ginger
Honey Syrup, 278
hormones, 12–13, 23, 24, 28,
341–42, 399
hospital bed rest, 357, 358

Hot and Sour Soup, 94–95
Huevos Rancheros, 40–41
human chorionic gonado-
tropin (HCG), 13
human placental lactogen
(HPL), 13
Hummus, 57
Hummus Pita Pocket, 82
hydration, with nausea, 15
hydrogenation of fatty acids,
386
hypoglycemia, 343

insomnia, 28
insulin, 341–42, 345, 348, 382
insulin resistance, 382–83
insulin therapy, bedtime
snacks with, 346–47
iodine, 397
iron, 21, 22, 23, 27, 395–96
iron deficiency anemia, 14,
334, 396
iron supplements, 23, 24
Italian Spinach and Egg Soup,
97

Jicama with Lime Juice and
Salt, 56
juicy foods, craving for, 19

Kale. *See* Greens
Kegel exercises, 28
ketones, 346
ketosis, starvation, 346
key nutrients
for first trimester, 15
for second trimester, 22
for third trimester, 27

lactase supplements, 326
lactose intolerance, eating
plan for, 326–33

lamb, caution about, 17
Leeks
  Couscous with Chickpeas and Greens, 212–13
  Greek Spinach Pie, 208–9
  Minestrone, 100–101
  Spanakopita, 208–9
  Winter Vegetable Couscous, 214–15
  Winter Vegetable Soup, 102
leg cramps, 28
Lemon juice
  Broccoli with Garlic and Lemon, 242
  Chicken, Lemon, and Olive Stew with Couscous, 174–75
  Chicken Soup with Egg and Lemon, 93
  Lemonade, Sparkling or Flat, 69
  Lemon Buttermilk Vinaigrette, 165
  Lemon Vinaigrette, 164–65
  Lemon Yogurt Vinaigrette, 165
  Snapper with Lemon, Capers, Oregano, and Olive Oil, 194
  Sole with Lemon, Capers, Oregano, and Olive Oil, 194
  Sole with Olive Oil, Lemon, and Scallions, 193
  Strawberries with Mint and Citrus Juice, 282
  Tabbouleh, Classic, 138
  Tabbouleh, Couscous, 139
  Wilted Spinach with Lemon Juice, 240

Lentils
  French Lentil Salad, Warm or Cold, 136–37
  Lentil Soup, 103
  Warm Lentil Salad with Goat Cheese, 137
lettuce leaves as wraps, 71
Lime juice
  Chicken Breasts with Indian Flavors, 170
  Jicama with Lime Juice and Salt, 56
  Limeade, Sparkling or Flat, 69
  Melon with Mint and Lime, 277
  Quinoa and Black Bean Salad with Lime Dressing, 140
  Strawberries with Mint and Citrus Juice, 282
lipids, 385. See also dietary fats
liquids, 15, 28
listeriosis, 29, 319
low-density lipoproteins (LDLs), 387–88
Low-Fat, High-Protein Quesadillas, 216–17
Low-Fat Mayonnaise, 64

macronutrients, 381–88. See also carbohydrates; dietary fats; dietary fiber; protein
macrosomia, 343
magnesium, 395
manganese, 15, 397–98
Mango Smoothie, 44
Marinated Carrots, 124
Mayonnaise. See Dressings
meals. See also eating plans
  regular, 14

meats, cold, warning about, 17
medical conditions, preexisting, 6
Mediterranean Chicken Stew, 172–73
Melon with Mint and Lime, 277
menus. See eating plans
Mexican Chicken Salad, 159
Mexican Chicken Soup with Zucchini, Chickpeas, and Tomatoes, 90–91
Mexican Scrambled Tofu, 37
micronutrients, 381, 388–99. See also minerals; phytochemicals; vitamin(s)
Microwave Oatmeal with Milk and Raisins, 31
Milk. See also Soy milk
  Banana Smoothie, 44
  Banana Strawberry Smoothie, 44
  Blueberry Frappe, 68
  Blueberry Peach Frappe, 68
  Bread Pudding with Apples or Peaches, 269
  Cherry Clafoutis, 274
  Chocolate Pudding, 270–71
  Corn Gratin, 250
  French Toast, 38
  human, quality of, 374
  Mango Smoothie, 44
  Microwave Oatmeal with Milk and Raisins, 31
  Peach Smoothie, 44
  Potato Gratin, 255
  Rice Pudding, 280
  Spinach, Broccoli, or Asparagus Flan, 228
  Strata with Tomatoes and Greens, 218–19
  Strawberry Smoothie, 45

Milk (*cont.*)
  Summer Vegetable Gratin,
    248
  unpasteurized, 17
  Winter Vegetable Soup, 102
minerals, 394–98. *See also specific minerals*
Minestrone, 100–101
Mint
  Melon with Mint and Lime,
    277
  Orange and Mint Salad, 281
  Pineapple with Mint, 277
  Strawberries and Peaches
    with Mint, 281
  Strawberries with Mint and
    Citrus Juice, 282
  Strawberry Orange Soup,
    282
  Yogurt Dip with Mint or
    Dill, 245
Miso
  Grilled Portobello and
    Cheese (or Miso) Sand-
    wich, 83
  Miso Soup with Tofu, 96
modified bed rest, 357
Molasses Bread, 53
molybdenum, 398
monounsaturated fatty acids,
  386
Monterey jack cheese
  Classic Quesadilla, 216
  Grilled Cheese Sandwich,
    84–85
  Low-Fat, High-Protein
    Quesadillas, 216–17
  Quesadillas with Black
    Beans, 217
  Quesadillas with Greens,
    217
  Quick Individual Omelets,
    Flat or Folded, filling, 36

mood swings, 13
"morning sickness," 13–14,
  15–17, 333–34
Moroccan Cooked Carrot
  Salad with Cumin, 123
motilin, 23
Mozzarella cheese
  Mozzarella or Goat Cheese
    and Roasted Peppers, 87
  Roasted Pepper and Moz-
    zarella Antipasto, 120
  Tomato, Mozzarella, and
    Basil Sandwich, 85
  Tomato and Mozzarella
    Antipasto, 120
Muesli, 33
Muffins
  Bran Muffins, 48–49
  High-Protein Muffins,
    50–51
multiple pregnancies
  eating plan for, 333–41
  nursing multiples and, 375
  weight gain for, 10
muscle cramps, 28
Mushrooms
  Baby Spinach Salad with
    Mushrooms, 111
  Grilled Portobello and
    Cheese (or Miso) Sand-
    wich, 83
  Hot and Sour Soup, 94–95
  Miso Soup with Tofu, 96
  Mushroom and Barley
    Soup, 104–5
  Pasta with Quick Tomato
    Mushroom Sauce, 205
  Pasta with Tomato Mush-
    room Sauce, 204–5
  Quick Individual Omelets,
    Flat or Folded, filling, 36
  Simple Homemade Pizza,
    210

Stir-Fried Chicken and
    Broccoli, 176–77
  Stir-Fried Tofu with Broc-
    coli and Mushrooms,
    226–27
  Wild Rice Stuffing, 187–88

Napa cabbage
  Asian Coleslaw, 128
nausea, 13–14, 15–17, 16, 333–34
niacin (vitamin B3), 391–92
Niçoise Salad, 150–51
noncooks, eating plan for,
    317–25
nonheme iron, 396
Noodles
  Asian Noodles, 262
  Asian Noodle Salad, 160–61
  Asian Noodle Soup with
    Spinach and Salmon, 92
  Asian Noodle Soup with
    Tofu and Spinach, 92
  Chicken Noodle Soup, 89
  Tofu Noodle Soup, 89
nursing mothers, 373–80
Nuts
  Banana Bread, 52
  Black Bean Tostadas, 234–35
  Brownies, 272
  Chalupas, 234–35
  Curried Mixed-Grain
    Salad, 142–43
  Flourless Orange Cake, 273
  Muesli, 33
  Spinach Salad with Chick-
    peas, Walnuts, and Feta,
    114
  Three Omega-3 Salad, 114

Oatmeal
  Microwave, with Milk and
    Raisins, 31
  Muesli, 33

Pear Crumble or Crisp, 275
older women, weight gain for,
    10–11
Olives
    Chicken, Lemon, and Olive
        Stew with Couscous,
        174–75
    Greek Salad, 115
    Simple Homemade Pizza,
        210
    Tomato and Arugula Salad
        with Feta Cheese, 116
omega-3 fatty acids, 27, 385,
    386
omega-6 fatty acids, 385–86
Omelets
    Individual, Flat or Folded,
        Quick, 34–36
Onions
    Gazpacho, 106
    Greek Salad, 115
    Mexican Chicken Soup
        with Zucchini, Chick-
        peas, and Tomatoes,
        90–91
    Minestrone, 100–101
    Simple Homemade Pizza,
        210
    Vegetarian Mexican Soup,
        91
    Winter Vegetable Couscous,
        214–15
Orange(s)
    Beet and Orange Salad, 117
    Couscous with Oranges
        and Dates, 32–33
    Flourless Orange Cake, 273
    Orange and Mint Salad, 281
Orange juice
    Dried Figs in Orange Juice,
        277
    Strawberries with Mint and
        Citrus Juice, 282

Strawberry Orange Soup,
    282
Oregano
    Snapper with Lemon, Ca-
        pers, Oregano, and Olive
        Oil, 194
    Sole with Lemon, Capers,
        Oregano, and Olive Oil,
        194
over-the-counter pharmaceu-
    ticals and vitamins, 6
overweight before pregnancy,
    6
ovo-lacto vegetarian eating
    plans, 305, 308–12

packaged foods, eating plan
    using, 317–25
Pancakes
    Buttermilk Pancakes, 39
Pan-Cooked Summer Squash,
    247
Pan-Cooked Tofu, 223
Pan-Seared or Grilled London
    Broil, 180–81
pantothenic acid (vitamin
    B5), 27, 392
Parmesan cheese
    Italian Spinach and Egg
        Soup, 97
    Tomatoes with Parmesan,
        86
Parsley
    Chickpea Salad, 133
    French Lentil Salad, Warm
        or Cold, 136–37
    Tabbouleh, Classic, 138
    Tabbouleh, Couscous, 139
    Warm Lentil Salad with
        Goat Cheese, 137
partially hydrogenated veg-
    etable oil, 386
Pasta. See also Noodles

Creamy Pasta with Broc-
    coli, 197
Creamy Pasta with Greens,
    198–99
Garlic Soup with Broccoli,
    98–99
Minestrone, 100–101
Pasta with Pesto and Green
    Beans, 199
Pasta with Tomato Mush-
    room Sauce, 204–5
Pasta with Tomato Sauce,
    201–2
Quick Spinach and Tomato
    Lasagna, 206–7
Summer Pasta with Toma-
    toes and Green Beans or
    Peas, 200
Tortellini with Broccoli and
    Sage, 203
Pâtés
    warning about, 17
    White Bean or Black-Eyed
        Pea Pâté, 58–59
    White Bean Pâté Sandwich,
        82
Pea(s)
    Basmati Rice Pilaf with
        Peas, 258–59
    Chicken Noodle Soup, 89
    Minestrone, 100–101
    Summer Pasta with Toma-
        toes and Green Beans or
        Peas, 200
    Tofu Noodle Soup, 89
    Wild Rice Salad, 144–45
Peaches
    Blueberry Peach Frappe, 68
    Bread Pudding with Apples
        or Peaches, 269
    Peach Smoothie, 44
    Strawberries and Peaches
        with Mint, 281

Peanut butter
  Crudités with Thai Peanut
    Sauce, 55
  Peanut Butter and Banana
    Sandwich, 78
Pears
  Pear Crumble or Crisp, 275
  Pears Poached in Ginger
    Honey Syrup, 278
pelvic area cramps, 28
Peppers. *See* Bell peppers;
    Roasted peppers
phosphorus, 395
phytochemicals, 399
phytoestrogens, 399
Pickles
  Quick Cucumber Pickles,
    126
Pineapple with Mint, 277
Pinto beans
  Quick Refried Beans, 231
  Refried Beans, 230–31
  Simmered Pinto Beans with
    Cilantro, 229
Pizza
  Simple Homemade Pizza,
    210
placenta
  hormones produced by, 13,
    24, 342
  weight gain due to, 11
Poached Chicken Breasts, 156
Polenta
  Easy Polenta, 260
  Polenta with Tomato Sauce
    and Beans, 261
pollutants, in fish, 17
polyunsaturated fatty acids,
    386
Pork
  Hot and Sour Soup, 94–95
  Roast Pork Loin with

Fennel-Pepper Rub, 184
  Stir-Fried Pork and Greens,
    185
potassium, 15, 22, 396
Potatoes
  Baked Potato Skins, 254
  Baked Russet Potatoes, 253
  Dry-Roasted Waxy Pota-
    toes, 253
  Minestrone, 100–101
  Mushroom and Barley
    Soup, 104–5
  Niçoise Salad, 150–51
  Potato and Green Bean
    Salad, 130–31
  Potato Gratin, 255
  Potato Salad, 129
  Steamed New Potatoes or
    Fingerlings with Herbs,
    252
  Warm Potato and Goat
    Cheese Salad, 132
  Winter Vegetable Soup, 102
preconception counseling and
    health care, 5–6
prepared foods
  eating plan using, 317–25
  risks associated with, 319
prescription drugs, 6
progesterone, 13, 23
protein, 22, 27, 384–85
protein powder in smoothies,
    45
protein turnover, 384
Prunes
  Cheese-Stuffed Figs or
    Prunes, 56
  Dried Fruit Compote, 42
  Scandinavian Fruit Soup, 43
pteroylglutamic acid (PGA), 5,
    393–94
Puddings

Bread Pudding with Apples
    or Peaches, 269
  Chocolate Pudding, 270–71
  Rice Pudding, 280
pyridoxal/pyridoxamine/pyri-
    doxine, 15, 27, 392–93

Quesadillas
  Classic Quesadilla, 216
  Low-Fat, High-Protein
    Quesadillas, 216–17
  Quesadillas with Black
    Beans, 217
  Quesadillas with Greens,
    217
Queso fresco
  Black Bean Tacos, Quick,
    232
  Black Bean Tostadas, 234–35
  Chalupas, 234–35
Quick Cucumber Pickles, 126
Quick Individual Omelets,
    Flat or Folded, 34–36
Quick Refried Beans, 231
Quick Spinach and Tomato
    Lasagna, 206–7
Quick Tofu Sandwich, Simple,
    79
Quinoa
  cooking directions for, 265
  Curried Mixed-Grain
    Salad, 142–43
  Quinoa and Black Bean
    Salad with Lime Dress-
    ing, 140

Raisins
  Bran Muffins, 48–49
  Bread Pudding with Apples
    or Peaches, 269
  Dried Fruit Compote, 42
  Microwave Oatmeal with

Milk and Raisins, 31
Molasses Bread, 53
Rice Pudding, 280
Scandinavian Fruit Soup, 43
Raspberries
Berry Cream, 271
raw foods, 17, 29
ready-to-eat foods, eating plan
using, 317–25
Red Snapper Fillets Baked in
Foil, 191
Refried Beans, 230–31
refrigerator, food safety and,
29
relaxin, 24
reluctant cooks, eating plan
for, 317–25
reverse peristalsis, 23
riboflavin (vitamin B2), 391
Rice. *See also* Wild rice
Basmati Rice Pilaf with
Chickpeas, 257
Basmati Rice Pilaf with
Peas, 258–59
Chicken Soup with Egg and
Lemon, 93
cooking directions for, 265,
266
Curried Mixed-Grain
Salad, 142–43
Fried Brown Rice and Veg-
etables, 222
Rice Pudding, 280
Zucchini and Rice Gratin,
249
rice-flour wrappers, 71
Ricotta cheese
Black Bean Tostadas, 234–35
Chalupas, 234–35
Cheese-Stuffed Figs or
Prunes, 56
Roast Beef Sandwich, 78

Roast Chicken, 171
Roasted Beets and Beet
Greens, 243
Roasted peppers
Chicken, Red Pepper, and
Avocado Sandwich, 73
Chicken Breast and Red
Pepper Sandwich, 73
Chicken Sandwich with
Lettuce and Tomato, 73
Mozzarella or Goat Cheese
and Roasted Peppers, 87
Roasted Pepper and Moz-
zarella Antipasto, 120
Roasted Red Pepper Salad,
119
Roast Pork Loin with Fennel-
Pepper Rub, 184
Roast Turkey, 186
Roquefort cheese
Cobb Salad, 154–55

Sage
Beans and Sage, 87
Tortellini with Broccoli and
Sage, 203
Salad(s), 108–63
Arugula or Baby Greens
and Beet Salad, 112–13
Asian Chicken Salad, 158
Asian Coleslaw, 128
Asian Noodle Salad, 160–61
Baby Greens Salad, 110
Baby Spinach Salad with
Mushrooms, 111
Bean Salad with Cumin
Vinaigrette, 134–35
Beef and Arugula Salad, 147
Beet and Orange Salad, 117
Broccoli and Chickpea
Salad with Egg, 141
Chickpea Salad, 133

Cobb Salad, 154–55
Coleslaw, 127
Creamy Cucumber Salad,
125
Curried Chicken Salad,
156–57
Curried Mixed-Grain
Salad, 142–43
Egg Salad, 146
French Lentil Salad, Warm
or Cold, 136–37
Frisée, Poached Egg, and
Bacon Salad, 148–49
Grapefruit and Avocado
Salad, 118
Grated Carrots in Vinai-
grette, 122
Greek Salad, 115
Guacamole, 121
Marinated Carrots, 124
Mexican Chicken Salad, 159
Moroccan Cooked Carrot
Salad with Cumin, 123
Niçoise Salad, 150–51
Orange and Mint Salad, 281
Potato and Green Bean
Salad, 130–31
Potato Salad, 129
Quick Cucumber Pickles,
126
Quinoa and Black Bean
Salad with Lime Dress-
ing, 140
Roasted Pepper and Moz-
zarella Antipasto, 120
Roasted Red Pepper Salad,
119
Spinach Salad with Chick-
peas, Walnuts, and Feta,
114
Tabbouleh, Classic, 138
Tabbouleh, Couscous, 139

Salad(s) (*cont.*)
  Tempeh and Sesame Salad, 162–63
  Three Omega-3 Salad, 114
  Tomato and Arugula Salad with Feta Cheese, 116
  Tomato and Mozzarella Antipasto, 120
  Tuna and Bean Salad, 152–53
  Tuna and Green Bean Salad, 153
  vegetarian, 307
  Warm Lentil Salad with Goat Cheese, 137
  Warm Potato and Goat Cheese Salad, 132
  White Bean and Basil Salad, 137
  Wild Rice Salad, 144–45
salad bars, 319
Salad dressings. *See* Dressings
Salmon Fillets Cooked in the Microwave, 190
Salsa. *See* Sauces
salty foods, craving for, 19, 21
Sandwiches, 70–87
  Avocado Sandwich, 75
  Barbecued Tempeh Sandwich, 81
  Black-Eyed Pea Pâté Sandwich, 82
  Bruschetta, 86–87
  Chicken, Red Pepper, and Avocado Sandwich, 73
  Chicken Breast and Red Pepper Sandwich, 73
  Chicken Sandwich with Lettuce and Tomato, 73
  Club Sandwich, 72
  Creamy Cucumber Sandwich, 125

  Egg Salad Sandwich, My, 77
  Grilled Cheese Sandwich, 84–85
  Grilled Portobello and Cheese (or Miso) Sandwich, 83
  Hummus Pita Pocket, 82
  Peanut Butter and Banana Sandwich, 78
  Roast Beef Sandwich, 78
  Sardine Spread and Cucumber Sandwich, 76–77
  Tofu and Spinach Pita Pocket, 80
  Tofu Sandwich, Simple, Quick, 79
  Tofu Sandwich with Avocado and Tomato, 79
  Tomato, Mozzarella, and Basil Sandwich, 85
  Tuna Sandwiches, 74–75
  vegetarian, 306–7
  White Bean Pâté Sandwich, 82
  wraps, 71
Sardine Spread and Cucumber Sandwich, 76–77
saturated fatty acids, 386
Sauces
  Creamy Garlic Dip, 245
  Curried Yogurt Dip, 61
  Fresh Tomato Salsa, 63
  Fried Eggs with Spicy Cooked Tomato Sauce, 40
  Salsa with Avocado, 63
  Soy Ginger Dipping Sauce, Simple, 60
  Tahini Soy Dipping Sauce, 60
  Teriyaki Dipping Sauce, 61
  Yogurt Cheese, 65

  Yogurt Dip with Mint or Dill, 245
Savoy cabbage
  Asian Coleslaw, 128
Scandinavian Fruit Soup, 43
Scrambled Tofu, 37
second trimester, 18–24
  blood volume during, 21
  calcium needs during, 22
  cravings during, 19, 20–21
  fetal development during, 18–19, 21
  iron needs during, 21, 22
  key nutrients for, 22
  maternal heart during, 21
  menus for, 364–69
  problems during, 22–24
  protein needs during, 22
  weight gain during, 18
selenium, 398
serotonin, insomnia and, 28
serum cholesterol, 387
serum ferritin test, 14
Sesame paste. *See* Tahini
Sesame seeds
  Asian Chicken Salad, 158
  Tempeh and Sesame Salad, 162–63
shellfish, caution about, 17
Simmered Black Beans or Pinto Beans with Cilantro, 229
sleep problems, 28
smoking cessation, 5
Smoothies
  additions, 45
  Banana Smoothie, 44
  Banana Strawberry Smoothie, 44
  Mango Smoothie, 44
  Peach Smoothie, 44
  Strawberry Smoothie, 45

snacks, 15, 28, 346–47
Snapper with Lemon, Capers, Oregano, and Olive Oil, 194
Snow peas
  Asian Noodle Salad, 160–61
sodium, 398
soft foods, craving for, 19
Soft Tacos or Tostadas with Chicken, Corn, and Avocado, 233
Soft Tacos with Tofu and Tomatoes, 211
Sole with Olive Oil, Lemon, and Scallions, 193
Soups, 88–107
  Asian Noodle Soup with Spinach and Salmon, 92
  Asian Noodle Soup with Tofu and Spinach, 92
  Chicken Noodle or Tofu Soup, 89
  Chicken Soup with Egg and Lemon, 93
  Chilled Cucumber Yogurt Soup, 107
  Garlic Soup with Broccoli, 98–99
  Gazpacho, 106
  Hot and Sour Soup, 94–95
  Italian Spinach and Egg Soup, 97
  Lentil Soup, 103
  Mexican Chicken Soup with Zucchini, Chickpeas, and Tomatoes, 90–91
  Minestrone, 100–101
  Miso Soup with Tofu, 96
  Mushroom and Barley Soup, 104–5
  Scandinavian Fruit Soup, 43

Strawberry Orange Soup, 282
  vegetarian, 307
  Vegetarian Mexican Soup, 91
  Winter Vegetable Soup, 102
sour foods, craving for, 19
Southern Italian–Style Broccoli Rabe, 241
Soy milk
  Banana Smoothie, 44
  Banana Strawberry Smoothie, 44
  Mango Smoothie, 44
  Peach Smoothie, 44
  Strawberry Smoothie, 45
Soy sauce
  Soy Ginger Dipping Sauce, Simple, 60
  Tahini Soy Dipping Sauce, 60
  Teriyaki Dipping Sauce, 61
Spanakopita, 208–9
Spinach. *See also* Greens
  Asian Noodle Soup with Spinach and Salmon, 92
  Asian Noodle Soup with Tofu and Spinach, 92
  Baby Spinach Salad with Mushrooms, 111
  Couscous with Chickpeas and Greens, 212–13
  Creamy Pasta with Greens, 198–99
  Greek Spinach Pie, 208–9
  Hot or Cold Spinach Frittata, 220–21
  Italian Spinach and Egg Soup, 97
  Pasta with Tomato Sauce, 202

Quesadillas with Greens, 217
Quick Individual Omelets, Flat or Folded, 35
Quick Spinach and Tomato Lasagna, 206–7
Spanakopita, 208–9
Spinach Flan, 228
Spinach Salad with Chickpeas, Walnuts, and Feta, 114
Stir-Fried Pork and Greens, 185
Strata with Tomatoes and Greens, 218–19
Three Omega-3 Salad, 114
Tofu and Spinach Pita Pocket, 80
Wilted Spinach with Lemon Juice, 240
Winter Vegetable Couscous, 214–15
Spreads
  Apple-Cinnamon Tofu Spread, 46
  Sardine Spread and Cucumber Sandwich, 76–77
  White Bean or Black-Eyed Pea Pâté, 58–59
  White Bean Puree, 62
  Yogurt Cheese, 65
Squash. *See* Summer squash; Winter squash
starches, 382
starvation ketosis, 346
Steak Fajitas, 182–83
Steamed Artichokes with Dips, 244–45
Steamed New Potatoes or Fingerlings with Herbs, 252

Stews
  Chicken, Lemon, and Olive Stew with Couscous, 174–75
  Mediterranean Chicken Stew, 172–73
  Stir-Fried Chicken and Broccoli, 176–77
  Stir-Fried Pork and Greens, 185
  Stir-Fried Tofu with Broccoli and Mushrooms, 226–27
  Stir-Fried Tofu with Red Chard, 225
  Strata with Tomatoes and Greens, 218–19
Strawberries
  Banana Strawberry Smoothie, 44
  Frozen Strawberry Banana Yogurt, 279
  Strawberries and Peaches with Mint, 281
  Strawberries with Mint and Citrus Juice, 282
  Strawberry Orange Soup, 282
  Strawberry Smoothie, 45
strict bed rest, 357
Stuffing
  Wild Rice Stuffing, 187–88
sugars, 382
Sugar-snap peas
  Asian Noodle Salad, 160–61
sulfur, 398
Summer Pasta with Tomatoes and Green Beans or Peas, 200
Summer squash
  Mexican Chicken Soup with Zucchini, Chickpeas, and Tomatoes, 90–91

Pan-Cooked Summer Squash, 247
  Summer Vegetable Gratin, 248
  Vegetarian Mexican Soup, 91
  Zucchini and Rice Gratin, 249
  Zucchini "Pasta," 205
Summer Vegetable Gratin, 248
Sunflower seeds
  Muesli, 33
sweet-and-sour foods, craving for, 19
sweet foods, craving for, 19, 20
Sweet potatoes
  Baked Sweet Potatoes, 256
Sweet Success, 348
swelling, 334
Swiss chard. See Greens

Tabbouleh
  Classic Tabbouleh, 138
  Couscous Tabbouleh, 139
Tacos
  Egg and Bean Tacos, 235
  Soft Tacos with Chicken, Corn, and Avocado, 233
  Soft Tacos with Tofu and Tomatoes, 211
Tahini
  Hummus, 57
  Tahini Soy Dipping Sauce, 60
take-out foods, 319
tart foods, craving for, 19
Tempeh
  Barbecued Tempeh Sandwich, 81
  Tempeh and Sesame Salad, 162–63
Teriyaki Dipping Sauce, 61
thiamin (vitamin B_1), 391

third trimester, 25–29
  fetal development during, 25–26
  key nutrients for, 27
  menus for, 370–72
  problems during, 26, 28
  weight gain during, 25
Three Omega-3 Salad, 114
Tofu
  Apple-Cinnamon Tofu Spread, 46
  Asian Noodle Soup with Tofu and Spinach, 92
  Broiled or Grilled Tofu, 224
  Hot and Sour Soup, 94–95
  Mexican Scrambled Tofu, 37
  Miso Soup with Tofu, 96
  Pan-Cooked Tofu, 223
  Scrambled Tofu, 37
  Scrambled Tofu with Herbs, 37
  Scrambled Tofu with Onion, 37
  Soft Tacos with Tofu and Tomatoes, 211
  Stir-Fried Tofu with Broccoli and Mushrooms, 226–27
  Stir-Fried Tofu with Red Chard, 225
  Tofu and Spinach Pita Pocket, 80
  Tofu Green Goddess, 67
  Tofu Mayonnaise, 66
  Tofu Noodle Soup, 89
  Tofu Sandwich, Simple, Quick, 79
  Tofu Sandwich with Avocado and Tomato, 79
  Tofu with Dipping Sauces, 60–61

Tomatoes
Avocado Sandwich, 75
Chicken Sandwich with
Lettuce and Tomato, 73
Club Sandwich, 72
Cobb Salad, 154–55
Fresh Tomato Salsa, 63
Fried Eggs with Spicy
Cooked Tomato Sauce,
40–41
Gazpacho, 106
Greek Salad, 115
Grilled Cheese and Tomato
Sandwich, 85
Grilled Tuna with Tomato-
Balsamic Salsa, 196
Guacamole, 121
Huevos Rancheros, 40–41
Mediterranean Chicken
Stew, 172–73
Mexican Chicken Soup
with Zucchini, Chick-
peas, and Tomatoes,
90–91
Minestrone, 100–101
Niçoise Salad, 150–51
Pasta with Quick Tomato
Mushroom Sauce,
205
Pasta with Tomato Mush-
room Sauce, 204–5
Pasta with Tomato Sauce,
201–2
Polenta with Tomato Sauce
and Beans, 261
Quick Individual Omelets,
Flat or Folded, 35
Quick Spinach and Tomato
Lasagna, 206–7
Quinoa and Black Bean
Salad with Lime Dress-
ing, 140
Salsa with Avocado, 63

Simple Homemade Pizza,
210
Soft Tacos or Tostadas with
Chicken, Corn, and Avo-
cado, 233
Soft Tacos with Tofu and
Tomatoes, 211
Strata with Tomatoes and
Greens, 218–19
Summer Pasta with Toma-
toes and Green Beans or
Peas, 200
Tabbouleh, Classic, 138
Tabbouleh, Couscous, 139
Tofu Sandwich with Avo-
cado and Tomato, 79
Tomato, Mozzarella, and
Basil Sandwich, 85
Tomato and Arugula Salad
with Feta Cheese, 116
Tomato and Mozzarella
Antipasto, 120
Tomatoes with Parmesan,
86
Tomato Gratin, 251
Vegetarian Mexican Soup, 91
White Bean and Basil Salad,
137
Toppings
Beans and Sage, 87
Mozzarella or Goat Cheese
and Roasted Peppers, 87
Tomatoes with Parmesan,
86
Yogurt Cheese, 65
Tortellini with Broccoli and
Sage, 203
Tortillas. See also Quesadillas;
Tacos; Tostadas
Chicken Fajitas, 182–83
Fried Eggs with Spicy
Cooked Tomato Sauce,
40–41

Huevos Rancheros, 40–41
Steak Fajitas, 182–83
as wraps, 71
Tostadas
Black Bean Tostadas, 234–35
Chalupas, 234–35
Tostadas with Chicken,
Corn, and Avocado, 233
toxoplasmosis, 29, 319
trans-fatty acids, 386
triglycerides, 386
trimesters. See specific
trimesters
Tuna and Bean Salad, 152–53
Tuna and Green Bean Salad,
153
Tuna for the Week, 74
Tuna Sandwiches, 74–75
Turkey
Club Sandwich, 72
Roast Turkey, 186
Turkey Burgers, 178
Turnip(s)
Minestrone, 100–101
Winter Vegetable Couscous,
214–15
Winter Vegetable Soup, 102
Turnip greens. See Greens
twin pregnancies. See multiple
pregnancies

unpasteurized fruit juices,
milk and milk products,
17
urination, frequent, 28

vegan eating plans, 305–6,
313–17
Vegetable(s). See also specific
vegetables
caution regarding, 17
Crudités with Thai Peanut
Sauce, 55

vegetable juices, 9
vegetable oil, partially hydrogenated, 386
vegetarian eating plans, 305–17
Vegetarian Mexican Soup, 90–91
Vinaigrettes. *See* Dressings
vitamin(s), 388–94
  fat-soluble, 15, 27, 389–91
  in human milk, 374
  water-soluble, 15, 22, 27, 391–94
vitamin A, 15, 27, 389–90
vitamin B$_1$ (thiamin), 391
vitamin B$_2$ (riboflavin), 391
vitamin B$_3$ (niacin), 391–92
vitamin B$_5$ (pantothenic acid), 27, 392
vitamin B$_6$ (pyridoxal, pyridoxamine, pyridoxine), 15, 27, 392–93
vitamin B$_{12}$, 393
vitamin C, 22, 27, 391
vitamin D, 390
vitamin E, 27, 390–91
vitamin supplements, 6

warm foods, craving for, 19
Warm Potato and Goat Cheese Salad, 132
washing of foods and hands, 29
Watercress
  Cobb Salad, 154–55
  Grapefruit and Avocado Salad, 118
weight gain, 7–11
  during first trimester, 13–14
  low, 7
  for multiple pregnancies, 10, 333
  prepregnancy weight and, 7–8, 10

during second trimester, 18
during third trimester, 25
for women over 40, 10–11
weight reduction, before becoming pregnant, 6
wet foods, craving for, 19
Wheat berries
  cooking directions for, 267
  Curried Mixed-Grain Salad, 142–43
wheat germ in smoothies, 45
White beans
  Beans and Sage, 87
  Tuna and Bean Salad, 152–53
  White Bean and Basil Salad, 137
  White Bean or Black-Eyed Pea Pâté, 58–59
  White Bean Pâté Sandwich, 82
  White Bean Puree, 62
Whole Trout Baked in Foil, 192
Wild rice
  cooking directions for, 267
  Wild Rice Salad, 144–45
  Wild Rice Stuffing, 187–88
Wilted Spinach with Lemon Juice, 240
Winter squash
  Winter Vegetable Couscous, 214–15
  Winter Vegetable Soup, 102
Winter Vegetable Couscous, 214–15
Winter Vegetable Soup, 102
Wraps, 71

Yogurt. *See also* Frozen yogurt
  Banana Smoothie, 44
  Banana Strawberry Smoothie, 44

Berry Cream, 271
Black Bean Tostadas, 234–35
Bran Muffins, 48–49
Chalupas, 234–35
Cherry Clafoutis, 274
Chicken Breasts with Indian Flavors, 170
Chilled Cucumber Yogurt Soup, 107
Coleslaw, 127
Creamy Cucumber Salad, 125
Creamy Cucumber Sandwich, 125
Curried Yogurt Dip, 61
Frozen Banana Yogurt, 279
Frozen Strawberry Banana Yogurt, 279
Herbed Yogurt Cheese, 65
High-Protein Muffins, 50–51
Low-Fat Green Mayonnaise, 64
Low-Fat Mayonnaise, 64
Mango Smoothie, 44
Molasses Bread, 53
Peach Smoothie, 44
Potato Salad, 129
Strawberry Smoothie, 45
Warm Potato and Goat Cheese Salad, 132
Yogurt Cheese, 65
Yogurt Dip with Mint or Dill, 245
Yogurt Vinaigrette, 165

zinc, 15, 27, 396–97
Zucchini. *See* Summer squash
zygote, 12